*L*iving *D*angerously
*A*re everyday toxins making you sick?

*L*iving *D*angerously

Are everyday toxins making you sick?

Pat Thomas

Newleaf

Newleaf
an imprint of
Gill & Macmillan Ltd
Hume Avenue, Park West, Dublin 12
with associated companies throughout the world
www.gillmacmillan.ie
© Pat Thomas 2003
0 7171 3600 0
Index compiled by Cover to Cover
Design and print origination by Carole Lynch
Printed by Rotanor, Norway

This book is typeset in Adobe Garamond 11pt on 14pt.

*The paper used in this book comes from the wood pulp of
managed forests. For every tree felled, at least one tree is
planted, thereby renewing natural resources.*

A CIP catalogue record for this book is available
from the British Library.

1 3 5 4 2

Contents

Acknowledgements

THIS MASSIVE UNDERTAKING COULD NOT HAVE BEEN EMBARKED upon without equally massive levels of support, both practically and emotionally. My agent Laura Longrigg is both a friend and an advisor, and I could not make progress without her. I am indebted to Eveleen Coyle, Michael Gill, Peter Thew and Cliona Lewis – indeed, all at Newleaf/Gill & Macmillan, who have never been fazed by my somewhat Cassandra-like spirit, but have instead striven to encourage it and give it voice.

This spirit has also been honed by my long and productive association with Lynne McTaggart and Bryan Hubbard at *What Doctors Don't Tell You, PROOF!* and *Living the Field,* who equally have never shied away from challenging the status quo. Thanks to them for remaining flexible with the extra demands on my time that my book-writing activities always entail. Grateful thanks also to Sharyn Wong, who brought intelligence and a keen eye to the copyediting of this work. To all my busy friends whose homes have provided ad hoc and reciprocal after-school support, and likewise to my family who give me support, even if they don't always understand or agree, love and deepest thanks. Finally, to my son, Alexander – you are my inspiration. When I grow up, I want to be just like you.

Introduction:
Poisoned and Confused

HOW ARE YOU FEELING? ARE YOU FULL OF VIM AND VIGOUR? DO YOU greet each day with enthusiasm and optimism? Or are you one of the growing millions of people throughout the world who are suffering from vague, ill-defined, but nonetheless debilitating health and emotional problems such as headaches, sinusitis, fatigue, depression, mood swings and digestive difficulties? Perhaps, more worryingly, someone in your family is ill with one of medicine's mystery illnesses such as cancer, diabetes or arthritis – diseases that appear to strike otherwise healthy people out of the blue and for no reason at all.

If you are looking for answers to these kinds of health problems, this book has plenty of practical advice. But on the pages that follow, you won't find the usual suspects of germs, genetics and the 'stress' of modern life being blamed for these debilitating health conditions. Instead, the evidence presented here proposes that such symptoms are the signs of a body that is slowly being poisoned and confused by environmental toxins.

Believe it or not, there is now a considerable body of evidence to show that fatigue, lack of vitality, pain syndromes and a range of other vague symptoms are the result of exposure to a multitude of environmental poisons. Unlike germs, which can produce an easily defined illness within a few days or weeks of exposure, chemical toxins are slow-motion poisons, stored in the body often for decades and causing subtle damage at a cellular level years before they begin to produce identifiable symptoms. Left unattended, these symptoms can, over time, develop into more serious diseases such as heart disease, autoimmune disorders and even cancer later in life.

So compelling is the evidence that a specialist field, environmenta medicine, has evolved to track and assess the impact of environmenta factors on health, and to treat those exhibiting symptoms o environmental illness.

A normal healthy body is a body where the internal systems are all in balance – a state known in medical parlance as homeostasis Environmental toxins profoundly disturb this balance. In response to these toxic exposures, and without our being aware of it, the body begins to expend an enormous amount of energy – energy that would otherwise be available for other areas of our lives – in the attempt to return to a state of balance. It is little wonder that one o the main early-warning signals of an environmentally poisoned body is the kind of profound exhaustion experienced by those suffering from chronic fatigue.

With prolonged or chronic exposure to environmental poisons the body also becomes 'confused' – a process profoundly illustrated by autoimmune diseases such as lupus, diabetes and arthritis – all o which have recognised environmental origins. When these disorder occur, it is because the body can no longer recognise what is 'self from what is 'not-self' and turns its immune forces against its own tissues.

Something similar happens in allergic disorders, when the body begins to overreact to substances that would normally not cause a reaction in a healthy person. Likewise, we know that exposure to substances that mimic or disrupt the body's natural functions such a heavy metals and hormone disrupters can cause similar kinds o problems. These substances can, for instance, initiate a confusing cascade of chemical reactions in the body – like switching off th mechanism that prevents cells from replicating out of control as the do in cancer – which have the potential to become the foundation for devastating diseases later in life.

The list of ways in which our modern environment confuses th body is as broad as it is frightening. The human body is electric, an is affected by the increasingly strong man-made electric fields in an around our homes and offices. Perfumes and other airborne pollutant can directly enter the brain and change the electrical impulses it produces, affecting our mood and behaviour in occasionally dramatic ways, resulting in depression one minute, and stimulation and euphoria the next. Some heavy metals can also act as mimics of thyroid and other hormones as well as disturbing the body's neurological functions.

These effects on human health have far-reaching implications for us as individuals, but also for society as a whole. First, they can make our bodies sick and, as anyone who has ever been very ill or who has lived with and cared for a chronically or terminally ill person knows, illness can deeply affect our quality of life and our relationships with those around us.

But the kinds of toxins we are exposed to also affect us in other ways that might not have been predictable even a few years ago. Disturbing evidence now links certain environmental toxins, such as heavy metals, with a range of emotional and behavioural problems[1] including violence, addiction, learning disabilities, hyperactivity, intolerance and lowered intelligence.

Autism, too, is believed to be predominantly an environmental illness stemming either from prenatal exposure to neurotoxins,[2] or from exposure very early in childhood to heavy metals – for instance, those contained in early childhood vaccinations – and other pollutants.[3]

In addition, toxins in the environment age us prematurely. Since we currently live in a society where the number of over-65s is at an all-time high, this has important implications for the longer-term health of a large proportion of the population. In 1900, 4 percent of the US population was over the age of 65. Today, that figure stands at 12 percent. If current projections are correct, the elderly will comprise approximately 20 percent of the US population by the year 2020. Projections for northern Europe suggest the figures there could be even higher. If these older people are suffering from many of the diseases we currently associate with old age – most of which, as this book will show, are preventable – the burden of care will place an enormous strain on our financial as well as emotional reserves.

Equally worrying is the emerging theory that the effects of toxic exposures don't begin and end with the symptoms in the exposed individual. There is growing evidence that the damage done by exposure to toxic chemicals, particularly reproductive toxins, may carry on through generations, effectively rewriting human DNA.[4]

The inference is profound since increases in emotional problems and the possibility of genetic rewiring take disease beyond the province of the humble GP and local health services and into the realms of social policy and politics.

This is important information that every citizen should have access to and yet, while doing the research for this book, it became clear that the general feeling among the scientific elite was that many of the topics covered in this book are the special preserve of scientists, that they are too complex for the average person to understand, and that most of us should simply leave the debate about their relevance to everyday life to the 'experts'.

Indeed, most people think of the scientific community as groups of ultra-intelligent individuals who have lots of important discussions with each other about their fields of expertise and who feed off of each other's discoveries for the betterment of humankind. In reality, scientists tend to be insular, rarely looking outside of their own fields of expertise or making links with discoveries in other fields. This is why scientific discovery in many areas, including the field of environmental health, can be such a slow process. It is not because there is little left to discover, but because we have lost the ability to imagine how all the pieces of the puzzle fit together and to ask the vital question "what if . . .?"

This book is essentially an exercise in connecting the dots – those disparate pieces of information about environmental toxins and their effects on health dug up by scientists around the world. If, for instance, an environmental toxin can affect your neurological system, it can then cause headaches, muscle twinges and poor concentration. In some vulnerable individuals, it can also eventually result in Alzheimer's disease and multiple sclerosis. Looking at it in this way as a potential progression, the link between the early, seemingly vague symptoms and the later more devastating disease seems both obvious and plausible.

Most people can grasp that there are things in the environment that are harmful to human health. And it seems a simple enough proposition to want to find out more about them and possibly find ways of protecting yourself from them. Yet, coming to grips with the sheer number of potentially toxic agents in our environment, in our food and water, and in the air we breathe – and the innumerable ways in which they can adversely affect human health – may prove to be one of the most challenging things you will ever do. In this field, there are no simple answers. There are no magic bullets, no Band-Aids and, ultimately, no short cuts on the path to better health.

What's more, once all the dots are connected, you may not like the picture it makes. It is both surprising and dismaying to realise that our greatest exposure to environmental toxins is in our homes, offices and schools. Yes, of course, factories, areas of high traffic and any number of anonymous industrial polluters also have a role to play. But for the most part, the toxins most likely to make us sick are the ones we unknowingly come into contact with every day in the places we generally consider the safest.

Another disturbing aspect of the study of environmental illness is the realisation that there is no such thing as a single pollutant. We are daily exposed to multiple pollutants that are toxic in and of themselves, but which also have the ability to combine with other types of toxins to create an even more powerful effect on the body. What this means is that it is not exposure to individual toxins that is the most important. Instead, it is our total exposure and, ultimately, our total body-load of toxins that is most influential.

In this respect, the advice in this book for avoiding specific types of toxins should not be taken as some sort of fundamentalist doctrine. No one can do all of these things at once. Instead, think of it as an *à la carte* menu of choices for lowering your total body-load of toxins that you can accept or reject according to your needs, your inclinations and your lifestyle. Some people may even reject the information and suggestions in this book entirely, reasoning that they may be knocked down by a bus tomorrow. Indeed, this is a guiding precept for many people.

For others, however, the idea of caution and guardianship, of long healthy lives on a healthy and unique planet, remains a powerful motivating force. For those people, this book will hopefully represent a strong and practical step forward into cleaning up their immediate environments. What's more, if enough individuals clean up their own environment, refuse to part with their hard-earned cash for products that pollute their bodies, their lives and the wider environment, and insist that employers and school governors ensure clean, safe working and learning environments, the knock-on effects cannot fail to be a healthier population, a better world for us all and a healthier future for generations to come. In the end, that is probably the most positive effort we can make in this lifetime, and the best example and legacy any of us can leave to future generations.

part one

What's Happening to Me?

1 Does This Sound Like You?

*"There's something going round"; "It must be stress";
"I think it's something I ate"; "It's probably the change
in the weather"; "I'm just run down".*

THESE ARE THE KINDS OF THINGS WE TELL OURSELVES WHEN WE FEEL ill, but can't figure out why.

At one time or another, most of us have had the experience of feeling vaguely unwell — not sick enough to take to our beds and certainly not sick enough to require a hospital visit, but uncomfortable and run down enough to consider a visit to the doctor. When you are feeling this way, your symptoms may come and go, may be severe one day and mild the next. Even more perplexing, they may seem completely unconnected with any type of illness you know of.

You may, for instance, be suffering from chronic sinus problems, headaches, occasional nausea, skin rashes, muscle twinges, fatigue, dizziness, stomach problems, constipation, menstrual irregularities, water retention, unexpected gain or loss of weight, depression, irritability, or poor memory or concentration. Clearly, a healthy person shouldn't have these symptoms, so you go to the doctor who, after examining you, says something like:

> *"I can't find anything wrong with you"; "There's something going round"; "It could be stress"; "It's probably something you ate"; "You're probably run down."*

And you leave the doctor's surgery none the wiser about your condition.

This feeling of vague unwellness is becoming more and more common. Usually, we (and our doctors) dismiss it as meaningless. Your physician may call it 'iatrogenic' – which means 'without a known origin'. In their frustration, some doctors will even blame the patient, suggesting that he or she is a 'hypochondriac', that the illness is psychosomatic, or all in the head.[1]

But the fact is, you don't get sick for no reason; and what if your symptoms were not only real, but also meaningful? What if they were tiny warning shots across your bow; your body's way of saying "take care of me before it's too late"? Would you take the hint and do something about it – even if it meant changing your lifestyle and letting go of some long-held assumptions?

Germs and Genetics

Everyone knows that germs and genetics govern our health and well-being. We learn this from a very early age from our teachers, our parents and the local GP. Get a cold and you are told there is a 'bug' going around. Develop a more serious disease and your genetic predisposition is at fault. But how much influence do genes and genetics really have?

The idea that germs are the cause of all human misery began in the late 1800s with Louis Pasteur – the father of the 'germ theory of disease'. Pasteur was emphatic that the most important determinant in the onset of an illness was the germ itself. Pasteur's theory is still widely taught in medical schools, and our fear of these microscopic foes is such that we regularly douse our homes and even ourselves with disinfectants. Our fear of germs has also led us to overuse germ-killing medicines such as antibiotics – a response which, ironically, has only served to make germs stronger, more resilient and more dangerous to human health.

Although Pasteur was one of the fathers of modern medicine, not all his contemporaries agreed with his views. Another eminent scientist of the day, Claude Bernard, was vehement that it was actually the 'milieu', or the environment, that was most important to the disease process. Microbes, he acknowledged, do change and evolve, but how they do so is a result of the environment (or terrain) to which they are exposed.

For example, the bacterium that causes pneumonia, *Streptococcus pneumoniae*, is a normal bug that resides in all of our throats, *all of the time*. Since we don't all get pneumonia from it, the determining factor cannot be the virulence of the bacteria. This microorganism multiplies without restraint only when our own defences become compromised.

Both men acknowledged certain aspects of each other's research but, even then, money, connections and shouting very loud, rather than logic or evidence, shaped the way medicine was practised. Pasteur was the stronger, more flamboyant character and a much more vocal opponent compared with the quiet Bernard. Pasteur also came from a 'good' family – he was wealthy and had the right connections. In his lifetime, he went to great lengths to disprove Bernard's view and eventually managed to convince the scientific community that his view alone was correct.

Ironically, on his deathbed, Pasteur finally acknowledged Bernard's ideas. Just before he passed away, he is rumored to have said: "Bernard was correct; the microbe is nothing, the terrain is everything."

It was a complete about-face, and one actually reflected in Pasteur's notes from his later work. Unfortunately, Pasteur forbade his family to publish these documents. However, upon the death of Pasteur's grandson in 1975, some 10,000 pages of laboratory notes became public, making it clear that, for an entire century, mainstream medicine, which had developed its theories of healthcare based on the annihilation of the germ, had been going down the wrong road.

Conventional science has partly caught up with the concept of 'terrain.' Few would argue that it is the overall health of the individual (reflected by the strength of the immune defences and the optimum function of all the internal organs), which is most important to continued good health. Alongside this, advances in personal hygiene, cleaner homes and better working conditions have greatly removed the threat of germs to our day-to-day health.

So, if it's not germs, what is it that produces this vague feeling of unwellness?

To assess the health of the nation, it is useful to look at broad trends in health. With our greater and more widespread affluence now, we should be healthier than at any other time in human history. But the evidence suggests otherwise. Diseases such as asthma and cancer are on the rise. So are learning disabilities and emotional and behavioural problems, such as depression, aggression and violence. These are all disorders that baffle scientists and doctors. Often, their causes are difficult to pinpoint and, in the search for an answer, many scientists have turned to the specialised field of genetics.

Our genes are both the building blocks and blueprints for the way we look, the way we behave, the way our bodies function, and our inherent biological strengths and weaknesses. For years we have laboured under the impression that all humans have the same genetic make-up. Those who deviate in some way from this basic blueprint are the ones, say scientists, who will be more prone to illness, disease or aberrations in behaviour.

Clearly, some genetic deviations do produce illness, and some of these – such as haemophilia, cystic fibrosis, Huntington's disease and sickle-cell disease – can be very serious. The ongoing human genome project seeks to unlock the secrets of genetic influences on human health and disease. Genetic medicine is already being practised. But so feeble is our understanding of the power of our genes that simply splicing healthy genetic material into the genetic sequences of 'faulty' individuals has met with disappointing results. Splicing healthy genes into humans, as scientists are discovering, is not as simple as splicing them into plants, and may have consequences for immunity somewhere else down the line. In addition, buried under every reported success story of genetic therapy in animals, there is a string of unreported (or only minimally reported in medical literature), often dismal, failures.

One of the most interesting findings of the human genome project, however, is that there are no genetically 'pure' types. We are all unique. We all deviate from previously perceived norms in some way.[2] As this has become apparent, scientists have been forced to reassess the true impact of genetics on health and disease.

The deeper we look into this issue, the more it becomes evident that genetic inheritance also plays only a minor role in many of the diseases we associate with modern life or with ageing.

Our genes, for instance, have very little to do with how we age or how long we live.[3] Similarly, for autoimmune disorders, such as arthritis, environmental factors may be more important than genetics.[4] New evidence also suggests that, for many years, studies estimating the lifetime risk of women with the BRCA1 and BRCA2 genetic mutation developing breast cancer, or having recurrent breast cancer, have overestimated such risks by nearly 100 percent.[5] Other factors, say the scientists, such as lifestyle and environment, are more influential.

Studies of identical twins, who have the same genetic make-up and therefore should have the same lifelong risk of cancer, have also shown that genetics, at best, play a supporting role in the development of cancer. What really counts is where and how you live, and what environmental stressors your body is exposed to.[6] Indeed, it is now acknowledged that as many as 70 percent of cancers have an environmental origin that is related to diet and lifestyle, but also to exposure to toxic substances.

Our focus on germs and genetics as the biological bad guys is a reflection of one of the major faults of medical science – the inability to see the bigger picture. It is this tunnel vision, along with the tendency to believe that what we currently know is all we need to know, that continues to distract us from important emerging evidence about other equally significant contributors to ill health.

Human Ecology

In the past, if you mentioned the subject of 'ecology' to most people, the immediate association was likely to be the impact that toxins had on wildlife and plants – an assumption based on man's superiority and separateness from nature. Now, we know that this assumption is an arrogant one and that humans are as profoundly affected by toxic substances in the environment as every other living thing.

For years, chronic exposure to low levels of poisons in the environment was associated primarily with allergies or 'intolerance' in humans – a catchall term used to describe a collection of seemingly unrelated symptoms. As research in this area progressed, it became clear that, with the rising level of environmental assaults on the body, the impact of environmental toxins was also expanding, resulting in a wide range of symptoms extending beyond allergies. New medical diagnoses, such as 'sick building syndrome'[7] and 'multiple chemical sensitivity',[8] began to emerge. The chemicals involved in these disorders were found to be neurotoxic and disruptive to the endocrine and immune systems. It took only a small leap of logic for physicians to begin to speculate that, left unattended, these initial vague symptoms could, over time, develop into more serious diseases later in life, including heart disease, autoimmune disorders and even cancer.

In general, popular books on health still promote the idea that there are simple 'magic bullets' that can help us fight the twin terrors of germs and genetics. Usually this involves taking something – vitamin or mineral supplements, herbs, designer foods and exotic exercises. While each of these things can be important to the overall picture of health, such advice may be limited in its effectiveness and even misleading in the face of an increasingly polluted world.

The magic-bullet theory of healthcare is certainly seductive. It promises that we can substantially change our lives with little thought or effort. But, in doing so, it ignores the major contribution that environment makes to ill health. Mounting and persuasive evidence suggests that it is toxic exposures in our day-to-day lives – most of which are the byproducts of our consumer-orientated society and difficult (at least emotionally) to let go of – that play the most vital role in the development of chronic illnesses and degenerative diseases.

We now know more than ever before about the things in our environment that have the potential to make us ill.[9][10] Typically, these include:

- *Airborne pollutants*, such as benzenes, xylenes and other solvents, and VOCs, commonly used in perfumes, petrol and other consumer products as well as in industrial fallout
- *Endocrine disrupters,* present in pesticides, plastics, toiletries, flame retardants and industrial pollution, including dioxins and PCBs (polychlorinated biphenyls)
- *Electromagnetic fields (EMFs)* that surround you every time you use electrical equipment such as TVs, computers and mobile phones
- *Pesticides*, found in and on foods, but also in our water supply (for instance, fluoride began life as a pesticide) and in the air
- *Heavy metals*, including the mercury found in dental fillings and some fish, food preservatives and cosmetics.

So compelling is the evidence that a specialist field, environmental medicine – or, more formally, clinical ecology – has evolved to assess the impact of these environmental factors on health and to treat those suffering from what is broadly termed 'environmental illness'.

The field of environmental medicine is largely acknowledged to have begun with the clinical observations of Dr Theron Randolph in the 1960s. Randolph is known as the founding father of environmental medicine, and many of his works remain standard references even today.[11] However, it is really only during the last decade that the field has burgeoned and penetrated into the wider consciousness. Today, it is a speciality practised by more than 3000 physicians worldwide, most of them in the US and Great Britain as well as in Canada and Australia.

While we all carry these toxins in our bodies to a greater or lesser extent, some groups such as children, women (especially pregnant women) and the elderly are more affected than others.[12] It seems incredible that we could be exposed to so many pollutants on a regular basis, but as the table below shows, you don't have to do anything more energetic than simply move through your day to be exposed to a multitude of environmental toxins.

24 Toxic Hours

Activity	Airborne Pollutants	EMFs	Hormone Disrupters	Pesticides	Toxic Metals
Morning					
Bedroom and other rooms furnished with MDF or wood-effect furniture	✓				
Radio alarm wakes you up		✓			
Switch on TV		✓			
Walking across carpeted floor	✓		✓	✓	✓
Cup of tea/coffee				✓	✓
Juice from plastic carton			✓	✓	
Hot shower/soak in the bath	✓		✓	✓	✓
Toiletries, including shampoo, soap, toothpaste, shaving foam, deodorant	✓		✓		✓
Hairdryer/electric shaver/electric toothbrush		✓			
Personal hygiene items, such as tampons/ panty shields/nappies			✓		
Use air freshener	✓		✓		
Hair spray, mousse, gel	✓		✓		
Fluorescent lighting in bathroom		✓			
Use microwave		✓			
Use blender, electric can opener, etc.		✓			
Breakfast, including cereal, toast, bacon, eggs, yoghurt, fruit			✓	✓	✓
Apply makeup/perfume/aftershave	✓		✓		✓
Put on clothes washed with perfumed detergent and/or fabric softener	✓			✓	
Put on dry-cleaned clothes	✓				
Check e-mails	✓	✓			
Travel to and from work					
Tube or bus	✓	✓		✓	✓
Bicycle	✓		✓	✓	✓
Walking	✓		✓	✓	✓
Car	✓	✓		✓	✓
Airplane	✓	✓		✓	

Activity	Airborne Pollutants	EMFs	Hormone Disrupters	Pesticides	Toxic Metals
Travel to and from work contd.					
Mobile phones, yours and other people's		✓			
Wearing a pager		✓			
Personal stereo use		✓			
Office					
Wood-effect furniture	✓		✓		
Polypropylene carpet	✓			✓	
Air-conditioning/heating	✓	✓		✓	
Use computer	✓	✓	✓		
Use other office equipment e.g. photocopier, franking machine, electric pencil sharpener	✓	✓			
Coffee/tea breaks, including drinks and snacks				✓	✓
Use toilet	✓	✓		✓	
Reapply makeup/perfume	✓		✓		✓
Eat lunch, including sandwich, pub lunch				✓	
Go to the pub	✓	✓	✓	✓	✓
Pick up dry cleaning	✓				
Sit under fluorescent lighting	✓	✓			
Use electric fans/heaters	✓	✓			
Use mobile phone		✓			
Evening					
Switch on lights		✓			
Switch on TV/stereo		✓			
Glass of wine/beer			✓	✓	✓
Reapply make-up/perfume to go out	✓		✓		✓
Go to the pub/club	✓	✓	✓	✓	✓
Use mobile phone					
Use gas stove/oven	✓				
Use electric stove/oven		✓			
Eat tinned food			✓	✓	✓
Heat food in plastic container			✓	✓	
Evening meal, including meat, vegetables, bread, grains, pulses, fruit, dairy			✓	✓	✓
Have a cigarette	✓			✓	✓
Use cordless phone		✓			
Switch on electric blanket or under-blanket		✓			
Sleep in bed with metal frame		✓			

Activity	Airborne Pollutants	EMFs	Hormone Disrupters	Pesticides	Toxic Metals
Evening contd.					
Wash dishes			✓	✓	
Walk across carpeted floor	✓			✓	✓
Make use of plastic storage for household goods	✓		✓		
Night lights		✓			
Sit on foam-padded furniture	✓			✓	
Clean house using conventional cleaners	✓		✓	✓	
Spray for ants/flies/wasps and other pests				✓	
Switch on gas-powered heating	✓				
Switch on electricity-powered heating		✓			

Polluted Bodies

In 2001, the US Centers for Disease Control (CDC) published the results of a study that had monitored levels of 27 toxic substances in the bodies of a general sample of 5000 American men, women and children. Twenty-four of these chemicals had never been systematically measured before, in spite of their widespread use and worries over their effects on human health. In addition, prior to this study, scientists had only ever measured the levels of many of these chemicals in air, water and food, and not the human body. The results were alarming and lead to the conclusion that levels of toxic metals, pesticides and plastics can be found in the blood and urine of most Americans.[13]

While the study confirmed that there had been substantial declines in exposure to tobacco smoke and lead since the early 1990s, exposure to other harmful substances, like mercury, particularly among women and young children, had risen.

The scientists also found that women of childbearing age are routinely exposed to phthalate, a chemical commonly used in plastics and cosmetics that has oestrogenic properties, and one that has been shown, in animal studies, to cause birth defects and reproductive problems.

When the second report by this group surfaced early in 2003,[14] it showed that things had not improved much. While lead levels in children continued to drop, and levels of PCBs and DDT had also come down for most of the population, the CDC investigators found that levels of metabolites (breakdown products) of the restricted pesticide chlorpyrifos are nearly twice as high in children as in adults – a good illustration of just how persistent some environmental pollutants can be. In addition, the report confirmed that women of reproductive age and children continue to have alarmingly high levels of hormone-disrupting phthalates in their bodies, and that up to 10 percent of American women are carrying mercury loads at levels considered harmful to the developing fetus. This ongoing study will be updated each year and will eventually provide data on human exposure to as many as 100 environmental toxins. It is also widely acknowledged as a yardstick by which people in other countries can judge their own toxic exposures.

Of course, the CDC surveys and others like it monitor only the most well-established poisons in the environment. New chemicals of unknown toxicity are being invented all the time and some which were thought harmless, even helpful, are now being found to be highly toxic. Stain repellents are a good example. In 2000, the US Environmental Protection Agency removed the stain repellent Scotchguard from the market because it contained chemicals known as perfluorooctane sulphonates (PFOS).

Perfluorinated chemicals (PFCs) are used as stain and water repellents in a range of products, such as clothes and soft furnishings, food packaging, cosmetics like shampoos, floor wax and some paper products, and in the production of Teflon. While Scotchguard is no longer on the market, a range of other fabric treatments such as Stainmaster and Gore-Tex remain widely available. Likewise, while Teflon pans are safe at room temperature, heated to broiling temperatures they emit PFCs into the air and, some believe, into your food.

According to the EPA, PFCs can cause birth defects and a variety of different cancers. Worryingly, a recent report by the US Environmental Working Group on one particular perfluorinated chemical, perfluorooctanoic acid (PFOA), revealed that this agent can be found in the blood of some 90 percent of US citizens – in some, at levels as high as those found in workers at factories producing perfluorinates.[15] PFCs do not break down in the environment and some observers believe that their effect on humans may make DDT look almost safe by comparison – a sobering thought for the next time you replace cookware or dress your children in 'practical' stain-repellent clothes.

Symptoms Associated with Environmental Pollutants

Nearly all our body systems and organs can be affected by environmental toxins, resulting in a number of seemingly unrelated symptoms. People who suffer from major diseases often acknowledge that they knew something was 'not right' years before their diagnosis, but simply couldn't put their finger on what it was.

If you are suffering from any of the following, without any other apparent illnesses, you might want to investigate an environmental cause.

System	Symptoms
Cardiovascular	Increased or irregular heartbeats; faster pulse; faintness; chest pain; tingling in the extremities; hand redness or blueness
Ear, nose & throat	Nasal congestion; sneezing; itchy runny nose; postnasal drip; sore, dry or tickling throat; itchy palate; hoarseness; hacking cough; pressure, ringing or popping in ears; earache; intermittent deafness; dizziness; loss of balance
Eyes	Blurred vision; pain in eyes; crossing of eyes; light sensitivity; twitching, drooping or swollen eyelids; redness and swelling of inner angle of lower lid
Gastrointestinal	Dry mouth; increased salivation; canker sores; stinging tongue; belching, reflux, difficulty in swallowing or heartburn; indigestion; nausea and vomiting; rumbling or pain in abdomen; cramps; diarrhoea; itchy or burning rectum
Genitourinary	Frequent, urgent or painful urination; poor bladder control; vaginal itching or discharge

Musculoskeletal	Fatigue; generalised muscular weakness; muscle and joint pain; stiffness; soreness; backache; neck and muscle spasm; generalised spasticity
Nervous	Headache or migraine; compulsively sleepy, drowsy, groggy, slow, sluggish or dull; depression, anxiety; mood swings; restlessness; head feels full or enlarged; feeling inebriated; floating; poor concentration, poor memory; feeling of separateness or apartness from others; stammering or stuttering speech
Respiratory	Shortness of breath; wheezing; cough; mucus formation in bronchial tubes
Skin	Itching, burning, flushing, pallor; warmth, coldness; tingling; excessive sweating; hives, blisters, blotches, red spots, pimples

In spite of this, many people believe they are immune or only minimally exposed to these types of environmental toxins. This kind of denial is an understandable and very human reaction to bad news. But it is also partly the result of misinformation campaigns by government and big business. When we are told that particular chemicals are safe, this is more often than not mere guesswork; there are no safety data at all on some 43 percent of the chemicals used worldwide today, and full safety data are available for only 7 percent of them. What's more, everything we have ever heard from 'official sources' about possible links between toxic exposures and human health has been based on misleading 'snap-shot' measurements; yet, this is often presented to the general public via the media in a falsely reassuring way.

The pesticide content of foods is a good example. When government agencies measure the presence of a pesticide in a single apple or carrot, detectable levels may be small. But we don't just eat a single apple or carrot each day. We consume many types of foods in combination and in quantity. Also, an apple or carrot may have residues of many different pesticides on it. Measuring one or two of these does not give a true picture of the total levels of pesticides on our foods. We are also exposed to pesticides in other ways, for instance, through our water, and in the air and dust in our homes. This total daily exposure cannot be accurately reflected in single measurements taken from single food items.

The same is true for figures relating to the safety of the toxic chemicals in cosmetics and cleaning products used in our office and home environments.[16] Levels in any single product may be low but, again, we use these things daily in combination and in quantity. The scent used in your laundry powder may not be high on its own but, combined with every other perfumed product you use, it can lead to significant levels of indoor air pollution with neurotoxic chemicals known to produce headaches, asthmatic reactions and even changes in brainwave activity.

There are many other examples that show up the fallacy of officialdom's reassurances that our environments are safe. For instance, your bedside lamp may only emit a small amount of radiation. But combined with the TV and video, computer, mobile phone, CD player, radio alarm, hairdryer, electric shaver, electric blanket and fan heater, the total amount of radiation you are exposed to each day can quickly become significant.

None of us lives the snap-shot life that regulating authorities use to calculate what they call the 'acceptable risk' of toxic exposures. Furthermore, when contemplating the idea of an acceptable risk, the obvious question – *"acceptable to whom?"* – remains stubbornly unanswered.

2 Who Says Your Environment Makes You Sick?

It seems incredible to most of us that everyday items such as carpets, plastics, cosmetics, garden pesticides, and even our food and air could contain chemicals capable of making us sick. Today, many doctors and government regulating authorities also have trouble with this concept and are therefore reluctant to acknowledge the increasingly large body of evidence showing the harmful and potentially lethal effects of industrial chemicals, electromagnetic radiation, and polluted air and water in our environment. This is partly because old ideas – such as the germ theory and belief in magic bullets – die hard.

But it is also because of the way that healthcare is marketed to the general public. Make no mistake, the idea of treating illness by taking (or buying) something – either conventional drugs or 'natural' herbs or vitamin supplements – generates billions in profits for the 'healthcare' business. The concept of having less, taking less and buying less as a potential form of 'therapy' is foreign to us and certainly not widely promoted. Indeed, many of the companies that produce the pesticides and other chemicals that pollute our bodies also manufacture the pharmaceuticals that we buy to repair the damage – a circle of profit that has no equal anywhere else in the corporate world.[1]

In spite of this resistance, most people do grasp the idea that there are certain things in our environment that can harm us, though few are aware of the extent of the problem, or how close to our own homes and lives these substance are.

The idea of toxins as harmful to health has also been enthusiastically promoted by the healthfood industry, where sales of antioxidant vitamins and herbs and 'detox' formulas are booming. Many people who buy and use these products, however, have only the faintest idea of what they are trying to protect themselves from.

Newspapers keep us similarly in the dark by reporting each new piece of the puzzle – industrial poisoning, contaminated food or consumer products, EMF-related cancer – as if it was an isolated and unique incident.

In fact, the bigger picture of environmental toxins and the threat they pose to health can be difficult to take in – even when all the evidence is in front of you. Interactions between industrial toxins are complex and unpredictable, and our understanding of the workings of the human body is still relatively crude.

In spite of all this, research linking a variety of environmental toxins with ill health is rapidly accumulating. Throughout the world, scientists working with well-known environmental groups such as Greenpeace, Worldwide Fund for Nature and Friends of the Earth have helped to put environmental health on the agenda for industry, government and the consumer alike.

A surprising number of studies in this field has emerged from the US, where there are several official agencies with the specific responsibility for monitoring and acting on disturbing trends in health. While the US system is far from perfect – indeed, it makes mistakes, misjudgments and oversights all the time – it towers above those currently in place in the UK and rest of Europe, and continues to provide useful and sometimes unsettling information on environmental health issues.

Among the government agencies in the US, the Environmental Protection Agency (EPA) has the specific remit to place restrictions on trade and industry if it finds that a particular practice is detrimental to human health. Similarly, the prestigious Centers for Disease Control (CDC) in Atlanta, Georgia, has recently established a nationwide tracking centre to identify and prevent health problems caused by environmental pollutants. This new agency is currently tracking what are called 'priority diseases', those known to be linked to the environment such as asthma, birth defects and cancers, and neurological diseases such as Alzheimer's, multiple sclerosis and Parkinson's. It is also tracking specific pollutants such as polychlorinated biphenyls (PCBs), dioxins, mercury, lead, pesticides, and air and water contaminants.

In addition, the US National Institute of Environmental Health Sciences (NIEHS), a branch of the National Institutes of Health (NIH), has the responsibility of monitoring the effects of environmental pollutants on human health. It has gone so far as to compile a list of known environmental illnesses.[2] This is by no means exhaustive, but it gives a good idea of the numerous ways in which a toxic environment is officially recognised to influence poor health. Included on the list are:

- Allergies and asthma
- Birth defects
- Cancer
- Dermatitis
- Emphysema
- Fertility problems
- Heart disease
- Immune-deficiency diseases
- Job-related illnesses
- Kidney diseases
- Lead poisoning
- Mercury poisoning
- Nervous system disorders
- Osteoporosis
- Pneumoconiosis

- Reproductive disorders
- Skin cancer
- Vision problems
- Waterborne diseases
- Yusho (PCB) poisoning.

In addition to research by government agencies, there is also the experience of environmental physicians worldwide to guide us. One particularly influential US group is the Greater Boston Physicians for Social Responsibility, which has produced several groundbreaking reports on environmental threats to health, including *In Harm's Way: Toxic Threats to Child Development* and *Generations at Risk: Reproductive Health and the Environment*. Their efforts have greatly contributed to a wider understanding of environmental illness.

Likewise, in the UK, the Environmental Medicine Foundation is a charity set up to promote and encourage medical research into the effects of the environment on our health, and to disseminate the results of that research. The EMF has worked tirelessly to improve our understanding of the causes of environmental illness.

Even so, there are many respects in which the UK lags behind the rest of the world in their commitment to environmental issues. The UK has no single department with the overall responsibility to monitor the impact of environmental toxins on human health, although the Department of Health (DoH), Department for Food and Rural Affairs (DEFRA) and the Pesticides Safety Directorate (PSD) do have responsibilities in this area. Each of these departments also has several advisory committees providing 'expert' specialist advice to the government on particular aspects of environmental concern. Unfortunately, these committees mostly comprise industry-friendly 'experts', whose information often serves to justify continued inactivity.

The UK's Environment Agency (EA) is responsible for regulating air, water and land quality. It has a role to play in implementing and enforcing laws relevant to these areas – though, like the DoH, it can be slow to react. The EA also acts as an information-providing service for both industry and government. Similarly, the core task of the

European Environment Agency (EEA) is to provide policymakers with the information needed to implement sound and effective policies to protect human health and the environment, and support sustainable development.

Most monitoring of the 'environment' in the UK is done at a local level. Many local authorities employ Environmental Health Officers (EHOs) and other environmental health professionals to work in specialised teams, the main focus of which is on food hygiene and safety (such as monitoring businesses that sell and store food), occupational health and safety (for example, monitoring local businesses to reduce job-related illnesses), private-sector housing (for instance, ensuring safety guidelines are adhered to), and noise and pollution control. While valuable, EHOs are not generally concerned with the broader spectrum of environmental pollutants and how they may be affecting human health.

Today, much of the responsibility for producing environmental laws and regulations has been given over to the European parliament. While there has been much talk of homogenising and harmonising rules and regulations throughout Europe, where the environment is concerned, there is still no clear consensus or way forward.

The shortcomings of the European system aside, there is a growing global awareness and acknowledgement of just how widespread environmental illness is becoming, and a greater demand on government agencies to take a more proactive and protective role where human health is concerned. This demand has been fuelled not just by the evidence of physical harm caused by environmental toxins, but also by disturbing evidence that these substances can also cause substantial, and sometimes irreversible, harm to our mental, emotional and behavioural health as well.

Nature, Nurture or Noxious Agents

"What's happening to the world today?" That's usually what people ask when presented with bewildering evidence that people are becoming more aggressive, more violent, more depressed and more emotionally unstable than ever before. Generally speaking, these emotionally disturbed individuals are treated with contempt by politicians and with sedatives by their doctors. Not surprisingly, the problem of our social decline is not getting any better.

It has long been assumed that the kind of people we develop into is largely the result of a combination of nature (our natural, genetic inclinations) and nurture (the emotional environment we grow up in). But with the advent of an increasingly toxic environment, this theory is rapidly breaking down. There is now a third element that may determine what kind of people we are – noxious agents.

Compelling evidence now links exposure to a wide range of environmental toxins with a number of emotional and behavioural problems[3] including violence, addiction, learning disabilities, hyperactivity, intolerance and lowered intelligence. These problems can cause tremendous difficulties within families, within communities and, some would argue, on an international scale.

Heavy metals are high on the list of personality-changing poisons. Exposure to lead, even at low levels, is associated with aggressive behaviour as well as learning disabilities.[4] Prenatal exposure to lead can also result in prematurity or low weight and a small head circumference at birth – an early indication for learning or behavioural deficits in the developing child. Chronic exposure to low levels of manganese has also been linked to violent behaviour.[5]

In fact, the effects of lead and manganese are also synergistic; they interact in such a way that individuals exposed to both show more profound effects than those exposed to either element on its own. Other aspects of lifestyle, such as alcohol and drug use (which are themselves associated with higher rates of violent crime), further increase the detrimental effects of toxic metals by reacting with them at a cellular level in the body and making their effects even more potent.

In addition, those on very poor diets are likely to be more affected than those receiving adequate nutrition. Brain cells, for instance, absorb more toxic metals when the diet is low in calcium, iron, zinc, vitamin D and other essential nutrients. Scientists have found that a poor diet on its own has an independent and deleterious effect on a child's behaviour and abilities.[6][7] But, when combined with exposure to toxic metals, the likelihood is increased that a child will develop some degree of attention-deficit disorder (ADD), hyperactivity or some other learning difficulty.

Industrial chemicals such as PCBs also make a contribution to behavioural problems. Research shows that children exposed to these chemicals while in the womb are prone to lowered IQs, hyperactivity and attention deficits that can persist well into adolescence.[8] Exposure to organophosphate pesticides has been associated with depression and anxiety in adults,[9] even at relatively low levels.[10] Similarly, exposure to solvents – the same as those found in perfumes, cleaning fluids and other petroleum-derived substances like plastics – is conclusively linked with mood swings, depression and anxiety.[11] Some observers even suggest that approximately 50 percent of individuals exposed to organic solvents at work exhibit the recognised symptoms of major mood disorders such as severe depression and bipolar disorder (manic–depression).[12]

Do Environmental Pollutants Make Cancer More Aggressive?

When most people think of the link between environmental agents and cancer, they think of how these substances can *cause* cancer. However, preliminary evidence from researchers at the Medical College of Wisconsin suggests that they also act on already established cancers.

The scientists first presented their findings at a meeting of the American Association for Research into Cancer, held in Philadelphia in 1999, and noted that aggressive prostate cancer cells were different in their genetic make-up from dormant cells, and that environmental pollutants – such as heavy metals, cigarette smoke, pesticides, or car and truck emissions – may trigger them to attack surrounding tissues and thereby spread more rapidly through the body. However, they also found that these same pollutants may also turn non-aggressive prostate cancer cells into killer cells.

Their research is ongoing and, amazingly, given what we know of the carcinogenic potential of environmental toxins, these scientists are the only ones currently studying the phenomenon.[13]

Such changes in human behaviour have enormous implications for the stability of societies throughout the world, so much so that a new discipline, 'biopolitics', has emerged to address them. The field of 'biopolitics' – which studies the interaction between the environment, health and government – is a relatively new science, but has some very important questions to put to our politicians.

For instance, the World Health Organization currently predicts that depression – yet another disorder that has been linked with toxic exposures and lowered immunity – is becoming an even bigger health problem than heart disease and may even surpass it as the number one cause of premature death by 2020. What does it mean to live in a society of emotionally unbalanced people? Similarly, how will social policy need to change if toxins are irreparably lowering IQs or increasing the tendency towards violence and aggression? Who are the politicians who will choose to preside over this sick society and how will they respond to the challenge of governing a population of unfocused, often violent individuals?

Once the link between polluting our planet and polluting our bodies and minds becomes apparent, it offers a clear way forward. If you want people to stop behaving in a polluted, dirty way towards each other, you need to ensure that regulations are in place to protect them from toxins that pollute both body and mind. If no such regulations are forthcoming, then people who wish to find out how they can reduce their own individual exposures to these toxins must be able to rely on good-quality information and advice from other sources.

The scientists who are forging this connection between biology and political policy are genuine pioneers. They understand that all things are connected and that, for us to move forward as a society, we must acknowledge the damage done by toxins. If we cannot, or will not, mediate it, at least we should consciously work with it.

Medicine's Denial of Environmental Illness

In spite of all that is known about environmental illness, many general practitioners refuse to take the idea seriously – a denial that often results in misdiagnosis and improper treatment.[14] Nevertheless, if you . . .

- Have consulted a GP who has not been able to explain the cause of your symptoms
- Are popping pills to relieve headache, digestive or muscular pain because a complete evaluation has failed to find the cause of your symptoms, or your doctor tells you that you have a condition such as arthritis, but only offers you a drug to suppress the pain and swelling
- Feel run down and depressed, and have been to see one or more doctors, who have offered little in the way of advice except a referral to a psychiatrist to treat your 'psychosomatic' problems
- Suffer from any of the problems listed on pages 14–15 and your GP can't do anything to treat them and the condition is deteriorating

. . . you may be suffering from environmental illness. Unfortunately, if you choose to take your symptoms to a conventional practitioner, you will need to be prepared for: a) the denial of any environmental links to your condition; and b) a struggle for recognition and treatment.

One reason for this is that the majority of physicians practising today were not taught about environmental illness in medical school. This situation is slowly changing and some of today's medical students are being educated about environmental health issues as part of their curriculum. But, in many cases, this only gives them an overview of basic problems encountered at work and at home – for example, the effects of tobacco smoke, poor hygiene and inadequate food storage.

Doctors who have been practising for many years may not have enough knowledge of environmental issues to detect environmental illness or even answer your most basic questions about environmental exposures. Worse, once they graduate and begin practising, few doctors have the time or the inclination to commit to an ongoing programme of education in this or other areas of health. New developments in everything from prescribing practises to surgical techniques and emerging theories of disease often pass the busy general practitioner by.

This is why more and more people are consulting environmental doctors – physicians who have been trained specifically in identifying environmental illnesses and who are able to advise on how best to treat them. Often, these physicians are conventionally trained doctors who have made this area their speciality. Sometimes, they are alternative medicine practitioners who have trained in various aspects of environmental medicine.

Some of the information in this book may help you to understand more about what makes you ill, and some of the advice will help you to reduce your exposure to the toxins that are making you ill. However, if you choose to consult a practitioner of any sort, you can help the process of diagnosis greatly if you are an active participant.[15]

- **Bring as much information as you can on the chemicals or other toxins that you believe you have been exposed to.** For home or work exposures from products, bring the actual product and/or a list of all its ingredients with you. This may mean contacting the manufacturer. In the US, manufacturers should be able to supply a Material Safety Data Sheet (MSDS), which should – but does not always – list health effects of ingredients. Most MSDSs are also relevant to the manufacture of products elsewhere in the world. If you are concerned about a community exposure, bring as much information about the chemical(s) involved as you can – what they were, the quantities released into the environment and how you were exposed (for instance, were they inhaled or ingested?).
- **Ask your practitioner to seek more information on health effects.** Physicians can sometimes obtain details of unlisted 'trade secret' ingredients that you cannot obtain yourself. If you are at all concerned, ask your doctor to do this. It will also help if you bring other information on health effects with you. Online databases such as the National Library of Medicine, the Clinical

Toxicology of Commercial Products and the International Chemical Safety Card (*see Chapter 11 Useful Contacts*) are good places to start.

- **Be prepared to dig deep into your past.** Make a list of any jobs you have done or places you have visited or lived in that might have exposed you to environmental pollutants or radiation.

On reading through the information in this book, it will become clear that the new healthcare paradigm needs to be based not on which magic bullets you take, but what toxins you choose to avoid. Tracking down environmental exposures in your day-to-day life can sometimes involve serious detective work. However, once the mystery is solved, you are then in a position to begin to do something positive to rid your life of these otherwise invisible threats to your and your family's health.

3 Silent Stress

THE EXPERIENCE OF FEELING STRESSED IS A FACT OF MODERN LIFE. The frayed nerves, the short temper, the anxiety, depression and fatigue that make up the emotional experience of stress are all too familiar in our day-to-day lives.

In our caveman past, our bodily responses to severely stressful situations – increased blood pressure and pulse, respiratory rate, energy requirements, muscle tone and perspiration, all triggered by the release of stress hormones – kept us safe when under attack from wild animals or warring tribes. These 'fight-or-flight' responses have been exquisitely honed over the lengthy course of human evolution. Their purpose was to preserve life by providing keener perception of potential dangers, greater strength in combat or other physical challenges and greater speed, enabling escape from potentially dangerous situations.

Most of us continue to equate stress with the physical and emotional experiences of everyday life although, today, these are more likely to entail bereavement, marriage, divorce, long working days, a new baby and unemployment rather than encounters with wild animals. But as humans have evolved, other sorts of stressors – physical, chemical, electromagnetic, nutritional, traumatic and even psychospiritual – have come into play. On a chemical level, the body does not differentiate between emotional stress and environmental stress. Anything that threatens to unbalance or harm the body can trigger its primitive fight-or-flight responses and cause the release of a flood of stress hormones.

There is even evidence that the 'low-dose effect' so common with environmental toxins also figures in our exposure to stress. Researchers in the Netherlands have discovered that small numbers of daily hassles can build up over the longer term and take their toll on our health.[1] Indeed, a body under constant stress – whatever the source – is a profoundly, chemically altered body drenched in hormones and other substances that are normally kept under tight control.

In the right proportions, stress hormones such as catecholamines (including dopamine, epinephrine [adrenaline] and norepinephrine [noradrenaline]), glucocorticoids such as cortisol and androgens such as dehydroepiandrosterone (DHEA) keep our bodies healthy. But too much or too little of them, and they become a form of slow poison, leading to a staggering list of stress-related disorders, including:

- allergies
- anorexia nervosa
- arthritis
- asthma
- atherosclerosis
- cancer
- constipation
- depression
- diabetes
- diarrhoea
- eczema
- fatigue
- headaches
- high blood pressure
- indigestion
- infections
- insomnia
- irritability
- irritable bowel syndrome

- loss of appetite
- muscle tension
- neck and back pain
- nutritional deficiencies
- peptic ulcer
- premenstrual symptoms
- psoriasis
- psychological problems
- sexual problems
- weight changes.

The human body is a vastly complex organism. It is finely tuned and adaptable. Indeed, it is this ability to adapt that helps us maintain our normal physiological state of balance. Your fight-or-flight responses are part of an in-built survival mechanism. Through a process referred to by doctors as allostasis[2] – the ability to achieve harmony and balance through change and adaptation – your body is constantly adjusting itself to prevailing conditions. The problem is that a body that is constantly adjusting itself to stressors is subject to a great deal of wear and tear. With all this overactivity, the adaptive mechanisms become worn out, leading to an inability to either adapt or shut themselves off (thereby reducing the levels of circulating stress hormones) once the stressful event has been resolved.[3]

The complex relationship between physical and psychological health is still not well understood. But we do know that the major body systems – nervous, endocrine and immune – are intricately linked. They share hormones, neurotransmitters and cytokines (substances which promote cell growth and division), a relationship that helps maintain the equilibrium necessary for a healthy body. However, in times of stress, one or more of these systems may be affected, and what disrupts the balance in one system can disrupt the others. The interactions between these systems have given rise to an entirely new branch of medicine – psychoneuroimmunoendocrinology. Study in this field has greatly enhanced our understanding of the intricate workings of the body.

Stress, whatever its origin, can also be a circular path. For instance, physical stress can lead to emotional stress and *vice versa*. When considering toxic exposures, the influence of stress should not be underestimated. A stressed-out body is a body less able to deal with poisons in the environment, and one that may, ultimately, become overwhelmed and less efficient at metabolising and excreting toxins. When your internal systems aren't working to excrete toxins, the body tends to limit the damage by 'diluting' toxins. It does this in one of two ways: by retaining water or, if the toxins are fat-soluble, storing them in fat. Not surprisingly, puffiness and weight gain, which are in themselves physically and emotionally stressful, are also associated with a body that is overwhelmed by toxic pollutants.

But there are other, even more subtle, stress reactions that link environmental toxins to higher levels of disease. The most important of these is the production of what are known as 'free radicals'. The damage caused by these substances is collectively known as 'oxidative stress'.[4]

The Impact of Free Radicals

Butter turns rancid, milk goes sour, apples turn brown, iron rusts. These are all everyday signs of decline caused by the presence of highly reactive molecules called free radicals.

In the field of environmental medicine, scientists and doctors have been investigating for many years the multitude of ways in which these toxic byproducts of metabolism can affect health.[5] Now, the term 'free radical' is beginning to seep into the wider consciousness. Nevertheless, most people still have only the sketchiest understanding of what these elements are and how they can harm health. Women's magazines, for instance, may write about free radicals in relation to the visible signs of ageing. But the damaging effects of these molecules go much deeper than crow's feet and sagging skin, in some instances causing irreparable damage to your internal organs.

Unlike other kinds of stress that produce recognisable emotional symptoms, free-radical stress is not immediately apparent. Instead, it is a gradual process that is ultimately associated with premature ageing and a range of diseases that have come to be synonymous with age, such as arthritis,[6] diabetes, heart disease,[7] dementia[8] and cancer.[9]

The free-radical theory of ageing has its roots in the 1960s when Dr Denham Harman, now professor emeritus of medicine and biochemistry at the University of Nebraska, published a paper implicating free radicals as a major cause of ageing and disease. Harman has since published numerous papers on this subject[10] and, although his theories were not at first taken seriously, they have since been proven to be sound, and now form the basis of much of our knowledge of health and disease.[11]

Simply put, free radicals are highly unstable molecules that can react quickly and aggressively with other molecules in the body to form abnormal cells. What makes these molecules unstable is the fact that they have an odd number of electrons – electrically charged particles – orbiting in their outer shell.

In general, electrons 'prefer' to exist in pairs. If for any reason the paired electrons become separated, the molecule becomes damaged and unstable. These damaged molecules are what we call 'free radicals', and will naturally 'search' for spare electrons to make them whole and stable again. In the body, they grab hold of any spare electrons that are floating around, but if there aren't enough spare electrons to go around, they attack body tissues and steal electrons from them.

Electrons are the nuts, bolts, rivets and screws of the body, keeping its molecular structure intact. The action of robbing electrons from body tissues is the basis of what is known as free-radical or oxidative damage. Furthermore, in the search for a mate, free radicals can infiltrate our DNA and damage its blueprint, resulting in mutated cells that can replicate out of control (as in cancer). They can also damage tissues and cause inflammation (as in arthritis), and impair our energy-producing pathways (and, as such, are implicated in symptoms of chronic fatigue).

We all produce free radicals as part of our normal physiology.[12] Simply eating, drinking and breathing creates free radicals in the body. Although we associate free radicals with tissue damage and decline, free radicals are not always harmful and can even serve useful purposes in the human body. For instance, white blood cells release free radicals to destroy invading germs as part of the body's defence mechanism against disease.

Are You Eating Stressed-Out Meat?

Animals are, of course, subject to the same stresses we are. Like humans, extremes in temperature, humidity, light, sound and confinement as well as excitement, fatigue, pain, hunger and thirst can stress animals out. So can environmental toxins such as sheep dip and pesticides in their food. Dairy cows[13] and sheep[14] living near EMF radiation also exhibit signs of greater stress and lowered immunity.

When an animal is under severe stress due to fear or pain, increased levels of stress-related hormones like epinephrine (adrenaline) and cortisone are found not only in the blood, but also in body tissues.[15] The stress experienced before slaughter is not only cruel, but it can cause undesirable effects on the quality of the meat, resulting in PSE (pale, soft, exudative) meat which, as the name suggests, is colourless and overly liquid, or DFD (dark, firm, dry) meat, which lies at the other end of the scale.

The quality of the meat may also be compromised in other, more important ways. As stress levels in animals go up, immunity goes down, making them more prone to bacterial and viral infections (and more likely to be given antibiotics and other medicines as prevention and treatment). These microbes and chemicals as well as all the other toxins, such as pesticides, remain in the fat and muscle of the animal and are passed on to humans when we consume conventionally reared meats. The human effects of this have not yet been properly evaluated. However, it may be an early and persuasive argument against eating commercially reared meats, reducing your overall meat intake or, for some, switching to a vegetarian diet.

Similarly, the highly reactive gas nitric oxide (NO) regulates all manner of neurological, vascular and immunological functions in the body, and even appears to act as an antioxidant under certain conditions. But too much NO is implicated in inflammatory diseases of the muscles and joints, glaucoma, diabetes and heart disease, to name but a few.

In a healthy body, levels of free radicals are kept in check by naturally antioxidant nutrients (such as vitamins A, C and E) taken in through our food and by protective enzymes (such as glutathione) generated in the body. These natural defence systems, however, can easily be overwhelmed by living in a toxic environment.

There is currently no test that can accurately measure levels of free radicals in your body.[16] However, by taking stock of your every-day exposure to environmental and dietary toxins, such as . . .

- Electromagnetic fields (EMFs)
- Heavy metals
- Pesticides
- Volatile organic compounds (VOCs)
- Petrochemicals
- Saturated and trans fats
- Cigarette smoke
- Over-the-counter and prescription drugs
- Food additives, preservatives and colourings
- Perfumes
- Alcohol
- Solvents, such as benzene and naphthalene

. . . you can get some idea of your level of risk. The more of these you encounter each day, the higher the level of free radicals in your body.

Interestingly, the overproduction of stress hormones such as cortisol and adrenaline also contributes to oxidative stress because, when they are metabolised, they also generate free radicals.

Food Sources of Important Antioxidants

Antioxidants are substances that help fight oxidative stress. More than 150 antioxidants can be found in food. The higher the quality of the food – if it is fresh and organic – the higher its antioxidant value is likely to be. Among the most important antioxidants are vitamins C and E, carotenoids (especially beta-carotene), lutein, lycopene and the mineral selenium. Natural sources of these include:

Vitamin C
Fruits (especially citrus); vegetables, including green and red peppers, tomatoes, potatoes and green leafy vegetables

Vitamin E
Vegetable oils such as soybean, corn and sunflower; vegetable-oil products like margarine; whole grains, wheat germ, nuts and seeds; apricots; green and leafy vegetables such as spinach and broccoli

Beta-carotene
Carrots, green peppers, apricots, tomatoes and tomato-based foods

Lutein
Spinach, kale, romaine and other lettuces, leeks, broccoli, celery, mustard greens, parsley, corn, kiwi fruit, egg yolk

Selenium
Cashew nuts, halibut, salmon, scallops, tuna

Lycopene
Cooked or processed tomatoes and tomato products (heating transforms lycopene into a more easily assimilated form), watermelon, guava, pink grapefruit, canned apricots.

In addition, supplementing with antioxidants has been shown to reduce the risk of a number of diseases, such as heart disease in both men and women[17] as well as a variety of cancers,[18] cognitive decline[19] and early death.[20]

Who is at Risk?

We are all at risk from a toxic environment. But some groups are more at risk than others. US researchers have found that some types of individuals – for instance, those on very low income, and those with other lifestyle risks such as excessive alcohol intake – are most vulnerable. Because the problems of poverty and broken families often coexist with inadequate diet, housing with lead paint and ageing water pipes, drug and alcohol abuse, smoking and exposure to industrial pollution as well as inadequate prenatal healthcare and low rates of breastfeeding, the poorest urban populations are those at the highest risk of health and behavioural disorders. In this group of individuals, symptoms often show up very quickly after exposure.

Nevertheless, the relatively affluent should not consider themselves immune. Our consumer-orientated society encourages us to buy and use a whole range of products that contain toxic chemicals, endocrine disrupters and heavy metals, all of which can cause similar health problems over the longer term.

Breastmilk: Toxic or Tonic?

Throughout the world, breastfeeding rates are falling. Healthy women who can breastfeed their children are now refusing to do so because the feminism of the day has convinced them that they must reclaim their bodies soon after childbirth or be lost forever. But bottlefeeding with commercial formulas, especially those based on soya, exposes infants to manganese levels that are four or five times higher than found in breastmilk. High levels of manganese can be neurotoxic and this may be one reason why studies show that breast-fed infants have IQ scores 2–8 points higher than comparable babies fed infant formulas.

While it is true that sometimes disturbing levels of pesticides and other industrial pollutants can be found in breastmilk, paediatricians and other experts nonetheless agree that breastmilk is still the only food truly suitable for young human infants. The benefits of long-term breastfeeding, in terms of intelligence, but also in terms of short- and long-term health, greatly out-weigh any risks, especially if the parents have done all they can to eliminate other environmental toxins from the baby's immediate environment. Mothers who are concerned about toxins in their breastmilk should do all they can to rid their bodies and environments of toxins before they become pregnant. Specialist groups such as Foresight can provide invaluable advice in this regard.

Women and children first

In the old days, the call for 'women and children first' was a protective gesture – designed to remove vulnerable people from dangerous situations. Today, it is a statement about those who are most likely to come to harm first upon exposure to environmental toxins.

Children are many times more vulnerable to the effects of toxic insults than adults. The worst effects of environmental poisons on children can clearly be seen in the increasing rate of childhood cancers.

According to medical scientists, the reason for the rise in child-hood cancers is something of a mystery. Indeed, some experts continue to decry that cancer is rare in children. Yet, statistics show that, after accidents, childhood cancer is the second biggest killer of children.[21] [22]

Just like adults, children can be prone to cancer at any site in the body, but two sites – the bones and the brain – are now particularly common. Figures from the US National Cancer Institute show that most childhood cancers are on the rise. Rates for acute lymphocytic leukaemia (ALL) have risen 10 percent in the last 15 years, and the incidence of central nervous system tumours is up by more than 30 percent.

Cancer is, of course, a multifactoral disease. But while scientists continue to focus their research on the genetic links to childhood cancer, important environmental triggers – in the form of mercury-containing vaccines, pesticides, food additives and electromagnetic radiation – are all but ignored.

The reason why children are at an increased risk from environmental pollution is in part because their response to toxic exposures is often very different from that of adults. Good examples of this are the paradoxical responses to phenobarbital and methylphenidate (Ritalin) in children compared with adults. Phenobarbital acts like a sedative in adults, but produces hyperactivity in children; Ritalin, a cocaine-like drug, is used as an anti-hyperactivity drug in children, but has a stimulant effect in adults.

There are many reasons for this paradoxical response. But perhaps the most influential is that infants and children are still growing and developing. During childhood, different systems and organs develop at different rates and in different phases. Growing tissue may be much more sensitive to toxic exposures than other tissue. Indeed, studies of exposure to cigarette smoke have shown that the risk of dying of breast cancer is greater for those who started smoking before age 16 than for those who started smoking after age 20.[23]

Studies on the effects of radiation also suggest an increased susceptibility in those exposed during childhood.[24] Among survivors of the atomic bombings of Hiroshima and Nagasaki at the end of World War II, susceptibility to leukaemia was greater for those who were under 20 years of age when exposed compared with those who were older when first exposed. Moreover, the type of leukaemia developed varied according to the age at exposure.

In addition to growing and developing, children differ from adults in a number of other ways that can increase their susceptibility to toxins.[25] For example:

- Their body systems have a less-developed ability to break down toxins[26]
- They eat, drink and breathe more for their weight than adults, which means they take in more toxins per kilogram than adults – for example, the air intake of a resting infant is twice that of an adult under the same conditions
- They crawl around on the floor near dust and other potentially toxic particles
- They are more likely to put things in their mouths and eat things that they shouldn't.

Children's bodies may also have less capacity to repair damage. In addition, the developing fetus is extremely sensitive to toxic chemicals. This is because the developing body is extremely sensitive to complex interactions of signalling chemicals (hormones). Disruption of these hormonal signals can permanently skew the body's development.

Women should watch out

Although it is not entirely clear why, women are also more vulnerable to environmental toxins. Like children, women tend to have smaller body frames and so their exposure per kilogram of body weight will also be higher than men's. In addition, women naturally carry more body fat than men and, since many toxic substances are stored in fat, this means that women carry potentially more toxins in their bodies. Some researchers also believe that women are more likely to use toxic products in everyday grooming and household cleaning. Many women also work in jobs that expose them to toxic substances and radiation.

Once again, trends in health and behaviour tell us something about how women are likely to be affected by these toxins. Rates of disorders such as diabetes,[27] arthritis and systemic lupus erythematosus (SLE or lupus)[28] are rising. So are reproductive disorders such as endometriosis,[29] polycystic ovarian syndrome (PCOS) and infertility. Many cancers, including those of the breast, endometrium, lung and skin, are becoming more common in women. Again, because cancer is multifactoral, it can be difficult to track its origins. But an examination into the rise in once-rare cancers such as non-Hodgkin's lymphoma can shed an entirely different light on the subject.

The term 'non-Hodgkin's lymphoma' is a catchall phrase used to cover several different cancers that develop from the lymphatic system, a complex network of cells and channels that runs throughout the body.

Scientists admit that they are baffled by the steady rise of this immune-system cancer, which now accounts for around 3 percent of all cancers. Yet, in the last 20 years, the incidence of NHL has increased by approximately 73 percent. A large proportion of that increase occurred between 1973 and 1987, when the incidence of NHL rose by a massive 51 percent.[30] Most (though not all) victims are women.

To understand how important is the link between toxins and immune-system cancer, it is helpful to know that the lymphatic system is one of the cornerstones of the immune system with a function primarily to clear debris and help defend the body. It is made up of thin tube-like vessels that branch out like veins into all parts of the body carrying lymph, a watery, colourless fluid, to the lymph nodes – small bean-shaped nodes found in clusters around the armpits, and in the pelvis, neck and abdomen. The lymph nodes produce infection-fighting cells like lymphocytes and antibodies, and also act like a filter and drain, sifting out foreign matter in the lymph fluid.

A number of significant associations between NHL and solvent exposure have been reported in the medical literature.[31] In 1976, an accidental release of large quantities of poisonous industrial byproducts called dioxins in Seveso, Italy, resulted in the exposure of more than 5000 local residents. Follow-up studies revealed elevated rates of non-Hodgkin's lymphoma and soft-tissue sarcomas – cancers of muscle, fat, blood vessels or any of the other tissues that support, surround and protect the organs of the body – among exposed residents.[32]

But chemicals such as pesticides in everyday use are also implicated in raising the risk of NHL by 50 percent.[33] Other studies put the figure higher. One investigation by the US National Cancer Institute (NCI) in 1986 found that farmers who used 2,4-D, the most common lawn pesticide, on more than 20 days a year were six times more likely to develop NHL compared with unexposed persons. Another found that individuals who frequently mixed or used herbicides themselves were eight times more likely to develop this type of cancer.[34]

Increased exposure to PCBs (polychlorinated biphenyls; found in flame retardants, plastics and insulation materials as well as in some detergents, hairspray and other personal-care items) has also been linked to the continuing rise in NHL.[35] Similarly, those exposed to the flame retardant tetra-BDE, such as professional car, bus and truck drivers, are also at increased risk.[36] Flame retardants are widely used in the vehicle-manufacturing industry.

NHL, however, is not just an occupational hazard. Women who use hair dye (particularly dark-browns or blacks and reds) may be increasing their risk of rare cancers, including NHL and multiple myeloma, by anywhere from two[37] to four times[38] over non-users. Nevertheless, this link, as well as the link with other cancers, remains controversial.[39]

Finally, there is research suggesting that exposure to electro-magnetic fields may be a risk for certain types of cancer, among them NHL. According to the available data, those exposed to EMFs on a regular basis may have 1.4–2.2 times the risk of non-exposed individuals of developing lymphatic cancer.[40]

Rare cancers, of course, are not the only effect of toxic exposures. Women are also at greater risk of menstrual disorders, mood swings, headaches, allergies and chronic fatigue. Part II of this book details the myriad ways in which environmental exposures to endocrine disrupters, radiation and heavy metals directly contribute to these problems. But women, of course, also have the responsibility of bearing children, and decades of research make it clear that a woman's fertility can be affected by pollution. Should she conceive, her child's level of health will be largely dependent on her own. Many of the environmental illnesses that children suffer from have their roots in toxic exposures in prenatal life.

The Elderly At Risk

Older people may also be at increased risk from environmental toxins. The process of ageing is accompanied by many changes in the physical state of the body that can predispose to damage from a toxic environment.

- Long-term environmental stress can lead to an increased production of stress hormones such as corticosteroids which, in turn, can lead to immune suppression and diminished healing capacity.
- The accumulation of free-radical damage, cellular 'garbage' and DNA damage due to, for example, radiation or environmental toxins can all result in mutations that make cells less resilient and more prone to disease.
- Natural ageing involves some decrease in bone mass and changes in certain systems, such as a decreased blood flow through the heart, and diminished pancreatic, thyroid and lymphatic functioning.
- Some of the disorders caused by these changes can result in diseases (such as atherosclerosis) that prevent the elderly from exercising and staying active, thereby exacerbating any health problems they may have.

It is also widely acknowledged that the elderly are generally overmedicated. Doctors who prescribe unnecessary medication to our elderly are not only compromising their health status, they are adding to the toxic burden of their bodies. Even more worrying, some medications and environmental toxins interact with each other, making their individual effects on the body even more powerful.

Breaking the Cycle

Most of us are unaware of the contribution of environmental factors to our stress levels. And yet, because they tend to bypass our conscious awareness, environmental and other stressors that are not emotional or psychological in nature are arguably the most harmful to our health. Certainly, in the face of the insidious poison of environmental hormones, indoor air infused with harmful gases or the web of electromagnetic radiation that surrounds us each day, the usual behavioural solutions for managing stress – such as reframing your perceptions of that stress to make them more positive or sharpening your coping abilities – aren't really effective. After all, there isn't anything inherently positive about being poisoned. In a body overwhelmed by environmental poisons, the usual recommendations such as relaxation and exercise may no longer be enough to completely counteract the effects of stress.

Few of us have the choice of living in an unpolluted environment. City dwellers are often obliged to travel and live in places where pollution from cars and factories is a fact of life. Many of us work and live in buildings so full of chemicals that they have come to be known as 'sick buildings'. Good evidence shows that many of the substances that we come into contact with each day are causing a health crisis in our bodies, and it behooves us to do what we can to reduce our exposure whenever and wherever we can.

To cope with environmental stress, you need to be aware of the environment and understand how it affects you even when you are not immediately aware of its influence. Once you know the sources of your environmental stress, the only way to 'cope' is to remove as much of it as possible from your life. You can also increase your intake of antioxidant foods and supplements (*see box, pages 34–35*) as well as follow the supportive advice in Chapter 10.

The following chapters provide good, often detailed, information on how specific environmental pollutants affect our health as well as what practical avoidance strategies to take that can make a substantial difference to your health.

part two

The Vitality Grabbers

4 Prudence and Precaution

WHO DECIDES WHAT RISKS YOU WILL TAKE WITH YOUR HEALTH AND your life? And on what information is that decision based?

Among human beings, there used to be common sense precepts that provided guidance, for instance, "Better safe than sorry" and "Look before you leap". To this day, doctors are still expected to uphold the ideal of "First do no harm". But if studies are correct, then doctors or, more specifically, the drugs they prescribe in vast quantities, are, in fact, the third leading cause of death in the US[1] (and potentially elsewhere in the West). It is reasonable to wonder just how many take the oath seriously anymore.

Although there is a prevailing trend in our culture towards less cautious life philosophies, at heart, most of us want to keep ourselves and our families safe from the deleterious effects of environmental poisons. Yet, there is still an erroneous belief that environmental toxins are things that are 'out there' – a belief that makes it difficult to get to grips with the idea that there are no longer any barriers between what is out there in the wider environment and what is polluting the immediate environment in your home, school or office.

Even if you do perceive the problems and risks of living in close proximity to toxins such as pesticides, persistent organic chemicals, man-made hormones and heavy metals, it can be hard to motivate yourself to speak up when you feel something is wrong. The potential risks of electromagnetic pollution are a good example of the way that some environmental pollutants present us with an emotional dilemma that can serve as a silencer. Electricity has long been sold to us as a 'clean' source of energy that makes life better for everyone. Indeed, we all benefit from the use of electricity in some way, and the experience of its benefits can make it very hard to take on board the idea that electromagnetic radiation can also be harmful.

Because of this, most of us simply go with the flow, taking the safety of the products we buy or services we use for granted – reasoning that such things would not be widely available to the public if they were not safe. While going with the flow can be a useful, even workable, philosophy in life, when it comes to today's environmental toxins, the flow you may be going with could be so toxic that it could eventually kill you.

Over the years, our lack of care for ourselves, our planet and the wellbeing of future generations has allowed manufacturers to get away with selling us everyday products, including food, cosmetics and household cleaners, that are laced with poisons. It has allowed industry and agriculture to get away with polluting our waterways and soil. Worse, it has allowed governments to get away with providing heavy subsidies to these polluters while at the same time refusing to fund studies into the cause and effects of pollution, and completely ignoring the impact this environmental onslaught has on the planet and its inhabitants.

As a result, we now live in a world overwhelmed with toxic substances. They are in our air, our water and our food. People who protest against such actions are inevitably labelled hysterics and scaremongers. We are told repeatedly that humans are healthier now that at any other time during our evolution. And yet, if we are so healthy, why are we popping so many pills? How is it possible that, in 2001, sales for the top 20 drug companies topped £155 billion – double their sales for 1997?[2] Why is the average American spending £354.80 per year on medicines, and the average Briton £124?[3]

For years, the environmental and public health movements have been struggling to find an idea that will give concerned individuals the opportunity pick up the threads of prudence and precaution again, a concept that acknowledges, but ultimately overrides, scientific uncertainty about cause and effect, and shifts the burden of proof of relative harm or safety from the consumer to the polluter.

The issue of scientific uncertainty is, in fact, an enormous barrier in the campaign to protect human health from the threat of a toxic environment. When environmental groups and individuals speak out against potentially harmful practices, they are inevitably asked to supply 'proof' of harm (in contrast, the polluters rarely have to supply data, in some cases not even safety data for the chemicals they produce or use). Yet, 'conclusive' studies – as defined by the medical and scientific communities – into the harmful effects of pesticides, electromagnetic radiation and other harmful substances are hard to find.

One reason for this is that not all of the current studies into environmental toxins conform to that 'gold standard' of medical research, the double-blind, randomised, placebo-controlled trial. Indeed, it may be impossible to construct such a trial around environmental toxins. Since we are all exposed to a greater or lesser extent, it would be impossible to find a large enough and healthy enough group of non-exposed individuals to compare results with. What's more, the ethics of exposing trial participants to known carcinogens to see how long it would take for them to become sick would be highly questionable. These difficulties have, for a very long time, worked in favour of polluters. However, readers should not fall into the trap of assuming that no clear-cut evidence of harm is the same as evidence of safety.

Likewise, as our understanding of the body grows, it becomes apparent that the harm caused by environmental toxins is initially very subtle. In contrast, most scientific research is constructed to measure the gross and obvious changes in people's health, and regulations and other actions to protect human health are usually implemented only after evidence of significant harm – for example, mass deaths and clusters of severe illnesses, usually accompanied by lawsuits – has been established.

Other hurdles stand in the way of our understanding of the harm caused by environmental toxins. When assessing the harm done by environmental toxins, many government agencies use what is known as 'risk analysis' to calculate levels of acceptable risk. Indeed, the idea of acceptable or low risk is enthusiastically sold to the public as a good reason to continue exposing ourselves to certain toxins, such as radiation or heavy metals.

In addition, when potential hazards are addressed by government agencies, they are usually addressed one at a time, even though none of us is ever exposed to pollutants one at a time. Broader issues, such as the need to promote organic agriculture, to de-escalate our addictions to shopping and to acquiring consumer goods, to encourage the use of non-toxic products and to phase out whole classes of dangerous chemicals are also rarely addressed.

To overcome all these barriers requires new thinking about the nature of 'evidence', but also about effective means of protection. In response to this need, a sophisticated version of the old adage "better safe than sorry" has evolved.

Known as the Precautionary Principle,[4] it is based on the idea of 'forecaring' and the knowledge that science, because of its limitations and uncertainties, is simply not able to provide an accurate prediction of future hazards. The Precautionary Principle does not call for an abandonment of science. Instead, it suggests that we:

- take action even in the face of uncertainty
- place the burden of proof of relative safety or harm on the proponents of an activity rather than on the potential victims
- explore alternatives to possibly harmful actions
- use democratic processes, including decision-making that involves the views of those who are most affected.

The Precautionary Principle stands in stark contrast to the acceptable risk or risk analysis model that is currently used by scientists to reassure the public of the safety of environmental toxins. Risk analysis – which evolved out of the world of engineering in the 1970s – was and is a good way of measuring things we can know, for instance, the weight a suspension bridge can bear. But it is a very poor method of calculating subtler, less quantifiable, human health risks, such as the effect of certain neurotoxic chemicals on a child's neurological development (which appears to have more to do with the timing of exposure than with the amount).

With risk analysis, whatever can't be quantified (that is, reduced to a numerical, statistical risk factor) is simply taken out of the equation as unimportant. But doing so creates large gaps in our understanding, and gives big corporations and government agencies a good excuse to continue moving forward with actions that may well be harmful to human health.

Perhaps most crucially, the Precautionary Principle acknowledges that the nature of what is considered scientific 'evidence' has to change. In these days, we must take into account all kinds of data – classical studies, case reports, consumer complaints and more – to arrive at reasonable conclusions.

The chapters that follow summarise some of the most common everyday pollutants and their effects on human health. Some of this information is not easy to read – nor was it easy to write. This is in part because we want and enjoy the benefits that many of the sources of these toxins bring. It is also because of the staggering realisation of just how widespread these poisons really are.

Much of this book is written with the Precautionary Principle in mind. Because of this, there will be inevitable criticism that it is somehow unscientific or unbalanced. Readers must decide for themselves whether this is true.

In putting this book together, a great deal of evidence from large-scale trials, smaller observational studies, case reports, consumer reports, and diverse philosophies and theories has been woven together. This should not be taken as a rejection of science; on the contrary, it would be wonderful to see more and better studies into the harmful effects of a toxic environment.

If there is a sense in which this book is 'unscientific', it is in the total rejection of our crude ideas of cause and effect as applied to the exquisitely sensitive and complex human organism, of the idea that the traditional methods of research are the best ways to study harm and predict risk, and of the belief that the scientific community is in a strong position to tell the average citizen what risks should and should not be taken. Indeed, given the shortcomings of modern scientific methods, and the tunnel vision that has come to be associated with scientific thought, the position of conventional scientists as 'experts', particularly in the field of environmental health, is particularly untenable.

Each of us has to make up our own minds, and each of us has to take the actions that we feel are appropriate to safeguard our own health. What a philosophy like the Precautionary Principle brings into the equation is the realisation that the average citizen has the power within their grasp to reject bland assurances of safety in favour of actual proof. It provides support for the idea that our own environments are our business, and that we can make changes for the better that could have a significant impact on our longer-term health as well as that of future generations.

Go ahead and look before you leap – it may well save your life.

5 Sick Buildings, Sick People

AIR IS LIFE. EVERY TIME WE INHALE, WE ABSORB OXYGEN THAT IS VITAL to the optimal function of every cell, tissue and organ in the body.

But along with life-giving oxygen, we are also absorbing a range of hazardous gases and minute particles of toxic dust. In fact, whatever is in our air is also in our bodies. So, the quality of air we breathe is vitally important.

For years, ecologists have warned that the poor quality of our outdoor air is having a profound effect on the health of the planet. The generally conservative medical press has likened the release of greenhouse gases to an act of 'biopolitical terrorism' against the citizens of the world.[1] Climate changes resulting from air pollution, say observers, will lead to increasingly severe global catastrophes such as storms, flooding and soil erosion, loss of animal and plant species, shifts in agricultural areas, and major threats to public health from air pollution, water scarcity and tropical diseases.

On a worldwide scale, pollution has been linked to holes in the ozone layer, global warming, acid rain and unpredictable weather patterns. It is also associated with higher rates of respiratory disorders such as asthma as well as lung and skin cancers. Recently, air pollution, which can block the sun's rays, has been linked to a depletion of vitamin D in the body, leading to a re-emergence of rickets among children and higher rates of osteoporosis in adults.

This is the kind of unsettling information that makes most of us want to hide away indoors. In fact, many parents keep their asthmatic children indoors on particularly polluted days to avoid pollution-triggered asthma attacks. Unfortunately, as evidence from the US Environmental Protection Agency (EPA) has shown, the air indoors – in our homes, offices and even schools – is far from safe.

In 1985, the EPA published the findings of one of the most famous and devastating studies into indoor-air quality. The Total Exposure Assessment Methodology (TEAM) study changed most of our cherished assumptions about the safety of indoor air.[2] The TEAM data showed that our greatest personal exposure to pollutants – in particular, carcinogenic and neurotoxic volatile organic compounds (VOCs) – is from air inside the home and not from outside air, as had previously been thought.

Oxygen Boosters?

There are many products on the market that purport to boost oxygen levels in the body. Often, these are vials of specially processed water that the manufacturer claims has been 'superinfused' with oxygen. Such cures for oxygen 'deficiency' have never been tested and never been proved to cure anything.

Claims that our atmosphere used to contain more oxygen than it now does should also be viewed with suspicion.

Some proponents of oxygenated water (and other oxygen-based therapies) claim that, once upon a time, our air contained 40 percent oxygen. Such claims ignore the fact that oxygen is a very flammable substance and, at that concentration, there is a risk that we could all spontaneously combust. It is not the lack of oxygen in modern air, but the build-up of other gases – VOCs, carbon monoxide, radon and ozone and, some believe, higher rates of positive ions due to electropollution (*see Chapter 7*) – that causes our air to be less healthy than it once was. The stubbornly shallow Western way of breathing also contributes to lower levels of oxygen in our bodies. A lack of oxygen is also linked with a lack of physical activity. So, want to get more oxygen in your lungs? Get in the habit of breathing more deeply, exhaling more fully and moving your body more.

The EPA scientists looked for the presence of 20 VOCs in samples of indoor air, outdoor air, personal air (the air very close to each individual, measured by monitors attached to clothing) and respired air (in the lungs) in a total of 780 people. Personal air samples contained the highest levels of VOCs – much higher than could have been predicted from any previous data. More worrying, levels of VOCs in the personal air space were much higher at night – when the body should be resting and repairing – and, once again, much higher than those measured outdoors during the same time periods.

Certain aspects of a person's lifestyle placed them at even greater risk from these gases. Smokers' lungs, for instance, retained more of these chemicals than those of non-smokers, a finding consistent with other research. Levels of benzene, xylene and tetrachloroethylene were also found to be higher in personal sample cartridges after a visit to the petrol station or the dry cleaners, suggesting that even with brief exposure, VOCs build up in the lungs.

People who work at a dry cleaners had much higher exposures than their customers; they also brought these chemicals home with them on their clothing and hair, and also in their lungs. Because of this, the homes of people who worked in dry cleaners showed significantly higher levels of tetrachloroethylene, leading to an increased exposure for the whole family – once again, a finding corroborated by other studies.[3]

Dichlorobenzene, commonly found in mothballs and air fresheners, was another solvent found in high concentrations in indoor air. Ten years after the TEAM study, another study found this pollutant in urine samples of 96 percent of all children in one US state and in 98 percent of 1000 selected adults from across the country, suggesting that the problem isn't getting any better.[4]

In the UK, the picture is much the same. In 1996, the Building Research Establishment in conjunction with the Medical Research Council's Institute for Environment and Health published data based on monitoring 174 homes in Avon, in the West of England. They found that levels of formaldehyde gas were 10 times higher indoors than outdoors. In addition, 12 homes exceeded World Health Organization recommendations for indoor-air quality. According to the researchers, the levels of indoor pollution were due to the cleaning agents used as well as gases generated by modern appliances, for instance, carbon monoxide, benzene and VOCs.[5]

Numerous studies conducted by the EPA since the TEAM results were released have shown measurable and, in some cases, disturbing levels of more than 100 known VOCs in modern offices and homes. In addition, reports from other countries, such as Australia[6] and Canada, also confirm that levels of VOCs and other harmful pollutants tend to be higher indoors than out.

All Buildings, All of the Time

If you dread going to work every day, it could be because you don't like your job. But it could also be that the environment you work in, with its mixture of gases, dusts and radiation, is literally making you sick. Likewise, if your children come home drained from school each day, it may be because they are spending six or more hours a day locked in a building that is little more than a toxic prison. Coming from a sick office or school to an equally polluted home may only make the problem worse – yet this is how most of us live.

Buildings are complex environments that can generate pollutants as well as trap and concentrate them. Nearly everything we use sheds particles or gives off gases, particularly when new. Clothing, furnishings, curtains and carpets, for instance, contribute fumes, fibres and other minute particles to the atmosphere. Office equipment, such as photocopiers, franking machines, printers and fax machines, give off a range of toxic gases, such as formaldehyde and benzene.

Cleaning processes such as sweeping, vacuuming and dusting may remove the larger particles, but often increase the levels of minute, easily inhaled, particles in the air. Chemicals used for cleaning and disinfecting are often toxic, and office and school supplies, such as pens, glues, and white-out fluids, may also give off harmful chemicals. Furthermore, people shed dead skin and hair all the time, adding to the already unwholesome mixture of toxins and allergens in the building's environment.

The presence of high levels of these indoor pollutants is in part due to the switch from working and living in buildings where open windows provided ventilation to working and living in more energy-efficient environments, where windows are sealed-up tight and the climate is controlled with heating and air-conditioning units. Indeed, sick building syndrome was originally called 'tight-building syndrome'.

This type of climate control has certainly made our working and living environments more comfortable in seasonal and geographical extremes of heat and cold. Also, it would not be so bad were it not for the fact that modern building, decorating and furnishing materials can give off such a wide variety and volume of toxic gases.

Soft-furnishing materials are a significant source of VOCs. Today, polyurethane foam and polyester fibrefill have replaced traditional upholstery fillers in sofas and chairs, and synthetic fabrics have replaced cotton, wool and silk in upholstery and draperies. Synthetic fabrics have also replaced natural wool in carpets. These new types of fabrics are generally treated with formaldehyde-based preparations to prevent them from wrinkling with regular use. In addition, vinyl- and plastic-coated wallpapers have replaced paper wall coverings.

Plastic items such as storage boxes, food containers and toys as well as paints, inks and adhesives are also found throughout our modern homes. These materials off-gas formaldehyde, benzene, xylene and other gases, and are often made with endocrine-disrupting plasticisers called phthalates (pronounced *thalates*) that can, under certain circumstances, leach into the environment. As more and more people follow the trend of working at home, office equipment such as computers, fax machines and photocopiers have added to the amount of ozone, plastics, fumes and VOCs as well as electro-pollution present in homes. Weatherproofing, double-glazing and other means of conserving energy and lowering heating bills ensure that these gases remain locked in our living environments.

Modern building materials are problematical too. Today, the use of standard plywood has given way to less-costly chipboard with a higher formaldehyde and VOC content. Plywood laminate beams, which may also off-gas considerable amounts of formaldehyde, have replaced solid wood beams. Flooring has changed from hardwood to plywood, and open-plan offices with their modular or cubicle landscapes contain hard-wearing synthetic carpets and partitions, laminated pressboard furniture and the usual office equipment, all of which give off formaldehyde, ozone, benzene and even a range of pesticides – sometimes at very high levels.

In extreme cases, some buildings have such high levels of these contaminants that they have come to be known as 'sick buildings' because, for the people who inhabit them, living and working there results in multiple and debilitating symptoms, collectively known as 'sick building syndrome' (SBS).

Although we tend to associate work-related illness with 'dirty' jobs – chemical factories, industrial workers, agriculture – many so-called 'clean' industries, everything from accountancy firms to microchip electronics industries and government offices – can produce significant work-related illness in their employees.

New or newly remodelled buildings, in particular, have a substantial amount of chemical off-gassing and can easily become sick buildings, producing symptoms of SBS in many of their inhabitants.[7]

Even carefully designed buildings can fall prey to the problems of SBS. In one well-known incident in the 1980s, the US EPA – the agency responsible for investigating environmental threats to health – moved its workers into a new building, only to find that they began to exhibit the symptoms of SBS. Detailed investigation of the problem led to the removal of 27,000 square yards of new carpet that was off-gassing a range of toxic chemicals.

Modern buildings lock these pollutants in but, even more crucially, those with automatic climate-control systems continuously recirculate a variety of unhealthy substances, including toxic gases, bacteria and dust. Evidence consistently shows that complaints about indoor-air quality and symptoms of sick building syndrome are significantly more prevalent in air-conditioned rather than naturally ventilated offices.[8]

We have yet to form a coherent picture of the long-term effects of living and working day after day, often for long years at a stretch, in sick buildings. However, the short-term effects – headache, dizziness, disorientation, difficulty concentrating, fatigue, and eye, nose and throat irritations – can be dramatic and debilitating enough, as the box below shows.[9–12]

Sick Building Symptoms

For convenience of diagnosis, the symptoms associated with 'sick buildings' are generally classified into one of two broad categories: sick building syndrome and humidifier fever. The former is usually associated with chemical off-gassing while humidifier fever is usually associated with overgrowth of bacteria in air-conditioning and humidifier units. These are further divided into type 1 and type 2 symptoms. Type 1 symptoms are similar to symptoms of colds and flu; type 2 symptoms tend to be more like allergic reactions.

Syndrome	Symptoms
Sick building syndrome (type 1)	Lethargy and tiredness; headache;dry, blocked nose; sore, dry eyes; sore throat; dry skin and/or skin rashes
Sick building syndrome (type 2)	Watery/itchy eyes and runny nose; symptoms similar to hayfever
Humidifier fever (type 1)	Flu-like symptoms, generalised malaise, aches and pains, cough, lethargy, headache
Humidifier fever (type 2)	Chest tightness, difficulty in breathing, fever, headache, wheezing, chest tightness, occupational asthma

---

As if working in a polluted environment isn't enough on its own, job stress – brought on through overwork or a lack of job satisfaction – can worsen or even bring on the symptoms of SBS, even in offices that appear to be clear of known toxins.[13 14] Those aspects of modern working practices known to make office workers more vulnerable to symptoms of sick building syndrome include:

- *Personal/emotional factors*, such as job stress and dissatisfaction, where an employee is in the office hierarchy
- *Occupational factors*, such as long hours, time spent on computers and other machinery such as photocopiers and franking machines, and handling carbonless copy paper

- *Psychological factors*, such as perceptions of comfort (for example, levels of lighting, seating, room temperature/humidity) and control, awareness of the general ambience of the office environment and personal interoffice relationships
- *Gender*, as women are more sensitive to SBS triggers than men.

What's in the Air?

Drawing from EPA and other data, the most common indoor pollutants can be divided into five broad categories:

- *Volatile organic compounds (VOCs)*: such as benzene, styrene, tetrachloroethylene and paradichlorobenzene
- *Combustion byproducts*: the result of incineration or burning
- *Breathable dust and particulates*: such as heavy metals, asbestos and fibreglass
- *Bioaerosols*: including microbes (bacteria, mould, fungi) and dander
- *Radiation*: energy emitted from electrical equipment as well as radon gas.

These categories can only be general because some pollutants are in the form of both gases and particulates (dust), or can be formed by off-gassing or as a result of combustion processes. Nevertheless, such categories offer a useful starting point for understanding the overpowering mix of chemicals in indoor air.

It is likely that, if you were to monitor the average building for the presence of these substances on any given day, levels could be low enough to be considered 'acceptable' or even 'safe', according to current guidelines. However, such guidelines ignore the way that VOCs behave in the environment (for instance, levels increase as temperature rises). In addition, while this chapter considers the effects of certain toxins on air quality, it should be noted that many of these are also present in our water and food.

Current safety guidelines also ignore the 'low-dose effect' – that is, the idea that even small doses of certain chemicals can have big repercussions on health in both the short and long term – which is beginning to receive a great deal of serious attention from scientists throughout the world.[15] The fact is, some people are extremely sensitive to even low levels of these chemicals. Whether these individuals are unusual or whether they are, as some suggest, the canaries in the coal mine remains to be seen.

Volatile Organic Compounds

The most common types of gases found indoors are volatile organic compounds (VOCs) – liquid or solid substances that turn into or emit gases at room temperature. This process is known as off-gassing. VOCs are bad news. They have no colour, smell or taste, yet they are potent neurotoxins that attack the body's central nervous system (the brain and spinal cord) and peripheral nervous system (the network responsible for relaying sensory information to the brain, but is also involved in controlling organs and muscles such as the heart, stomach and intestines).[16]

Depending on their level of volatility – that is, their ability to leapfrog about in the air, not just across rooms but, once outdoors, across county and state lines as well as oceans and continents – VOCs can either float around of their own accord until they are inhaled, or stick to solid surfaces until something (for instance, a footstep on a carpet) stirs them up and makes them more easily inhaled. VOC molecules are also very small – so small that they can easily leach out of sealed containers.

VOCs include a vast range of individual substances, such as hydrocarbons (for example, benzene and toluene), halocarbons (such as chlorofluorocarbons [CFCs] and hydrofluorocarbons [HFCs]) and oxygenates (chemicals added to fuels to increase their oxygen content such as ethyl alcohol and methyl tertiary butyl ether [MTBE]).

Individuals exposed to high levels of VOCs can experience a range of neurological symptoms, including diminished thought processes and perception of current events, poor memory, slower reaction time, reduced hand–eye and foot–eye coordination, and disturbances in balance and gait. Exposure can also lead to mood disorders, the most common of which are depression, irritability and fatigue. When the peripheral nervous system is affected, numbness in the extremities, tremors and an inability to handle small objects or do fine work with the hands are common. VOCs have also been implicated in kidney damage,[17] immunological disorders and increased cancer rates.[18]

A closer look at some of the more common VOCs shows just how harmful to human health they can be.

Benzene

Benzene is used in many solvent cleaners, and is also found in every-day items such as petrol, inks, oils, paints, plastics, petrol, detergents, tobacco smoke, synthetic fibres and rubber. In addition, it is used in the manufacture of detergents, explosives, pharmaceuticals and dyes.

How you could be affected: Chronic exposure to even relatively low levels causes eye, nose and throat irritation, headaches, loss of appetite, loss of coordination, drowsiness, nervousness and psychological disturbances. In animal tests, inhalation of benzene has led to cataracts and blood disorders (such as anaemia, leukopenia [abnormally low numbers of leukocytes in the blood] and thrombocytopenia [abnormally low numbers of blood platelets]), and lymphatic as well as bone marrow diseases such as leukaemia. Moreover, it has been shown to be mutagenic (capable of causing DNA mutations), and has caused cancer and birth defects in some studies.

Ethanol (ethyl alcohol)

Ethanol is widely used in paints and protective coatings, printing and duplicating inks, industrial solvents and cleaners, paint and varnish removers, as a de-icer in fuels and automotive brake fluids, in electronics manufacturing and in the production of plasticisers. In the home, it can be found in perfume, hairspray, shampoo, fabric softener, dishwashing liquid and detergent, laundry detergent, shaving cream, soap, mineral oil-based lotions, air fresheners, and nail polish and remover.

How you could be affected: Ethanol is on the EPA's 'hazardous waste' list. It can cause dermatitis, liver damage and intoxication. It causes central nervous system disorders, and is irritating to the eyes and upper respiratory tract even at low concentrations. Inhalation and ingestion cause mostly the same symptoms, including an initial stimulatory effect followed by drowsiness, impaired vision, loss of muscle co-ordination and stupor.

Formaldehyde

One of the most common and devastating contaminants in indoor air, formaldehyde is found in hundreds of different sources, including urea-formaldehyde foam insulation (UFFI), wood products such as hardwood panelling, particle board and fibreboard, furniture made from pressed-wood products, various plastics, synthetic fibres in rugs, durable-press drapes, ceiling tiles, carpet glue as well as glues for tiles and panelling, pesticides and paint. Factory-finished radiators give off significant amounts of formaldehyde from their enamelled coatings, especially when heated. It is also emitted from electric stencil-cutting machines, and is present in heating and cooking fuels like natural gas and kerosene, and cigarette smoke. Levels of emission increase as room temperature rises.

Consumer paper products that have been treated with urea-formaldehyde (UF) resins include grocery bags, waxed papers, facial tissues and paper towels. UF resins are also used as stiffeners, wrinkle resisters, water repellents, fire retardants and adhesive binders in floor coverings, carpet backings, and permanent-press clothes and furnishing fabrics. Many common household-cleaning agents and toiletries contain formaldehyde-forming agents.

How you could be affected: The symptoms of low-grade formalde-hyde exposure include ear, nose and throat irritations, skin rashes, headaches and persistent flu-like symptoms. Indoor air levels of both solvents and formaldehyde are closely associated with lower respiratory tract symptoms (such as wheezing), and increased rates of asthma and chronic bronchitis, especially in children.[19] It has also been shown to cause poor sleep, impaired memory and lack of concentration, nausea and menstrual irregularities.

Formaldehyde exposure also increases the risk of several types of cancer, including cancers of the lung, throat and nose.[20]

Hydrocarbons

Solvents such as benzene and the related compound toluene can release highly reactive chemicals called hydrocarbons (*see also Polycyclic aromatic hydrocarbons, pages 72–73*). These can be found in various sources, including paints, solvents, synthetic materials and vehicle-exhaust fumes. Some automotive chemicals (gasoline additives, fuel-injection cleaners, carburetor cleaners) as well as some water repellents containing mineral spirits used for decks, shoes and sports equipment, general-use household oils and gun-cleaning products containing kerosene also give off hydrocarbons.

Household products that contain hydrocarbons include any product based on petroleum or mineral oils such as floor and furniture polishes, cleaning solvents (wood-oil cleaners, metal cleaners, spot removers, adhesive removers), baby oils, sunscreens, nail-enamel dryers, hair, bath, body and massage oils, and makeup removers. At room temperature, many of these products can release hydrocarbons into the air, even from within sealed containers. In the US, many of these products (especially those that are thin and flow easily) must now have safety caps to prevent children from ingesting or inhaling them.

How you could be affected: Common reactions to hydrocarbon exposure include respiratory, skin and eye irritation, nausea and headache. However, with long-term exposure, they can cause central and peripheral nervous system damage, and cancer. Ingestion of products containing hydrocarbons can lead to a fatal form of pneumonia.

Hydrogen chloride

Hydrogen chloride is used in the production of chlorides (such as pesticides and household bleach), and in cleaning fluids, fertilisers and dyes. It is also used in tanning leather, in electroplating and electric stencil-cutting machines, and in the photographic, textile and rubber industries. Hydrogen chloride can also be formed during the burning of many plastics. Upon contact with water, it forms hydrochloric acid. Both hydrogen chloride and hydrochloric acid are corrosive.

How you could be affected: Short-term exposure to hydrogen chloride may cause eye, nose and respiratory tract irritation and inflammation. Prolonged exposure to low concentrations may also cause dental discoloration and erosion. Chronic (long-term) occupational exposure has been reported to cause gastritis, chronic bronchitis, dermatitis and photosensitisation in employees.

Methanol (methyl or wood alcohol)

An organic solvent widely found in antifreeze, perfumes, windshield-washer fluid, Sterno canned heat, shellacs, various paints, paint removers, varnishes, duplicating fluids, petrol additives and solvents, and sewage treatments. It is also used in the production of formaldehyde as well as in the manufacture of cholesterol, streptomycin, vitamins, hormones and other pharmaceuticals.

How you could be affected: Methanol causes irritation to the eyes, respiratory system and skin. Symptoms of low-to-moderate levels of exposure include headache, nausea, vomiting, vertigo, lethargy and confusion. Blurred vision, decreased visual acuity and photophobia (sensitivity to light) are also common complaints.

Ozone

Ozone is naturally present in the air as a result of ultraviolet (UV) light acting on oxygen in our atmosphere. About 10–15 percent of ground-level ozone is transported from the stratosphere (the layer of atmosphere lying between 7–30 miles above the earth's surface). The rest is 'man-made' ozone, a major constituent of smog and the result of the action of sunlight on pollutants such as VOCs and nitrogen dioxide. Ozone can also be produced by electrical discharges, and is emitted by some items of electrical equipment, such as photocopiers and electrostatic precipitators (devices used to 'clean' the air by removing dust). Amazingly, ozone is sometimes added to air-conditioning systems to 'sweeten' the air and counteract smells. This is a poor and dangerous substitute for fresh air.

How you could be affected: Ozone is a dangerous gas that mimics the effects of ionising radiation (X rays and gamma rays) and, as such, can cause genetic damage. The symptoms of low-level ozone exposure may include cough, respiratory irritation, shortness of breath, headache, fatigue and eye irritation. These symptoms usually subside within two to four hours of cessation of exposure. Those suffering from asthma and other respiratory disorders may be most easily affected, but healthy people are not immune to the effects of ground-level ozone. No one should work in the same room as a photocopier that is in constant use or employed for long runs as, particularly if the room has no proper ventilation, this can produce high levels of ozone that can result in chest pain, coughing, nausea and impaired lung function.

New Cars: Tantalising But Toxic

Reports from Australia have shown that poor air quality is not limited to buildings. In one incidence, a Melbourne lawyer became ill for several days with a headache and lung irritation after picking up a locally built new car and driving it for only 10 minutes. In another case, an Australian government worker fell ill due to driving new government cars during the first six months after their delivery.

According to the Commonwealth Scientific and Industrial Research Organisation (CSIRO), the Australian government's research branch, there have been several reports of this type of problem relating to new cars built in Australia and abroad.[21] Their studies have shown that high levels of toxic air emissions remain in new cars for as long as six months after they leave the showroom. Their measurements show that levels of VOCs such as benzene (a known human carcinogen), acetone (a mucosal irritant), cyclohexane (a possible human carcinogen), ethyl benzene and MIKB (systemic toxic agents), and xylene (a fetal toxin) are unacceptably high in new cars. Even after four months, their levels in some cars were four times those considered safe for humans.

Take a look inside your car and you will see why. Plastics such as PVC predominate, as do fabrics treated with stain-resisting chemicals. Carpets, too, contain synthetics and are treated with pesticides. Driving for any amount of time sealed in this environment can produce eye, nose and throat irritation, headache and a worsening of existing neurological complaints. More dangerously, it can also cause an inability to concentrate, fatigue and drowsiness.

PCBs (polychlorinated biphenyls)

The manufacture and use of these dangerous chemicals, which include dioxin and dibenzofuran, are now banned in many countries, including the US and UK, but they may still be found in older electrical appliances, and may leak from ageing visual display units and fluorescent lights (*see Chapter 8 for more information on PCBs*).

How you could be affected: PCBs cause skin rashes but, more seriously, they can also cause cancer, damage to reproductive organs, birth defects, and damage to the liver and kidneys.

Pesticides

The word 'pesticide' covers a range of lethal chemicals such as insecticides, fungicides, herbicides and rodenticides, to name but a few. Pesticides can contain VOCs as both active and inactive (or 'inert') ingredients. Pesticides are used inside buildings for many reasons: to kill fungi, beetles, fleas, ants, booklice, silverfish, rodents, and plant and timber pests. They are also regularly used on buses, trains and planes, where they affect the air quality inside these vehicles. The pesticides used as wood preservatives often leach out into the air over a number of years.

All pesticides are harmful to humans (though some are more harmful than others). Treatment with these substances is sometimes carried out during working hours, with little apparent concern for the health of the people in the immediate environment. Even when spraying is carried out in buildings overnight or over the weekend, unsafe levels of pesticides will still be circulating in the atmosphere when employees return to work.

Pesticides are also used outdoors on city streets and parks, where they can be tracked indoors on shoes, and find a welcome home in carpets and indoor dust. This can be inhaled with other minute particulates when the dust is stirred up (for instance, every time you walk across a carpeted floor).

Pesticides may be also added to air-conditioning and ventilation systems to reduce biological contamination, although this is not an effective way to kill microbes. Only proper cleaning and maintenance can do this. Adding pesticides to the air-conditioning system only serves to circulate these toxins throughout the building.

How you could be affected: The hazards of pesticides depend on their chemical constituents (one product will often contain a 'cocktail' of chemicals). But, in general, these include cancer, fetal damage, liver and nerve damage, skin problems, and irritation to the eyes and respiratory system (*see Chapters 6 and 8 for more details*).

Solvents

Solvents are a major source of VOCs, and are widely used in adhesives, glues, cleaning fluids, paint and felt-tip pens, perfumes, paints, varnishes, pesticides, petrol, and household cleaners and waxes. Solvents such as toluene, acetone and trichloroethane are found in white-out fluids and thinners. The US Environmental Protection Agency's National Human Adipose Tissue survey in 1982 showed that four solvents – xylene, dichlorobenzene, ethylphenol and styrene – were present in 100 percent of tissue samples tested across the country,[22] confirming that these substances are not only very common, but also linger on in the body.

How you might be affected: Solvents are potent neurotoxins.[23] Exposure may cause headaches, dizziness or eye, throat and skin irritation as well as mood disturbances, loss of motor control, confusion and impaired memory. But the effects don't end there. Solvents have been found to decrease levels of the male sex hormone testosterone and the female luteinising hormone (one of the hormones regulating the menstrual cycle).[24] As a result, solvents have been associated with infertility,[25] decreased sperm count,[26] and increased rates of miscarriage[27] and fetal malformation.[28]

A wide range of solvents, including benzene, styrene, tetra-chloroethylene, carbon tetrachloride, carbon disulphide and formaldehyde, have also been associated with blood disorders such as leukaemia,[29] increased death rates from heart problems[30] and increased levels of insulin in the body.[31] Another study examining the cancer risk for house painters showed a 95 percent increased incidence of multiple myeloma, a 52 percent increase in bladder tumours, and a 45 percent increase in kidney and other urinary tract tumours.[32] Trichloroethylene, used as a dry-cleaning solution, but also in spray adhesives and some types of stencil machines, can cause liver cancer and damage to the lungs and central nervous system.

The safety record isn't much better for solvents used in medicines and cosmetics. Applied to the skin, beauty products containing the industrial solvent propylene glycol can cause dermatitis.[33] Case reports continue to show that intravenous propylene glycol – found in medicines such as phenytoin, phenobarbital, diazepam, digoxin and etomidate – can be toxic.[34] Its use is associated with seizures, liver and kidney damage[35] as well as haemolysis (destruction of haemoglobin from red blood cells), central nervous system damage, hyperosmolality (increased cellular permeability) and lactic acidosis.[36] How safe it is in our foods is anyone's guess.

Styrene

Styrene can enter the atmosphere from industrial emissions and tobacco smoke, but it is also emitted from synthetic carpets, and plastic and vinyl products such as vinyl floor coverings, blinds, textiles, synthetic rubber underlay, fillers and paints. It can also be found in some cleaning solutions.

How you could be affected: The International Agency for Research on Cancer (IARC) has classified styrene as a probable human carcinogen. Once in the body, it can cause damage to the liver and kidneys. It can also trigger central nervous system damage as well as skin and respiratory irritation.

Trichloroethylene

Trichloroethylene (TCE) is a commercial product with a wide variety of industrial uses. Over 90 percent of the TCE produced is used in the metal-degreasing and dry-cleaning industries. It is also added to printing inks, paints, lacquers, varnishes and adhesives.

How you could be affected: In 1975, the US National Cancer Institute reported that an unusually high incidence of liver cancer had been observed in mice given TCE through stomach tubes. The agency now considers this chemical a potent liver carcinogen. Over the longer term, workers exposed to trichloroethylene have a higher risk of cancers of the stomach, liver, prostate and lymphatic system[37] as well as an increased risk of death from these cancers.[38]

Vinyl chloride

Vinyl chloride is found in plastic products (as in polyvinyl chloride [PVC]) such as pipes, wire coverings and light fixtures, and in upholstery and carpets. The construction, furniture, automobile, plastics, rubber, paper and glass industries also rely on vinyl chloride for many of their products.

How you could be affected: Vinyl chloride is classified by the EPA as a human carcinogen. Short-term exposure to high levels can result in central nervous system effects such as dizziness, drowsiness and headaches. Long-term exposure can cause liver cancer in humans.

Perfume

Most of the toxic chemicals that pollute the air in our homes and other buildings can be found in a single bottle of your favourite perfume. Indeed, perfumes are among the nastiest pollutants in our indoor environment. First and foremost, they are nasty because they are poisonous. But they are nastier still because of the way they are marketed as luxury beauty items that enhance our bodies, our sexuality and our environment.

Most people, especially women, would find that statement provocative. Yet, consider that, of the several thousand different chemicals used in fragrance manufacture, 95 percent are derived from petroleum. Of the less than 20 percent of these that have actually been tested for safety, most have been found to be toxic to humans.[39] These chemicals include industrial solvents such as benzene derivatives and aldehydes, and many other known toxins and sensitisers capable of causing cancer, birth defects, central nervous system disorders and allergic reactions.[40] Some, like acetone, ethanol and methylene chloride, are classified by the EPA as 'hazardous waste'.

In addition to being used in perfumes, fragrance chemicals are increasingly being used in an ever-wider variety of products, including cosmetics, hygienic products, drugs, detergents and other household cleaners, plastics, industrial greases, oils and solvents, foods and tobacco products.

How you could be affected

In 1986, the US National Academy of Sciences targeted fragrances as one of the six categories of chemicals that should be given high priority for neuro-toxicity testing. This recommendation placed perfume ingredients right up there with insecticides, heavy metals, solvents and food additives as primary disease-causing agents.

There is ample evidence that inhaled fragrances can cause immediate side-effects. The fragrance portion of laundry products and cosmetics, for instance, is the number one cause of allergic and irritant skin reactions to those products. These are mostly local reactions caused by the product coming into contact with the skin. However, skin rashes can occur in sensitive individuals without the fragrance ever coming into direct contact with the skin.

There is nothing to stop the chemicals you inhale from entering your bloodstream and reaching your brain. In fact, they quickly and easily breach the 'blood–brain barrier' – the tightly tiled lining of the brain's vascular system that allows energy-giving glucose to pass, but not most other substances – and find their way to the limbic system – the control centre for many bodily functions, including emotion, instinct, voluntary movement, sleep, hormonal secretions and the interpretation of senses other than smell.

Perfumes can produce longer-term problems such as asthma as well as neurological and skin disorders.[41] Since most perfumes are primarily composed of solvents, their neurotoxic effects are similar to those for people exposed to the solvents in glues, varnishes, paints, paint strippers, nail-polish removers and petrol. Chronic problems associated with exposure to fragrance chemicals include:[42]

- agitation
- anaphylaxis
- anxiety
- asthma
- bronchitis
- confusion
- coughing
- depression
- difficulty breathing
- difficulty swallowing
- disorientation
- dizziness
- double vision
- ear pain

- eczema
- fatigue
- flushing
- headaches
- hives
- hypertension
- incoherence
- irregular heart beat
- irritability
- laryngitis
- lethargy
- mood swings
- muscle/joint pain
- muscle weakness

- nasal congestion
- nausea
- poor concentration
- rashes
- restlessness
- seizures
- short-term memory loss
- sinusitis
- sneezing
- spaciness
- swollen lymph glands
- tinnitus
- vertigo
- watery or dry eyes

In addition to being toxic on their own, perfume ingredients can react with other substances to become even more noxious. Most recently, US scientists have found that limonene, a component of the scent portion of lemon- and pine-scented products like air fresheners and furniture waxes, can react with indoor ozone to quickly form the kind of harmful particulates known to cause lung and heart disease.[43]

Fragrance free – and about time

There are now urgent calls for second-hand scent to be considered in much the same light as second-hand smoke. Indeed, scent may, in the end, prove to be even more of a health hazard as it produces immediate and debilitating symptoms in people exposed to it. The seeds of a fragrance-free movement have already been planted in the West.

In 1996, the American magazine *People* received a stack of complaints because of the inclusion of perfume strips among its pages. Similar protests occurred in Canada when *Canadian Geographic* and *Readers Digest* inserted scent-strip advertising. Such was the outcry that their publishers (perhaps in conjunction with their lawyers) had a rethink about these insertions in their publications and decided not to include them again.

Today, in the US and Canada, many women's magazines now offer subscription-only versions of their magazines without perfume strips. Several environmental groups have also led the way towards a scent-free environment by requesting that delegates at their conferences adhere to a fragrance-free policy. Some individuals now issue invitations to their homes with a request to come fragrance-free.[44] However, it is the local government in Halifax, Nova Scotia, Canada, that has taken this trend to its logical conclusion by implementing fragrance-free policies in all public offices and many private businesses. In doing so, they have managed to achieve what even the US Food and Drug Administration and the Environmental Protection Agency could not – an almost total ban on fragrances in public places.

Combustion Byproducts

As the term suggests, combustion byproducts are produced by burning things. Incineration can release a wide range of gases as well as particulates – minute and easily inhaled particles of dust that float around in our outdoor atmosphere and leach into our indoor air. Cigarette smoke is one of the main ways these toxic particulates get into our indoor atmospheres. Even human metabolism is a combustive process – the simple act of breathing in and out releases carbon dioxide into the air.

Carbon dioxide

Carbon dioxide is present in the unpolluted atmosphere at a concentration of about 0.03 percent but, since about 5 percent of the air we breathe out is carbon dioxide, levels can increase dramatically in inadequately ventilated areas. Carbon dioxide also comes from outside sources such as vehicle-exhaust fumes, nearby smoking chimneys or other exhausts.

How you could be affected: Too much carbon dioxide can initially bring on headache and lethargy, followed by breathlessness, sweating, visual impairment and tremor. In extreme cases, carbon-dioxide inhalation can lead to unconsciousness and even death. Indeed, excessive levels of carbon dioxide are thought to be a contributing factor to sudden infant death syndrome (SIDS).

Carbon monoxide

The major source of carbon monoxide is vehicle-exhaust fumes. However, any process of combustion can produce carbon monoxide, so this gas is produced by tobacco smoking, gas cookers, and gas or oil heaters. We all exhale a small amount of carbon monoxide in our breath. Carbon monoxide can also be emitted from combustion engines (as used in automobiles and gas-powered lawn mowers, for example), poorly ventilated kerosene or space heaters, furnaces, wood-burning stoves, gas cookers and fireplaces.

How you could be affected: Carbon monoxide inhibits the distribution of oxygen in the blood to the rest of the body. Depending on the amount inhaled, symptoms can include fatigue, headache, weakness, confusion, disorientation, nausea and dizziness. These symptoms are sometimes confused with flu or food poisoning. Children, the elderly, and people with heart and respiratory illnesses are particularly at high risk for adverse health effects of carbon monoxide. Smokers have significantly higher levels of carbon monoxide (and, thus, lower levels of oxygen) in their blood. However, non-smokers who spend their working day in an atmosphere containing high levels of carbon monoxide will have low blood-oxygen levels comparable to those of smokers and possibly the early symptoms of carbon-monoxide poisoning. Long-term exposure to carbon monoxide is associated with heart disease, and extremely high levels can cause death.

Nitrogen dioxide

Nitrogen dioxide is formed as a result of the oxidation of the air pollutant nitric oxide. It is emitted from vehicle exhausts, tobacco smoke, and gas heaters and cookers. Most nitrogen-dioxide emissions are traffic-related, so levels are generally highest in urban rather than rural areas. Nitrogen dioxide also plays a major role in the atmospheric reactions that produce ground-level ozone and acid rain.

How you could be affected: Exposure to nitrogen dioxide can result in shortness of breath and chest pain. It can exacerbate existing respiratory disorders such as asthma and bronchitis. Relatively short exposures of 15 minutes can begin to impair the normal transport of gases between the blood and lungs in healthy adults.

Polycyclic aromatic hydrocarbons (PAHs)

This is a large group of highly carcinogenic hydrocarbons that are released when certain substances are burnt. Most people are exposed to PAHs when they breathe in smoke (including cigarettes, but also from barbecues and bonfires), auto emissions or industrial exhausts. Mothballs, blacktop and creosote wood preservatives also contain PAHs. They can also enter our environment in unforeseen ways. For instance, some medicated skin creams and shampoos containing coal-tar ingredients contain PAHs. Likewise, burning incense can release significant amounts of carcinogenic PAHs into the air.[45]

How you could be affected: PAHs can be absorbed through the skin, and can contaminate water and soil. General effects of exposure include respiratory, skin and eye irritation, nausea and headache. Over the long-term, PAH exposure can cause central and peripheral nervous system damage, and cancer.

Sulphur dioxide

The most common natural source of sulphur dioxide is volcanoes. The single largest man-made source of sulphur dioxide is coal burning, which accounts for about 50 percent of annual global emissions. Oil burning accounts for a further 25–30 percent. Common industrial sources of sulphur dioxide include smelting, production of elemental sulphur and sulphuric acid, conversion of wood pulp to paper and incineration of refuse.

How you could be affected: Exposure to sulphur dioxide causes respiratory irritation, runny nose and cough. Long-term exposure can lead to chronic bronchitis, lung damage and altered sense of smell. It can mix with other pollutants to increase the carcinogenic effects. Research has shown that asthmatics may be more sensitive to sulphur dioxide than other individuals.

Tobacco smoke

Burning tobacco releases a complex mixture of particles and more than 4000 chemicals into the air. Forty-three of these are known to induce cancer in both humans and animals, and many of the others can induce cancer when combined with other substances. Cigarettes contain highly addictive nicotine and carcinogenic nitrosamines. But they also contain:

- **Arsenic,** used in rat poison
- **Acetic acid,** a hair dye and photo developer
- **Acetone,** the main ingredient in paint and nail-polish remover
- **Ammonia,** a common ingredient in household cleaners
- **Benzene,** found in glues and paints
- **Cadmium,** found in batteries and artists' oil paints
- **Carbon monoxide,** a poison
- **Formaldehyde,** often used to embalm dead bodies
- **Hydrazine,** a component of jet and rocket fuels
- **Hydrogen cyanide,** a poison used in gas chambers
- **Naphthalene,** a carcinogen found in explosives, mothballs and paint pigments
- **Nickel,** used in the process of electroplating
- **Phenol,** used in disinfectants and plastics
- **Polonium,** a radioactive metal absorbed from phosphate fertilisers
- **Toluene,** found in embalmer's glue.

In addition, cigarette manufacturers often add neurotoxic perfumes (aromas) to the tobacco to make it smell less like tobacco – a cynical gesture intended to make second-hand smoke less objectionable to non-smokers in the vicinity of the smokers. At present, upwards of 600 different aromas have been added to cigarettes.

How you could be affected: Many of the substances found in tobacco have toxic or irritant properties that cause symptoms similar to those of sick building syndrome – such as eye and nose irritation, coughing, breathing difficulties, sore throat and hoarseness, headache, nausea and dizziness – in both smokers and non-smokers. However, the long-term effects of involuntary exposure to second-hand smoke are the most worrying.

Second-hand smoke is a powerful toxin that affects us all. In the 1980s, several scientific committees and national organisations concluded that exposure to environmental tobacco smoke (also called 'passive smoking') is a cause of lung cancer in non-smokers.[46–49]

More recent reviews have concluded that non-smokers living with smokers have a 24 percent greater risk of contracting lung cancer than those living in a smoke-free household. The more a partner smokes, the higher the spouse's risk.[50] People exposed to workplace smoke are also at greater risk. A joint report of the Trades Union Congress (TUC) Action on Smoking and Health (ASH) and the Chartered Institute of Environmental Health (CIEH) in the UK in 2003 produced figures to show that there are three times as many deaths from passive smoking at work than the total number of deaths from workplace injuries. The report's author notes that more people died in 2002 from passive smoking at work in the UK than were killed by the great London smog of 1952.[51]

Non-smokers are also more at risk from heart disease if they live with smokers. A 1997 study published in the BMJ found that, by age 65, the risk of developing heart disease if you live with a smoker was 30 percent greater than if you didn't. This was a surprisingly high figure – roughly equivalent to just under half the risk of smoking 20 cigarettes per day, even though the relative exposure to tobacco smoke is only 1 percent that of a smoker.[52]

Breathable Dusts and Particulates

Dust is a fact of life. While we think of it as just dirt, its composition can be much more complex than that. Incineration and other industrial processes can produce minute particles (particulates) of a whole range of toxic substances, light enough to be carried on the air and into our homes, offices and schools. Likewise, ordinary house dust can absorb or be contaminated with heavy metals, pesticides and other toxic substances present in the indoor environment. These minute particles are small enough to be easily inhaled[53] and, once in the lungs, they tend to stick there, causing a range of respiratory problems. Bear in mind that some processes, such as combustion, produce gases as well as particulates. Thus, gas-burning stoves, fireplaces and cigarettes can also contribute toxic gases and particulates to the household air. Fine particles are also formed when you use any kind of aerosol.

Particulates are largely invisible, but devastating, pollutants. Some estimates suggest that they are responsible for up to 10,000 premature deaths in the UK each year. To follow are some of the most worrying particulates present in indoor air.

Asbestos

Asbestos is the name given to any one of six different fibrous minerals. Asbestos minerals have separable long fibres that are strong and flexible enough to be spun and woven, and are naturally heat resistant. Because of these characteristics, asbestos has been used for a wide variety of manufactured goods, mostly building materials such as roofing shingles, ceiling and floor tiles, paper products and asbestos cement products, as well as duct insulation in air-conditioning systems. The inevitable deterioration of asbestos products over time means that respirable fibres (those small enough to be inhaled) are released into the air. Fibres can also be released if these building materials are cut or damaged.

Asbestos is also used in friction products such as the clutch, brakes and transmission parts in automobiles, and in heat-resistant fabrics, packaging, gaskets and coatings. Some talc products, including the talc coating on children's crayons, also contain asbestos.[54]

Although asbestos use throughout the world is declining, problems still remain mostly because asbestos is big business. It took until 1989 for the EPA to finally ban all new uses of asbestos in the US. However, the Canadian government has fought all efforts to ban or control the use of this material. Canada is the world's second-largest exporter of asbestos and, when the US ban came into force, the Canadian government sued the EPA, challenged its European allies (many of which had also recommended the ban) and financed questionable science to prove that asbestos, especially Canadian asbestos, wasn't really dangerous. US asbestos manufacturers joined the fight and, supported by the governments of Canada and Quebec province, also sued the EPA. In October 1991, the US ban was overturned. As a result, it still remains legal to mine, import and sell asbestos in the US – a fact that did not receive much fanfare or press attention. Indeed, many US citizens still believe that it is illegal to use asbestos and that they are protected by law from its harmful effects.

In the UK, the use of some types of asbestos, such as amosite (brown asbestos) and crocidolite (blue asbestos), was banned in 1985. But it took until August 1999 to ban chrysotile (white asbestos), one month after the European Union (EU) ban of the same substance came into force. Australia has one of the highest rates of mesothelioma (a rare form of lung cancer caused by asbestos inhalation) in the world, yet the Australian government only banned importation of raw asbestos and products containing the deadly substance in 2003, with a view to completely phasing out existing products containing the deadly fibres by 2010.

How you could be affected: Many of us still inhabit buildings that contain asbestos in some form, and this means that asbestos is still an issue and still a killer. Asbestos is a confirmed human carcinogen, and all types of asbestos – blue, brown and white – can cause mesothelioma, cancer and fibrosis of the lung.

Asbestos mainly affects the lungs and the membrane that surrounds the lungs. Breathing high levels of asbestos fibres for a long time may result in scar-like tissue in the lung and in the pleural membrane (lining) surrounding the lung. This disease is called asbestosis and is usually found in workers exposed to asbestos, but not in the general public. People with asbestosis have difficulty breathing, often a cough and, in severe cases, heart enlargement. Asbestosis is a serious disease that can eventually lead to disability and death.

Breathing lower levels of asbestos may result calcifications (called 'plaque') of the pleural membranes. Pleural plaques can occur in workers and sometimes in those living in areas with high environmental levels of asbestos. Effects on breathing due to pleural plaques alone are not usually serious, but higher exposure can lead to a thickening of the pleural membrane that may restrict lung expansion and, thus, breathing.

Chemicals in the Carpet

The carpeting in your home is one of the major sources of neurotoxic VOCs such as 4-phenylcyclohexene, tetrachloroethylene, benzene, xylene, toluene, styrene and methylbenzene. It is also a reservoir for pesticides, tobacco smoke and heavy metals.[55]

To find out just how prevalent these chemicals are in carpets, one laboratory in the US tested more than 400 carpet samples of varying age. They found these chemicals present in more than 90 percent of the samples tested.[56] Even samples 20 years old or more were still giving off neurotoxic and potentially fatal VOCs.

However, it's not just VOCs that lurk underfoot. Carpeting and house dust also harbour pesticides. In 1993, the EPA-sponsored Non-Occupational Pesticide Exposure Study (NOPES) was published.[57]

This study also confirmed that indoor air was more toxic than outdoor air but, instead of looking for VOCs, the NOPES looked at pesticide levels. The researchers noted that, corresponding with the seasonal patterns of pesticide use, concentrations of pesticides in indoor air were highest in summer and lowest in winter. The most commonly detected pesticides were heptachlor, chlorpyrifos, aldrin, dieldrin, chlordane, atrazine, DDT, orthophenylphenol, propoxur, diazinon and carbaryl (*for more information on these, see Chapters 7 and 9*).

Recently, a report from the University of Exeter in the UK found that new carpets contain significant levels of the hormone-disrupting, brominated flame retardant BDE-209, the pesticides permethrin (implicated in the debilitating symptoms suffered by Gulf War veterans) and tributyltin (an immune- and reproductive-system toxin), and formaldehyde.[58]

Those most at risk from the pesticides in carpets are toddlers and infants, who spend much of their time on the floor and who tend to put things that have been in contact with the carpet into their mouths. According to the NOPES, this route of exposure provides infants and toddlers with nearly all of their non-dietary exposure to the neurotoxic, immunotoxic and endocrine-disturbing pesticides DDT, aldrin, atrazine and carbaryl.

Detergent dust

The dried residues of detergent, for instance, those used in carpet cleaning, can be liberated into the air every time you walk through the office.

How you could be affected: Detergent residues can cause respiratory irritation such as cough, dry throat, breathing difficulty, nasal congestion and headache. The severity of the effect often depends on the type of detergent and its formulation (for instance, whether it includes pesticides or formaldehyde-releasing stain guards).

Fibreglass

Fibreglass is the fine filament or fibre formed by forcing molten glass through small holes. The resulting 'glass wool' is generally used for heat and acoustic insulation, in fire blankets, and as reinforcement in plastics and mouldings.

How you could be affected: Dust and airborne fibres can be released when fibreglass-reinforced plastics are cut, ground or sanded. These thin fibres can irritate the skin and lungs. However, the biggest hazard may be from the epoxy or resin used to bind sheets of fibreglass to each other or to other materials. Some of these may contain styrene and so may cause irritation to the eyes, nose, throat and skin.

Fibreglass insulation can also indirectly contribute to indoor pollution since it prevents buildings from breathing, and encourages the growth of bioaerosols such as moulds, fungi and bacteria.

Toxic metals

Examples of the toxic metals commonly found in dust include lead, mercury, arsenic and cadmium. In their elemental form, these metals tend to be too heavy to ride on the wind. But once reduced to microscopic particles, they become mobile. Toxic metals are used in a variety of products, including light fixtures, pesticides and wood preservatives. They can be found in cosmetics such as eyeshadow and mascara, and can be emitted from industrial incineration and tobacco smoke.

How you could be affected: Toxic metals do not dissolve, evaporate or decompose. They have no function in the body and some are highly poisonous. Immune deficiency, lowered intelligence, aggression, violence and birth defects are just some of their effects. (*For a detailed discussion of toxic metals and their health effects, see Chapter 9.*)

Bioaerosols

The term 'bioaerosol' refers to both living and non-living biological air contaminants. These can include moulds or mildew (fungi), bacteria, viruses, algae, animal dander, dustmite allergens and pollen. These contaminants travel through the air and are often invisible. The most common indoor bioaerosols are bacteria and fungi. Given the right conditions, they can multiply, causing a range of symptoms and diseases in humans. According to environmental lawyers, toxic moulds are the asbestos of the new millennium, primarily because fungi – such as *Penicillium, Stachybotrys charcarum, Aspergillus* and *Altemaria* – can produce poisonous substances called mycotoxins, which are harmful to humans and animals if inhaled, ingested or absorbed through the skin, as well as VOCs. Some bacteria also produce both toxins (called endotoxins) and VOCs.

Many indoor air-quality problems begin as moisture problems, such as leaks, floods or excessive humidity. These moist conditions allow organisms like mould and mildew to grow rapidly and in many locations, including bathrooms, damp or flooded basements, wet appliances (humidifiers and air conditioners), and even carpets and furniture. Mould, mildew and other biological contaminants can also grow in poorly maintained building-ventilation systems. These systems then distribute the contaminants throughout the building to the occupants.

Microorganisms can also get indoors through the heating, ventilation and air-conditioning systems, doors, windows, cracks in the walls or the potable drinking water supply, or be brought in on the shoes and clothes of people working in or visiting the building. Water, humidity, temperature, nutrients (such as dirt, wood, paper and paint), oxygen and light determine whether and how well microorganisms will grow in the indoor environment. The most common microorganisms found indoors are fungi and bacteria.

Bioaerosols other than those from microorganisms (for instance, pollen and animal dander) get indoors in the same way as microorganisms. But these do not multiply, and generally only become a problem if allowed to accumulate.

Even the cleanest building can have bioaerosol problems. Indeed, levels of fungi and bacteria are thought to be increasing in offices and homes as well as in hospitals and other apparently 'clean' places because of a combination of artificial ventilation, weatherproofing and the overuse of antibacterial cleaning solutions.

How you could be affected: Bioaerosols enter the human body through the lungs, so the diseases they cause usually affect the respiratory system and generally fall into two categories: hypersensitivity diseases and infectious diseases.

Hypersensitivity (or allergic) diseases result from exposure to materials in the environment called antigens – substances that stimulate an allergic response by the body's immune system. Once an individual has developed a hypersensitivity disease, even a tiny amount of the antigen may cause a severe reaction. Hypersensitivity diseases – which include building-related asthma, humidifier fever, allergic rhinitis and hypersensitivity pneumonitis – account for most of the health problems caused by indoor bioaerosols.

Infectious diseases are due to the invasion and proliferation of harmful organisms into the human body. Some examples of infectious diseases caused by indoor bioaerosols include legionnaires' disease (a type of bacterial pneumonia) and Pontiac fever (a milder form of legionnaires' disease that produces only flu-like symptoms). Fungal infections such as histoplasmosis and cryptococcosis may occur when contaminated bird droppings enter the indoor environment.

Radiation

Energy waves of varying intensity and frequencies surround all of us all the time. The most powerful and damaging natural radiation is from the sun, but tends to be filtered out by the earth's atmosphere before it reaches the ground. But some types of natural radiation, for instance, naturally occurring radioactive gases, can become substantial problems indoors. The man-made electricity that powers our computers, TV sets, lights, heaters, air conditioners, telephones (both land lines and mobiles), microwave ovens, electric shavers, hairdryers, radio alarms and stereos also adds to the abundance of radiation in the indoor environment.

Electromagnetic fields

Electromagnetic fields (EMFs) are created by all electrical equipment, by the wiring in our buildings and by the overhead cables that transmit power across the country. Electromagnetic fields consist of an electric and a magnetic field, and scientists are divided on which component is more harmful or whether they are both equally risky. (*For a full discussion on EMFs, see Chapter 7.*)

How you might be affected: EMFs have been linked to higher rates of cancer, depression, suicide and chronic fatigue-like symptoms. They may add to the production of cell-damaging free radicals, depress immune function and have reproductive effects. Some authorities suggest that EMFs may also concentrate air pollution and other toxins, especially around sources of high-voltage emissions such as power lines – but also computer screens and TVs – causing a range of disorders associated with air pollution, including asthma and other respiratory problems as well as skin cancer.

Radon

Radon is a naturally occurring gas produced by the radioactive decay of the uranium present in all earth materials such as rocks, soils, brick and concrete. Outdoor air has some radon in it, but this gas is generally only a problem in confined spaces. Indoors, radon gas can seep into buildings such as offices, schools and homes through cracks or other openings in the foundation and, if ventilation is inadequate, concentrations can build up to much higher levels than outdoors. Radon also decays into other radioactive elements (such as polonium) that cling to the lungs, once inhaled.

How you could be affected: Radon is second only to smoking as a cause of lung cancer in the US and elsewhere. In addition, there is evidence that radon is much more dangerous to smokers than to non-smokers – due to the fact that it enhances the already damaging effects of tobacco smoke.

Cleaner Petrol? Don't Hold Your Breath . . .

Most people believe that, when lead was removed from petrol, our cars became cleaner and greener. But the truth is that unleaded petrol is still a carcinogenic, neurotoxic cocktail. While air-lead levels have declined, levels of all the other toxic substances in petrol have remained high. Some have even increased and some entirely new ingredients, introduced to make unleaded petrol run even cleaner, have proven to be highly toxic to humans. Some of the toxins in your tank include:

Hydrocarbons: unleaded petrol contains benzene, toluene, xylene and 1,3-butadiene. Not all these hydrocarbons are burned up in the engine, which means that some are released into the air. There are no safe levels of exposure established for these chemicals. Benzene is associated with a range of diseases, including cancer, leukaemia and anaemia. Catalytic converters can help reduce hydrocarbon emissions, but the effect doesn't kick in until they are warmed up.

Sulphur dioxide: exacerbates bronchitis and causes tightening of chest – a real problem for children and asthmatics.

Nitrogen oxides: tighten airways and exacerbate asthma. Levels are on the increase because of the increasing number of motor vehicles on our roads.

Carbon monoxide: deprives blood of oxygen and can lead to drowsiness, headaches, dizziness and symptoms of chronic fatigue. Inhaling too much causes death.

Breathable particles of lead, other metals and petroleum in the form of coke or soot can induce neurological dysfunction.

Methyl tertiary butyl ether (MTBE) is a petrol additive/lead substitute and known carcinogen used to enhance engine performance. According to the UK's Environment Agency, 14 million gallons of MTBE-enriched petrol are sold each year in the UK alone and, as in the US, this carcinogenic chemical is now thought to have penetrated deep into the country's water table.

The Influence of Ions

Apart from toxic gases and contaminated dusts, there are other aspects of modern buildings believed to contribute to ill health, stress and emotional distress. Whether indoors and outdoors, our air is charged with ions. These electrically charged particles are produced by the action of cosmic rays moving through our atmosphere, during lightning storms and from radon emissions from the earth's crust. During such phenomena, atoms can either gain or lose an electron, giving them either a positive or negative charge. The predominance of either positive or negative ions has, according to some observers, important implications for health.

All living things need ions to survive. When scientists in the former USSR tried to raise small animals (mice, rats, guinea pigs, rabbits) in air containing no ions at all, they all died within a few days. Similarly, experiments of plants growing in air deprived of ions produced stunted growth. From a health perspective, however, not all ions are created equal.

An atmosphere charged with negative ions is reputed to be associated with feelings of calmness, alertness and wellbeing, with quicker recovery from exhausting exercise, more appetite, sounder sleep, fewer bodily aches and pains, and fewer respiratory complaints. In natural environments such as near waterfalls, in forests or along a rocky coastline, the air is rich with negative ions which, some believe, make you feel energised.

Natural phenomena, such as certain types of weather and winds, can also produce an excess of positive ions, and this is thought to be a contributing factor in seasonal affective disorder (SAD). When positive ions predominate in the air, they are believed to increase levels of serotonin and histamine, producing a reaction not unlike hayfever, asthma and other breathing disorders. Other symptoms associated with a high level of positive ions are headaches, irritability, insomnia, hot flashes, tension, nausea, aching joints, depression, anxiety, lethargy, suicides, crimes and hospital admissions. Office equipment can also give off an excess of positive ions, making people feel sleepy and fuzzy-headed.

Some observers believe that some of the symptoms of sick building syndrome are linked to the greater levels of positive ions resulting from all the electrical gadgets and equipment in buildings. It is also thought that when we breathe in these positively electrically charged particles, they have a greater chance of becoming trapped in our (negatively charged) lungs. Since ions also attract particles of pollution, our lungs also retain more pollutants than if they were not attached to ions.

Most studies into negative ions and health are small, but the results are interesting. For instance, ionisers (machines that produce negative ions) have been used to kill bacteria[59] and reduce indoor levels of microbial air pollution. In one study, levels of microbes in the air of a dental clinic were reduced 40–50 percent with the use of an ioniser.[60]

Evidence from one of the few controlled human experiments carried out in the UK showed that increasing the number of negative ions in a computer-operating area reduced complaints of headache, nausea and dizziness, and resulted in a significant improvement in the rating of environmental quality. The workers, especially those on the night shift, reported feeling more comfortable and alert.[61]

There is evidence that raising the level of negative ions in the atmosphere by using an ioniser can improve SAD[62] and improve people's ability to cope with stress.[63] It should be noted, however, that there is also evidence that ionisers make no difference at all.[64]

Why is Indoor Air Negative Ion-Deficient?

A typical air-conditioned office in the city has only 50 negative ions (and 150 positive ions) per millilitre of air compared with 1000 negative ions (and 1200 positive ions) in the same volume of clean, outdoor, country air. A typical urban environment has 500 negative and 600 positive ions per millilitre of air. Reasons for the low ion level indoors include:

- *Humidity and heat:* Negative ions seem to become less effective as the ambient temperature increases above 22° C and when the humidity is relatively high
- *Ducted air conditioning:* Metal air ducts attract charged particles, thereby stripping ions out of the air as it passes through the ductwork. Electrostatic filters have a similar effect on ion levels
- *Static electricity:* In air-conditioned buildings, especially those with low humidity, static electrical charges can build up on carpets, furniture, wall fabrics, clothing and, in particular, on electrical equipment such as VDU screens. Ions in the room are then attracted to these static charges
- *Smoke and contamination:* Smoke and dust particles can act like a sponge, mopping up ions from the air
- *Overcrowding:* People remove ions from the air just by breathing, and each of us carries an innate amount of static electricity.

How to choose an ioniser

There is some evidence that ionisers reduce indoor air pollution, but much of what we know of the benefits of ionisers in the home is based on intelligent guesswork rather than comprehensive human research. Indeed, most of the claims for the benefits of ionisers have been made on the basis of animal studies or extrapolated from studies on the influence of weather on health.[65] [66]

Logically, such devices should have an effect and, on some people, this may be significant. But not everyone is sensitive to changes in air-ion concentration. Around 25 percent of people notice no difference when the proportion of positive to negative ions is changed. Women seem to respond more to ion depletion in the atmosphere than men and also respond more favourably to an ion-enriched environment.

Ionisers can vary enormously in quality and ability to charge the air, and you will certainly get what you pay for. That £29.99 special may seem to cheap way to enhance health but, at best, it may be ineffective at charging your room with negative ions – at worst, it may produce ozone that may make your condition worse.

Well-made ionisers should have controls that allow you to change the setting according to your needs. In addition, when choosing an ioniser, look for those that provide the maximum amount of technical information about their product. Look for:

- A minimum concentration of 1000 ions per cubic centimetre of air, believed to be the minimum necessary to produce a therapeutic response in the body. A good-quality ioniser will produce significantly more than this
- A statement from the manufacturer that their ioniser produces little or no ozone. A badly designed ioniser can produce high levels of ozone and, with it, nitrous oxide. The 'accepted' level of ozone output from ionisers is 0.1 parts per million (ppm) and this should be stated among the product details.
- The type of apparatus the ioniser uses to emit negative ions, which can be needles, brushes or coils. Of these, needles are probably the most efficient. They should be extremely sharp and precise in order to create small, breathable ions of oxygen. The needles used to emit the negative ions are subject to wear and tear – so make sure yours are replaceable.

Improving Indoor Air

Many people claim that family life is deteriorating and lay the blame at the feet of TV, video games and lack of basic social values. But what if there was another explanation? What if being locked up all day and night in toxic buildings was simply leaving us too tired and ill to interact with others in any meaningful way?

Making the air in your office or school healthier may be an uphill struggle. Fortunately, you are almost totally in control of the air inside your home, so a good place to start is by cleaning up your act there. Nevertheless, you also have rights at work and, likewise, your children have the right to expect a clean learning environment at school. A combination of practical measures and activism may be the best approach to ensure that, outside of your home, you are not exposed to unnecessary pollutants that can impact on your health.

Open a window. The best form of air conditioning is an open window that allows fresh air in and toxic air out. An open window is better for getting out smells than any number of fabric sprays, air fresheners, scented candles and incense sticks. And given that candles and incense are both expensive and potentially toxic, opening a window will have less of an impact on your purse as well as your health.

Make use of indoor plants. A number of common household plants have been found to act as air purifiers, removing VOCs from the air.[67] Boston ferns can detoxify 1000 microgrammes of formaldehyde from the air in one hour. Other useful plants include palms, peace lily, philodendron, English ivy, drachea and chrysanthemum (*see Chapter 10 for more details*).

Go fragrance-free. Our love affair with fragrance has allowed advertisers to pull the wool over consumers' eyes for years by linking fragrance with desirable qualities such as love, sexiness, freshness, innocence and a wild, independent spirit. Don't buy into it. Each of us has the capability to reduce the number of synthetic fragrances we come into contact with on a daily basis. Get out of the habit of using air fresheners and fabric softeners, and save perfume or aftershave for special occasions. Buy fragrance-free toiletries whenever you can. If magazine scent strips annoy you, write to the publisher to register your complaint.

Quit smoking. You will certainly be healthier for it. If you cannot or will not quit smoking, at least be respectful of those who choose not to smoke. Never smoke around children, and smoke outside of the house or office when you can so that the carcinogens from your cigarettes do not coat the furniture and walls. Where they are available, use designated smoking areas.

Vacuum and dust regularly. This will help keep levels of breathable particles down. Dust mites, pollens, animal dander and other allergy-causing agents can be reduced, though not eliminated, and pesticide residues and heavy metal levels can be kept to a minimum, through regular cleaning.

Use safe cleaning fluids. This will help you avoid exposure to harsh solvents and antibacterials. When cleaning your home, use only those detergents that are made from vegetable sources, and do not include bleaches or other pesticides. Simple cleaning solutions can be made from basics like vinegar and baking soda.[68]

Consider the problems of electropollution (*discussed in Chapter 7*).

Don't use aerosols. These concentrate fine droplets of toxic materials in the air that are easily inhaled into your lungs and, from there, enter your system. Aerosols can also be expensive and serve little useful purpose. So, the next time you go to the store, consider replacing aerosol products with liquids (or, at a pinch, pump-spray formulations – but be aware that fine pump sprays can also form toxic aerosols).

Redecorating? Look for organic paints, and solvent-free paint strippers and brush cleaners. These are now becoming more and more common in the shops. Where appropriate, use natural pigments – but don't rely on all natural pigments as being safe. Some, like vermilion, are highly toxic. At the very least, use low- or, if you can find them, zero-VOC, water-based, latex paints rather than oil-based paints. Not only will you then eliminate the hazards from the solvents in the paint, you will avoid the need to use additional solvents to clean the paintbrushes. If you do use solvent-based paints, wear protective gloves. When cleaning fresh oil-based paint from your skin, try massaging with a few drops of vegetable oil, butter or margarine instead of white spirit. Wipe dry, then wash with soap and water. Ensure adequate ventilation and, whenever possible, paint outdoors.

At work, take frequent breaks. Go outside, get some fresh air. Eat lunch away from the office environment.

Buy an ioniser. But remember, these are not magic bullets. Taking steps to minimise the amount of static electricity in the environment, using natural rather than synthetic fibres wherever possible, controlling humidity and temperature, removing pollutants and dust at source, making sure that all VDUs and other equipment in the office likely to build up a static charge are properly earthed, and ensuring that offices are not overcrowded may be a more efficient way of dealing with the problem of too many positive ions in the air.

Keep humidity to a minimum. This will discourage the growth of moulds and fungi. Aim to keep the relative humidity level in the house between 30–50 percent. Dry off wet surfaces and correct water problems. Thoroughly clean and dry water-damaged carpets and building materials (within 24 hours if possible) or consider removal and replacement. Ventilate the attic and crawl spaces to prevent moisture build-up. In kitchens and bathrooms, install and use exhaust fans that are vented to the outdoors. Vent clothes-dryer air to the outdoors as well.

Is radon a problem? Radon levels in homes vary during the day and from season to season. They are generally higher at night and during the winter. Although radon enters homes all the time, some is carried away by natural ventilation. Increasing the ventilation, especially on the ground floor, will help keep radon levels low (*see Chapter 10 for advice on monitoring radon levels*).

Speak to your employer about the state of the office environment. Given that ill health represents a significant loss in time and money, most employers are willing to consider any measure that will improve the health and productivity of employees. You could, for instance, suggest that cleaning staff use less toxic methods for cleaning, that air fresheners be banned in the office and that guidelines for fragrance-free workplaces are drawn up. Ban smoking in the office. Site electrical equipment as far away as possible from employees' work-stations. If you do not feel confident enough to approach your employer directly and you have a union representative, discuss these matters with him or her. Most health and safety executives publish guidelines on healthy office environments. Consider getting hold of a copy for your own information.

Clean up our schools. Get together with other concerned parents and let the school know that you care about the environment your child is learning in. Children are required by law to go to school, so our schools house a captive audience. This can make school governors and local councils somewhat less attentive to the problems of ventilation and toxic emissions. Children are unlikely to stay away from school if there isn't proper air conditioning and heating, and parents rarely demand it as a basic requirement; yet it can make the difference between lethargy and a disruptive attitude, and a peaceful class full of attentive children.

6 The Bug Stops Here

PESTICIDES. THE PRINCIPLE SEEMS SIMPLE ENOUGH. KILL THE BUGS that eat our crops and there will be more left for us. Keep bugs off our domestic garden plants and away from our houses, and our living environment will be cleaner, more beautiful and healthier. But it is not that simple, and there are good arguments in favour of the idea that our use of pesticides is both irrational and ineffective, and has very serious consequences not only for human health but, indeed, for the entire ecosystem of the planet.

It is almost impossible to talk about the folly of pesticide use without at least some nod in the direction of Rachel Carson and her now classic 1963 book *Silent Spring* – an eloquent and devastating look at where the overuse of agrochemicals, especially DDT, was leading us.[1] Carson's disclosures were a catalyst in the advent of the modern environmental movement and, although others before her had drawn upon the same metaphor, it was her book that really drove home the point that the massive use of pesticides after World War II amounted to a 'war on nature' with devastating consequences for mankind.

Forty years on, it is dismaying to see just how little impact her views – indeed, the views of ecologists everywhere – have made on the agricultural world. If anything, the use of pesticides has become more widespread, moving from the field to the high street to the home, without much apparent enquiry into appropriateness or safety or, more crucially, alternatives. DDT, of course, has been banned from use on crops, but it is so poisonous that it still lingers in our soils. Worse, in a kind of perverse spirit of 'waste not, want not', it is still being used to control mosquitoes in both developing and developed countries.

It is equally discouraging to see that pesticides have not removed the threat of pests from our crops – though they have been effective in producing highly resistant varieties of pests (in much the same way that overuse of antibiotics has produced highly resistant strains of bacteria). What's more, the use of pesticides on our produce doesn't stop at the farm. At every step from field to table, our fruits and vegetables are sprayed repeatedly with a variety of insecticides and fungicides.

Moreover, throughout their lifetime, animals bred for their meat are regularly treated with 'preventative' medicines – injections and oral medications containing pesticides to keep internal parasites at bay, and external applications such as sheep dips, warble-fly dressings and tick treatments. Their living quarters are also regularly sprayed to keep levels of flies and other insects low. The meat from our animals is invariably contaminated with these persistent chemicals.

Pesticide use in our homes and gardens, and in many public areas has also increased. Railway lines, waterways, embankments, city and suburban streets are regularly doused with bug-zapping chemicals. Even underground electric cables are treated with insecticides such as aldrin and chlordane to discourage any pests that may make the mistake of munching on them.

Grocery stores, restaurants, hotels, hospital cafeterias, some schools, and many apartment buildings and nursing homes are routinely sprayed and fumigated. Wooden playground equipment, decking and picnic tables are treated with a variety of substances, including arsenic (*see Chapter 8 for more information*). Every year, in our irrational bid to remove all traces of the humble dandelion from the earth's surface, we spray tons of toxic chemicals on parks, playgrounds, golf courses and other recreation grounds not because dandelions are inherently evil or health-threatening, but purely for aesthetic reasons.

Sources of common household pesticides, too, are becoming more common. These include bathroom- and kitchen-cleaning solutions, wallpaper pastes, paint, wooden furniture (especially if made from recycled railroad ties), insecticides for wood (such as woodworm treatments) and woollens (mothballs), roach, fly and wasp sprays, pest strips, sprays for indoor plants, head-lice and intestinal-parasite treatments, swimming-pool and spa disinfectants and algaecides, and pest- and weed-killers used in the garden. Our irrational fear of 'bugs' has also led to soft furnishings, carpets and mattresses being pretreated with powerful pesticides such as permethrin (the same pesticide implicated in the symptoms of Gulf War syndrome).

It is therefore not surprising that US scientists have concluded that pesticide overexposure – once an occupational hazard of agricultural and factory workers – is now everybody's problem. Their data show that 80 percent of all human pesticide exposure is actually *indoors* – in our homes, offices and schools – with measurable levels of up to 12 different pesticides found in the air of the average household. Home application, and the tracking-in of dust and dirt from outdoors are major sources of household pesticide pollution. But in one 1995 survey, somewhere in the region of 85 percent of American homes were found to have at least three to four different pesticide products in them, including pest strips, bait boxes, bug bombs, flea collars, pesticide-containing pet shampoos, aerosols, granules, liquids and dusts.[2]

Things aren't much better in the UK. According to the Pesticide Action Network (PAN) UK, in the year 2000, British householders doused their homes and gardens with £35 million worth of pesticides with a combined weight of 4306 tonnes. Home and garden sales showed a marked increase of 38 percent between 1999 and 2000. Worse, as much as 20 percent of these pesticides was disposed of by householders by pouring them down the drain. In response to this, the Pesticide Action Network announced its intention to mount a countrywide survey on household and garden pesticide use.[3] Results are not available at the time of writing but, with such intense use of pesticides in the home and garden, it is inconceivable that UK homes have lower levels of pesticides in the atmosphere than homes elsewhere in the developed world.

Flying Nasties

Airlines and other modes of public transport make use of pesticides for the same reason householders do – for 'disinfection'. Most airlines are keen to get rid of insects looking for a free ride. But according to some scientists, this practice endangers the health of both passengers and flight staff. The Northwest Coalition for Alternatives to Pesticides (NCAP), an environmental group based in Eugene, Oregon, points out that pesticides, while dangerous on land, have the potential to be particularly harmful when used on planes because up to 50 percent of the air inside the cabins is recycled. This means that passengers can sometimes find themselves sealed for hours at a stretch in a poorly ventilated chamber that has recently been gassed with no escape from the chemicals in the air. This brings up the intriguing question of whether severe jet lag – the symptoms of which are similar to pesticide poisoning and which often seems unrelated to distances travelled – is solely down to time differences and internal clocks, or whether it may also have something to do with long hours spent in a flying flea bomb.[4]

Quality Versus Quantity

These days, farmers and politicians alike are worried about producing enough food to meet global demands. Indeed, feeding the world is a major preoccupation and many agricultural practices, including the prodigious use of pesticides, are employed in the belief that they help maximise food yields and help the farmer meet increasing consumer demand. Government authorities and industry representatives continue to assure us that the substantial benefits associated with the use of things like agrochemicals far outweigh any risks.

What we do know for certain is that nutritious food is the cornerstone of good health. It is our backstop – the thing that holds us up, bolsters our immunity, fights free radical damage and maintains our energy cycles in the face of an increasingly polluted world.

While fruits, vegetables and whole grains are commonly thought to be high in essential nutrients, the majority of today's produce and grains are grown in depleted soil, doused with pesticides and stored for long periods of time (all the while being sprayed with more insecticides and fungicides) before being sold. They may be stored for an even longer time after purchase before being eaten or used in cooking.

In the developed world, this system has meant that few of us feel the pangs of hunger. But even if modern agricultural practices do meet our needs in terms of quantity, they fall desperately short of meeting our needs in terms of quality. This has moved some modern nutritionists to posit that, in the midst of all this plenty, we are still starving – for the basic nutrients that were once in our everyday food.

Conventional farmers are caught in a vicious circle of production. They add chemical fertilisers to the soil in the hope of increasing crop yields, but doing so ultimately increases many plants' susceptibility to pests. So more pesticides are used. But the pesticides they use can also affect the soil's capacity to sustain and generate fertility. Pesticides such as benzene hexachloride (BHC), DDT, DDD, aldrin, lindane and heptachlor all prevent nitrogen-fixing bacteria from forming the necessary root nodules on leguminous plants (such as beans, peas, clover and alfalfa). This soil effect happens quickly (often within a matter of weeks) after application.

Using synthetic fertilisers to make plants grow in otherwise depleted soils has other disturbing consequences. For instance, while the fertiliser will stimulate the plant to grow in the absence of any of the usual protective nutrients the soil should contain, the plants will also take up more of the heavy metals in the soil such as aluminium, mercury and lead, and these, in turn, are passed on up through the food chain.

All the while, the nutritional value of our food is plummeting.

In 1940, British chemists Robert McCance and Elsie Widdowson published the first of what would be their periodical examinations of the nutrient content of food.[5] When the fifth edition[6] of this tome – which has over the years become a standard reference work on the subject – was published in 1991, the British geologist-turned-nutritionist David Thomas undertook the work of comparing the values as published in the first and last editions of the book.

He examined the data for 28 raw vegetables and 44 cooked vegetables, 17 fruits and 10 types of meat, poultry and game,[7] and his findings make frightening reading. In today's foods:

- *Potatoes* have 30 percent less magnesium, 35 percent less calcium, 45 percent less iron and 47 percent less copper
- *Carrots* have 75 percent less magnesium, 48 percent less calcium, 46 percent less iron and 75 percent less copper
- *Broccoli* (boiled) has 75 percent less calcium
- *Spinach* (boiled) has 60 percent less iron and 96 percent less copper
- *Swedes* have 71 percent less iron
- *Spring onions* have 74 percent less calcium
- *Watercress* has 93 percent less copper
- *All meats* contained 41 percent less calcium and 54 percent less iron
- *All fruits* contained 27 percent less zinc
- *Apples and oranges* had 67 percent less iron.

Among Thomas' other worrying findings was that seeding the soil with only certain minerals (sodium, phosphorus and potassium) has greatly altered the natural mineral profile of our foods. Thus, swedes now contain 110 percent of the phosphorus they once did. Humans who eat this nutritionally altered food cannot help but experience an alteration in their natural mineral profiles as well.

Thomas' findings were not unique. In a 1997 study published in the British Food Journal, researchers documented a similar historical decline in the mineral contents of 20 common fruits and vegetables between 1930 and 1987.[8]

Modern potatoes, for instance, were shown to have 40 percent less potassium than the older ones. Carrots contained nearly half the calcium they once did and 75 percent less magnesium. Tomatoes contained 90 percent less copper. Among the fruits, apples contained two-thirds less iron than in 1930, as did oranges and apricots.

A similar exercise was carried out in the US in 1999 when nutritionist Alex Jack compared nutrient values in the current US Department of Agriculture (USDA) handbook with those published in 1975. He discovered a number of mineral deficits as well as the fact that cauliflower had 40 percent less vitamin C than it did in 1975. He wrote to the USDA for an explanation, but it declined to comment. The magazine *Organic Gardening* championed his efforts and published an open letter to the USDA, demanding that they answer Mr Jack. Embarrassed by the publicity, the USDA did eventually reply – with a letter full of the kind of bureaucratic doublespeak that always stands in the way of knowledge and progress, and mostly blaming unreliable methods of testing back in the apparent Dark Ages of 1975.

While it is true that testing methods have changed over the years, the methods used in 1975, while more time-consuming, were no less accurate than those used today.

In March 2001, *Life Extension* magazine also took up Mr Jack's cause[9] and, with his help and again using USDA nutrient tables (this time from 1963), ran their own comparison. The results? The vitamin C content in a serving of peppers has plummeted from 128 mg then to 89 mg now. The vitamin A in apples has dropped from 90 mg to 53 mg. Broccoli and collards (greens) have lost half their total vitamin A content, and cauliflower's vitamin C content has also declined by 50 percent.

The influence of pesticides

Depleted soil is not the only threat to our food and our health. Many classes of herbicide can alter plant metabolism and, thus, nutrient composition. For example, herbicides that inhibit photosynthesis (such as triazine or phenoyacetics) produce effects similar to growing a plant in low-light conditions. Under such conditions, the carbohydrate, alpha-tocopherol and beta-carotene content of a plant is reduced, and protein, free amino acid and nitrate levels are increased.[10] Equally, bleaching herbicides can reduce beta-carotene levels by inhibiting carotenoid production,[11] and sulphonylurea herbicides are known to inhibit the synthesis of branched-chain amino acids (which humans need to maintain muscle tissue).[12]

In a recent report published in the online journal *Conservation Ecology*,[13] researchers at the University of Guelph, Canada, have discovered yet another problem with the use of pesticides. They have found that a global shortage of bees and other insects that pollinate plants is destroying crops and could, if left unchecked, lead to a worldwide shortage of foods, and higher prices for fruits and vegetables in the shops.

Pollinators such as bees, bats, butterflies and birds play a key role in agriculture as they transfer pollen from one plant to another. It is a vital step in the production of most fruits and vegetables as well as for a handful of nuts and, of course, honey. Without sufficient pollination, apples, for instance, are usually smaller and less flavourful. In recent years, pollinator populations – both indigenous and those that are bought in to do the job (usually because local populations have been devastated) – have been hit hard by increased pesticide use, and much of their natural habitat, such as dead trees and old fence posts, has been destroyed to make room for more farmland.

Although concerns about pollinator shortages date back at least to biblical times, this report was unique because it tried to quantify the problem with the kind of bottom-line language that grabs people's attention. For instance, according to the Canadian Honey Council, honeybees – one of the most affected species – are responsible for one billion Canadian dollars' worth of produce each year. But it's not just industry that will lose out. If the trend continues, say the researchers, plant foods that require pollination to survive could become prohibitively expensive for consumers. In the worst-case scenario, instead of paying 30 pence for an apple at the supermarket, you might end up paying £1.50 for it.

Food to die for

The most comprehensive testing for the presence of unwanted chemicals in food is the ongoing US Total Diet Study (TDS), conducted by the Food and Drug Administration and updated yearly. The TDS looks for the presence of many different chemicals in food, but its findings on levels of chlorinated pesticides have been particularly distressing. In its 1988 report,[14] DDE (a close relative of DDT) was found in every single sample of raisins, spinach (fresh and frozen), chili con carne (beef and beans), and beef.

DDE was also found in 93 percent of processed cheese, hamburger, hot dogs, Bologna sausage, collards (spring greens), chicken, turkey and ice-cream sandwiches in the US. It was also present in 87 percent of lamb chops, salami, canned spinach, meatloaf and butter, and in 81 percent of sauces and creamed spinach.

Since DDT and DDE have been banned in the US since 1972, it is likely that some of this contamination is from produce imported from other countries that still use these chemicals. But some of it is also because of the persistence of these chemicals in our soil.

In the intervening years, things haven't got much better. The 1999 TDS showed that, among the foods sampled, 17 different pesticides were found in butter, 32 different ones in cherries, 29 in strawberries and 27 in apples. The baked-potato samples contained 23 pesticides and hamburger 22. Milk-chocolate samples contained 18 different pesticides.[15] Once again, DDE/DDT was the residue most often found, with chlorpyrifos-methyl, malathion, endosulfan, dieldrin and chlorpyrifos also being very common.

In the UK, the 1999 Annual Report by the Working Party on Pesticide Residues (WPPR) found that 27 percent of the full range of foods tested had pesticide residues.[16] Among them, DDT (which is banned in the UK) was found in beef slices, corned beef and lamb's kidney, and 2,4-D (also banned in the UK) was found in over half the oranges tested. Oranges, pears, lettuces, chocolate and apples contained the highest numbers and levels of residues. Three-quarters of the chocolate samples contained lindane (a relative of DDT), and one in eight jars of baby food was also contaminated. Surveys in Australia[17] and New Zealand[18] have found similarly high levels of pesticides in foods – though government representatives continue to decry detected levels as being well within the limits of legality and acceptable risk. Consumers, however, should not be lulled into a false sense of security – 'legal' does not necessarily mean 'safe'.

If the Nicotine Doesn't Get You . . .

Phosphate fertilisers don't just deplete the soil. They also contain high levels of radioactive metals. The phosphate in this type of fertiliser is taken from apatite – a rock that naturally contains radium, and the radioactive elements lead-210 and polonium-210. Indeed, the radioactivity of common fertiliser can easily be verified with a Geiger counter.[19]

All plants growing in soil that has been 'improved' with phosphate fertilisers will naturally absorb some of this radiation,[20] but tobacco plants appear to absorb more than most.

In trying to put the dose of radiation smokers receive into perspective, scientists have estimated that smoking a pack-and-a-half a day would be equivalent to a radiation dose of anywhere from 300 to 800 chest X-rays per year.[21]

Because of the electric and magnetic properties of metals, once in the lungs, these radioactive metals tend to clump together in tiny hot spots. These hot spots may be one reason why rates of lung cancer from smoking appear to have increased dramatically since the 1930s.[22]

Regulation, Shmegulation

Although official agencies claim that our ingestion of pesticides through food is low, a report in *Science* magazine estimated that, if you follow a conventional diet, you will be ingesting about 150 microgrammes of pesticides each day.[23] This seems a relatively small amount until you realise that there is no acceptable safe limit for human pesticide ingestion and, over the course of a year, a decade or a lifetime, the pesticides you ingest each day will build up in your organs and fatty tissue.

The direct human cost of controlling pests with chemicals is slowly being revealed to us in a legacy that includes higher rates of cancer and neurological disorders as well as lowered immunity. Under the circumstances, it would be reasonable to expect regulations to be brought in to protect us from pesticide exposure, especially in our food and in our homes. Yet, the current approach to pesticide regulation throughout the civilised world is slap-dash and full of shortcomings.

- **Regulations are based on the conviction that people are exposed only to single pesticides throughout their lifetime.**
  Safety testing is done one pesticide at a time, and regulations for individual pesticides are set on the assumption that each of us consumes only this one pesticide throughout our lifetime – an assumption that is, as the TDS data cited earlier shows, at odds with the reality of our lives. Other data also highlight the folly of this assumption. A study by the Environmental Working Group (EWG) in the US found 67 pesticides or metabolites in sources of drinking water sampled in the Midwest between 1987 and 1994.[24] More recently, another EWG study found nine pesticides and metabolites in a single glass of tapwater in one US state,[25] and the US Department of Agriculture found nine different pesticides on a single sample of apples.[26] Also, we don't simply ingest pesticides, we breathe them in as dust, pollution and vapour, and we absorb them through our skin – and each of these exposures contributes to our total exposure.

  Clearly, regulations must take into account the multiple pesticides we are exposed to every day since it is this total exposure that is likely to have the greatest impact on our health.

  What's more, there is emerging evidence to suggest that combinations may have more potent effects than single pesticide exposures. In June 1996, the journal *Science* – considered by many to be the conservative voice of mainstream science – reported the results of a study of pesticide combinations that found that the dangers of these chemicals when used in tandem were vastly underestimated.[27] In this study, chemicals such as endosulfan, dieldrin and chlordane were examined for their oestrogenic properties – that is, their ability to mimic oestrogen. Since the body already produces adequate oestrogen levels, such excess can lead to breast, uterine and testicular cancers, lowered sperm counts and malformation of male sex organs (*see Chapter 8*). Singly, these chemicals have a weak oestrogenic effect, but combined, their toxicity may increase 500- to 1000-fold.

The implications of this study are staggering and, not surprisingly, many scientists balked at the findings. However, if proved to be right, regulatory bodies could simply no longer afford to keep turning a blind eye to the issue of real-life exposures.

- **They do not adequately protect infants and children**.
  Children are not 'little adults'. A developing child may be many times more sensitive to the effects of pesticide exposure than an adult. Current standards ignore the fact that young children have a more rapid metabolism, and eat and drink far more than do adults in relation to their size. In addition, their organ systems (particularly the reproductive, endocrine and nervous systems) are still developing and, thus, are more vulnerable to toxic damage. In spite of this, no explicit adjustments are made in setting lifetime pesticide limits on food or water in relation to children.

  Many of the tests for pesticide safety, particularly those looking at long-term effects such as cancer or chronic nervous system toxicity, use animals. This is bad enough – the tests are cruel and may be inaccurate predictors of the effects in humans. But worse, these studies do not usually expose animals to pesticides during a period of life equivalent to human fetal development or infancy. Nevertheless, according to a series of independently reviewed studies, when fetal or infant animals are exposed to chemical carcinogens, cancer rates do rise and the latency period (that is, the period between exposure and development) for cancer in these animals is substantially shortened.[28]

  In addition, safety data ignore the fact that young children don't just ingest pesticides from food. The tracking in of pesticides from outdoors is a substantial source of indoor pollution. Putting toys and other items that have been in contact with the floor into their mouths is one of the major sources of pesticide ingestion among young children.[29]

- **Pesticides contain secret, inert ingredients that are not only toxic in themselves, but can enhance the toxic potential of the active ingredients.**

  All pesticides contain mixtures of both active and inert ingredients, though only the active ingredients are listed on the label. In many cases, these so-called inert ingredients make up more than 90 percent of the pesticide product, yet all of these ingredients are considered trade secrets. This means that the farmer and the housewife alike will never know what's really in the product they are using.

  Many inert ingredients allowed by the US Environmental Protection Agency are extremely toxic, including human carcinogens like formaldehyde, and endocrine modifiers like nonylphenol and bisphenol-A (this in addition to the many pesticides classified as probable human carcinogens).[30]

  In 1991, the Inspector General of the EPA issued a report on inert substances in household pesticides.[31] The report listed four categories of inert ingredients:

  - *Generally recognised as safe.* This category includes 300 substances such as dextrose, ethanol, fish meal, lard, olive oil, water and wintergreen oil
  - *Potentially toxic.* There were only 68 of these, including petroleum hydrocarbons, toluene, xylene and methyl bromide
  - *Toxic.* These 56 ingredients all show evidence of causing cancer, adverse reproductive effects, neurotoxicity or other chronic effects, or birth defects in laboratory animals or humans. This list includes aniline, asbestos, benzene, carbon disulphide, chloroform, formaldehyde, hexachlorophene, lead, cadmium and mercury oleate
  - *Unknown toxicity.* This was by far the biggest category with 1300 substances in it. According to the report, the EPA "knows little or nothing about the adverse effects of most of these inert ingredients". Examples include barium sulphate, epoxy resin, styrene acrylic copolymer, sodium nitrite, thymol, lithium chloride, naphthalene, polyethylene terphthalate,

D & C red number 37, malathion, kerosene, coal tar, asphalt, freon-114 and sulphuric acid.

Gathering information on the health effects of inert substances is a low priority for most official agencies, including the EPA. Nevertheless, the report concluded that most pesticide users are ignorant of the fact that pesticide products contain potentially toxic inert ingredients and that "the use of these pesticide products may be jeopardizing human health and the environment".

Know Your Pesticides

There are many different types of pesticides, each made from different starting materials and each with its own particular effects on the body.[32] However, some of the main classes of pesticides that are useful to know about include:

Organochlorines
The main representatives of chlorinated pesticides are aldrin, dieldrin, chlordane, heptachlor, transnonachlor, DDT and its metabolites (DDE, DDD), endrin, hexachlorobenzene and lindane (alpha, beta, delta, BHC). This group of chemicals also includes polychlorinated biphenyls (PCBs), originally used as electrical coolants, but which have also been used as pesticides. These have been used extensively in agriculture, in forestry and even in households over the last 20 years. Some organochlorines have been banned in Canada and the US due to their persistence in the environment. However, they are still manufactured in these countries and exported to developing countries for use in agriculture there. Chlorinated pesticides are hormone-disrupting and can cause various pathological conditions in humans, including cancer (see Chapter 8 for more information on this group of pesticides). PCB exposure can result in neurological disorders, malignant melanoma and liver cancers.

Organophosphates
Organophosphate pesticides, such as malathion, dursban, diazanon and carbonates, constitute 40 percent of all pesticides used. These chemicals are mainly used inside buildings. They disappear from the body within 24 hours but, even so, they have been found to cause delayed neurotoxicity involving the cerebral cortex, brain stem, spinal cord, peripheral nerves, muscles and eyes.

Carbamates
Including aldicarb, bendiocarb, carbaryl, propoxur and thiophanate methyl, carbamates are used extensively in agriculture, forestry and gardening. The immediate effects of exposure include muscle weakness, altered perception,

headache, nausea, vomiting, abdominal pain, visual problems and muscle twitches. Over the longer term, these compounds are carcinogenic, with reproductive effects including damage to testes, sperm and DNA, and behavioural effects.

Phenoxys

In this group of toxic chemicals, the most well known are 2,4-D and 2,4,5-T which, when proportionately mixed, constitute Agent Orange. Extensively used in the control of terrestrial broadleaved plants, they have been proven to cause leukopenia and non-Hodgkin's lymphoma. Agent Orange exposure has recently been linked to the development of type II diabetes.

Thiocarbamates

This group of fungicides includes the EBDCs (ethylene bis-dithiocarbamates), mancozeb, maneb and metiram. EBDC use is becoming more widespread. When EBDCs are used on stored produce, and also when such contaminated fruit and/or vegetables are cooked, its active ingredients break down into a chemical known as ethylenethiourea (ETU). ETU can cause goitres (enlargement of the thyroid gland), birth defects and cancer in exposed experimental animals. It has been classified by the EPA as a probable human carcinogen.

What's in the Water?

Water is one of the most essential nutrients to the human body, ranking second only to oxygen in terms of sustaining life. Humans can't live without water. It is necessary for carrying essential nutrients to the body's cells; it helps transport waste to the kidneys and lungs for excretion; it carries hormones and disease-fighting cells through the bloodstream; it is involved in digestion and metabolism, regulates our body temperature and our bowels, and cushions and lubricates our tissues and joints.

To a large extent, our health depends on the quality of the water we drink. And yet, drinking a glass of water is increasingly becoming an act of faith.

Any chemical we use will eventually wind up in our water supply. Although this fact escaped many of us for most of the last century, it was brought into sharp focus in 1971, when the Ralph Nader Study Group in the US reviewed over 10,000 documents acquired through the Freedom of Information Act. It was able to confirm that US drinking water contained more than 2100 toxic chemicals that could cause cancer.[33] Things haven't really improved much since then.

The sorts of chemicals most likely to be found in our water include pesticides such as carbamate insecticides (aldicarb and others), the triazine herbicides (atrazine and others) and fertilisers (such as nitrate nitrogen).[34] In addition, our water contains solvents (such as benzene, xylene and trichloroethylene), toxic metals (such as lead, mercury and arsenic) and radionuclides (such as radium). Long-term ingestion of these contaminants has been linked to liver or kidney dysfunction, cancer and reproductive problems.[35]

Most recently, a new class of water pollutants has been discovered.[36] Pharmaceutical drugs, including antibiotics, hormones, strong painkillers, tranquillisers and chemotherapy chemicals, are now being detected in our surface water, groundwater and drinking water.[37] German scientists have reported that some 30 to 60 drugs can be measured in a typical water sample in concentrations similar to those of pesticide contamination.[38] Many of these drugs are specially formulated not to be water-soluble, which means that they will remain intact in our rivers, streams and reservoirs until they are consumed by animals and humans, and become stored in the fatty tissues of their and our bodies.

Of course, we don't just drink this water – we bathe and shower in it as well, thus inhaling minute quantities of these chemicals into our lungs. Indeed, it has been suggested that the amount of volatile chemicals inhaled during a 15-minute shower with contaminated water is equivalent to drinking about eight glasses of contaminated water.[39] In addition, many industrial contaminants can easily pass through the skin into the body during showers, baths and dish-washing, more than doubling the amount of chemicals that pass into your body.[40]

In addition to being polluted with high levels of toxic chemicals, our water also contains harmful microbes. Studies by US water authorities have shown, for instance, that colonies (known as cysts) of *Giardia* can survive for up to three months in cool or cold water, while *Cryptosporidium*, now the leading cause of waterborne illness, can survive in such conditions for 12–18 months. Most of the parasites that live in our water supply have evolved resistance to our attempts at disinfection. In fact, *Cryptosporidium* can grow and thrive in solutions of chlorine bleach.[41] Perhaps not surprisingly, in the US, more than 80 percent of surface-water samples and 28 percent of drinking-water samples have been found to be contaminated with this parasite.[42]

Once again, government scientists assure us that levels of these contaminants in our water are low and do not pose a risk to health – or only pose an 'acceptable risk'. And once again, this reassurance reflects a belief that water is the only source of such toxins. While all of the chemicals in our water are cause for concern, two pesticides – one added for disinfection, the other for medication – are particularly worrying.

Killing bugs

Drinking water is disinfected with chlorine to kill microorganisms such as parasites, bacteria and viruses. Chlorination of drinking water has virtually eliminated typhoid fever, cholera and many other waterborne diseases from the Western world. However, this achievement has come at a price.

Once in the water, chlorine reacts with organic matter, such as sewage, animal waste, and soil and plant material that comes from a combination of agricultural run-off and urban sprawl, to form trihalomethanes and other harmful chlorine byproducts (CBPs). Our drinking water accounts for a major part of our total exposure to all these disinfection byproducts, followed by air and then food.[43] In addition, chlorination, which kills bacteria, also kills body cells. According to the EPA, chronic exposure to chlorine and chlorine byproducts may cause liver, kidney, heart and neurological damage as well as affect unborn children. Some of these byproducts are also known carcinogens.[44]

In 2002 in the US, the first-ever nationwide assessment of CBPs in drinking water, released by the Environmental Working Group

(EWG) and the US Public Interest Research Group (US PIRG), found that more than 100,000 women are at elevated risk of miscarriage or of having children with birth defects because of chlorination byproducts in the municipal tapwater.[45] This estimate, however shocking, squares with the results of other studies.[46]

In one, women who drank five glasses per day of cold tapwater containing trihalomethanes had an 80 percent higher risk of miscarriage.[47] In another, which reviewed more than 80,000 births between 1985 and 1988, women who regularly ingested water with a high level of CBPs were more likely to give birth to babies with low birth weight and various abnormalities. In addition, high levels of carbon tetrachloride in the water were associated with low birth weight, fetal death, and central nervous system, neural-tube and oral-cleft defects. Other abnormalities, including central nervous system, neural-tube and oral-cleft defects, were linked to high levels of dichloroethylenes and trichloroethylenes.[48]

Adult health is also affected by the presence of CBPs. There are studies that show an association between ingestion of CBPs and bladder cancer.[49] [50] One, published in *Journal of the National Cancer Institute* in 1997, found that people who drank eight cups (an otherwise 'healthy' amount) of chlorinated tapwater each day for 40–59 years had a 40 percent greater risk of bladder cancer than those who drank less tapwater or unchlorinated water. People who drank eight cups of chlorinated tapwater for 60 or more years had an 80 percent greater risk of bladder cancer.[51]

Fluoride: rat poison in your mouth

One of the greatest scams in the history of water pollution is certainly the addition of fluoride to the water supply. Unlike chlorine, which is added for purposes of disinfection, fluoride is added to drinking water for medication (to prevent tooth decay). In fact, fluoride is the only chemical added to water for this purpose.

Like most of today's toxic substances, fluoride has its roots in World War II research into weapons of mass destruction. Massive quantities of fluoride were essential for the manufacture of bomb-grade uranium and plutonium for nuclear weapons throughout the Cold War. Post-WWII, fluoride was a popular form of rat poison. However, as production of this product began to greatly outstrip its use as a rodenticide, scientists were spurred on by industry and the government to find other uses for it.

Today, fluoride is routinely added to the water supply of around 10 percent of the UK population (though this figure is set to rise in the coming years) and more than 60 percent of the US population. These figures are in stark contrast to the 98 percent of Western Europe that has rejected fluoridation on the grounds that it does not work and that it is morally reprehensible to forcibly medicate whole populations of people.

While we have been brainwashed to believe that fluoride protects teeth, research does not bear this out. Most studies into the benefits of fluoride are based on calcium fluoride rather than the more toxic form that is added to our water supply. Indeed, there are significant differences between naturally occurring calcium fluoride and the industrial waste – namely, hydrofluorosilicic acid, a byproduct of the phosphate-fertiliser industry – that is added to our water, and known to contain human carcinogens in a toxic mix of arsenic, beryllium, lead, cadmium, mercury, silicon and other major contaminants, including radioactive polonium (*see also box on page 101*).

It is possible that some people might reason that small quantities of these toxins are worth the risk if it means better teeth. But the largest dental survey ever conducted in the US (by the National Institute of Dental Research [NIDR] and involving more than 39,000 children) found virtually no difference in the incidence of tooth decay between children living in fluoridated and non-fluoridated areas.[52] In addition, several review papers have attested to the fact that dental decay does not increase when communities stop fluoridation.[53]

Instead, fluoridated water is responsible for increased rates of fluorosis (where teeth become white-spotted, yellow, brown-stained or pitted). In the US, 25 percent of school children are thought to be affected with fluorosis.[54] Studies show that the highest incidence of fluorosis is in areas where the water is naturally fluoridated, followed by areas where the water supply is deliberately dosed with fluoride. The lowest incidence of fluorosis is where the water is not fluoridated.[55]

However, what's in the water is not our only problem. Our exposure to fluoride is augmented by fluoride from other sources, including those not intended for ingestion, such as toothpaste.

Fluoride accumulates

While it has long been believed that fluoride has a half-life of 3.5 hours (the time it takes to clear from the body), studies into fluoride poisoning suggest that it takes much longer than that. When a community in Alaska was poisoned with fluoride due to a malfunction in the fluoridation-equipment system, blood fluoride levels did not return to normal within 24 hours, as would be expected. In fact, 19 days after the poisoning, the average level of fluoride in exposed individuals was still nearly three times the level of the few non-poisoned individuals residing in the same community.[56]

As a general rule, approximately half of each day's fluoride intake is retained. The rest is absorbed into calcified tissues, like bones and teeth, as well as some organs. Indeed, fluoride has a particular affinity for bones, and overexposure has been widely linked to the development of osteoporosis and a higher rate of hip fractures.[57] An accumulation of fluoride that begins in infancy can reach the lower levels of toxicity needed to produce bone damage after only 38 years. In fluoridated communities where the level of fluoride in the water is 4 parts per million (ppm; the maximum allowable in water and far below that for toothpaste), many people will be storing enough fluoride in their bones to cause damage by that age.

So, how much fluoride is too much? Since the 1950s, proponents of fluoridation have maintained that fluoridation of water at 1 ppm represented a minimal risk – between 2250–4500 times less than required to kill an adult and 250–500 times less than required to kill a child. However, several more recent reports show that what is known as the 'probably toxic dose' (PTD) of fluoride – that is, the ingested amount that would require therapeutic interventions and hospitalisation – is actually much lower, between 32–64 mg of fluoride per kg of bodyweight, administered in one dose.[58]

As these figures refer to pure fluoride, they do not reflect ingestion of toothpaste that contains compounds of fluoride – for example, sodium fluoride is a mixture of sodium and fluoride. You would need to take in 5–10 g of sodium fluoride to reach a lethal dose. Nevertheless, current toothpaste formulations do contain sufficient fluoride to exceed the PTD for young children. For instance, a 10-kg child who ingests 50 mg of fluoride (roughly equivalent to one-third of a tube of toothpaste containing 1500 ppm or one-half of a tube of 1000-ppm toothpaste) will have ingested a probably toxic dose.[59]

To put this in perspective, this means that there is enough fluoride in half of the average 100-mg tube of toothpaste to kill a small child. In the US, fluoride-containing toothpastes now come with a health warning and information on how to contact your local poisons control office in the event of accidental ingestion.

Health Effects of Pesticides

Pesticides deplete our soils, steal nutrients from our food and pollute our water, but their effects don't end there. There are other, equally worrying, effects (*see Chapter 8 for the influence of certain pesticides on the endocrine [hormone] system*). Pesticide use is also associated with neurological effects, decreased immunity, and reproductive and developmental abnormalities. What's more, these effects are not new.

By the late 1950s, a number of commonly used pesticides, including DDT and arsenates, had been linked with a range of disorders from leukaemia to skin cancer. In 1955, rising rates of hepatitis in the US were being linked to the increasing use of DDT and other chlorinated pesticides.

Every year, millions of people worldwide (mostly in developing countries) suffer severe poisonings from pesticides. Many more are exposed to levels that are considered low, but are still dangerous to health.[60] There has also been increasing concern among farmers in the US about their own higher-than-average rates of cancer.[61]

There are, however, many who dispute the theory that pesticides kill people as well as bugs. Some dissenters, for instance, refer to a 1996 report by the National Academy of Sciences which concluded that, as both synthetic and naturally occurring pesticides (those produced by the plants themselves; *see box, pages 122–123*) are consumed at such low levels, they pose little risk to health.[62] Others note that a 1997 panel of experts from the US and Canada, on reviewing more than 50 studies, likewise concluded that the benefits of eating fruits and vegetables far outweigh the potential risks from pesticides.[63]

Yet, more than 350 man-made toxic substances, many of them from residues in food, have been found in breastmilk and body fat. According to the report *Chemical Trespass – A Toxic Legacy*, produced by the World Wildlife Fund in the UK,[64] breastfed infants may be ingesting up to 42 times the WHO tolerable daily intake of dioxin-like compounds. Nevertheless, paediatricians still believe that the benefits of breastfeeding a baby still far outweigh the risk of toxicity.

Eating your vegetables brings undeniable benefits. Breastmilk is undeniably the only food truly suitable for human infants. But these facts cannot be taken to mean that consuming pesticide-laden food is safe. Such an assumption flies in the face of mounting evidence of the genuine harm that contact with pesticides from food as well as other sources can do to human health.

Children at risk

Concern over children's increased risk from pesticide exposure is not new. In 1989, the US Natural Resources Defence Council (NRDC) alleged that some 5500–6200 children might develop cancer later in life due to exposure to just eight pesticides during their preschool years.[65] That same year, the Environmental Protection Agency released a preliminary report suggesting that between 15,000 and 50,000 infants and children in the US each day run the risk of getting sick from potatoes on which the insecticide aldicarb has been used. But, as always, it is the link between pesticide exposure and the development of childhood cancer that has grabbed most of the headlines.

Childhood cancer

In spite of the objections of major chemical companies, the evidence linking pesticide exposure to childhood cancer is firmly established,[66] though not all show that it is ingestion of pesticides that poses the greatest risk. Research has shown that pesticide use in the home – for instance, to get rid of termites, flies and wasps, and in the form of no-pest strips, flea collars, and garden insecticides and herbicides – resulted in a significant increase in childhood brain cancers.[67]

Other reports and studies have linked pesticide exposure to a wide range of malignancies in children, including leukaemia, neuroblastoma, Wilms' tumour of the kidneys and non-Hodgkin's lymphoma as well as cancers of the brain, colorectum and testes.[68]

In a 1987 National Cancer Institute study, the risk of childhood leukaemia increased nearly four times when pesticides were used within the home at least once a week, and increased by more than six times when garden pesticides were used at least once a month.[69]

In another 1995 study involving 474 children, those living in homes where no-pest strips embedded with insecticides were used had up to a threefold greater risk of developing leukaemia than those living in homes without the strips. Even worse, children under 14 had four times the normal risk of tumours of connective tissue if their gardens at home were treated with pesticides or herbicides.[70]

Otherwise rare cancers can also become more common with exposure to pesticides. One study at the University of Southern California found that children whose mothers used pesticides in the home once or twice a week were nearly two-and-a-half times as likely to develop non-Hodgkin's lymphoma. Those whose mothers used pesticides on a daily basis were seven times more likely to have the cancer.[71]

In the same study, pregnant women exposed to the pesticides used by professional exterminators in their homes were three times more likely to have a child with non-Hodgkin's lymphoma, and children directly exposed to pesticides by professional exterminators were more than twice as likely to develop the disease.

Child development and intelligence

There is also ongoing concern regarding the toxic effects of pesticides on the developing brain and nervous system.[72] German researchers, for example, report that early exposure to polychlorinated biphenyls (PCBs), which are sometimes found in pesticides, can interfere with early childhood development.

The researchers looked at both pre- and postnatal exposure of 171 otherwise healthy infants, and measured their development at 7, 18, 30 and 42 months. At all of these timepoints, there was evidence that PCB exposure could retard mental and motor development. The only good news in the study was the fact that, where the mother breastfed her infant for longer (even if her breastmilk was a source of PCBs) and in families where parents provided a stimulating home environment, the damage done by the PCBs was significantly less.[73]

In another study, children exposed to a variety of pesticides in an agricultural community in Mexico showed impaired stamina, co-ordination, memory and capacity to represent familiar subjects in simple drawings.[74] Yet another study showed that children exposed to PCBs during fetal life had IQ deficits, and hyperactivity and attention deficits when tested years later.[75]

Mad-Cow Disease: Prions or Pesticides?

Mad-cow disease – formally known as bovine spongiform encephalopathy, or BSE – is widely believed to be a disease caused by prions. At the height of the BSE crisis, proponents of the prion theory believed that feeding cattle with sheep meat transferred the sheep disease scrapie, via infectious prions, to the cattle and this, in turn, was passed on to humans.

More detailed research proved that the role of prions was much more complex than that. Prions are a type of protein found in the membranes of normal cells. The prions thought to be involved in BSE are called 'metallo-proteins', as they are chemical compounds comprising protein molecules and metal ions. About a third of the proteins in the body are metalloproteins, including haemoglobin – the iron and oxygen-carrying component of red blood cells.

One theory that emerged from this was that scrapie was a form of chemical poisoning. Sheep are regularly dipped in pesticides to kill parasites. During this process, their heads are submerged and they inevitably swallow some of the toxic dip. This pesticide soup may have damaged normally benign prions in some sheep to such an extent as to cause neurological damage. In this scenario, it is the pesticides, not the prions, that were passed on to the cattle and eventually caused BSE.

How can this be?

Sheep meat has been fed to cattle for decades and, although it is an objectionable, unnatural diet, it did not produce any ill effects in cows or in humans until 1981. This is when the meat-rendering industry began using a non-solvent process to retrieve meat from carcasses. When solvents were in use, fat-soluble pesticides were 'dry cleaned' out of the meat. However, the new non-solvent process doesn't fully remove these toxins. Organophosphate pesticides in particular can have a very damaging effect on the nervous systems of animals, and it is believed that the symptoms of BSE – and of Creutzfeldt–Jakob disease (CJD) in humans – are related, at least in part, to our increasing ingestion of pesticides.

However, there is more to this complex argument than pesticides.

BSE belongs to a complex family of neurological disorders called 'transmissible spongiform encephalopathies' (TSEs). This family also includes CJD and variant CJD (vCJD), Gerstmann–Sträussler syndrome (GSS) and kuru in humans, scrapie in sheep, chronic wasting disease (CWD) in deer and elk, and feline spongiform encephalopathy (FSE) in cats. The symptoms of TSEs also mirror those of manganism (*see Chapter 9*) and, according to British scientist Mark Purdey, even if the prion theory is correct, it needs a radical rethink.[76] His research shows that the prions thought to cause BSE are not normally harmful until they bond with the manganese in animal feeds (in the 1980s at the start of the BSE crisis, British cows were fed poultry manure, which is high in manganese) or mineral licks. Bonding with manganese creates 'rogue' prions (essentially free radicals) that eventually cause the neurological degeneration seen in BSE.[77] Free-radical damage is, of course, not infective, which may be why attempts to induce BSE in other animals have not been successful.

Adults at risk

Among adults exposed to pesticides, there are three major areas of concern: cancer; reproductive effects (ranging from sterility, infertility and subfertility to birth defects, stillbirths and miscarriage); and effects on the brain and central nervous system (neurotoxicity). It is highly likely that the link with adult diseases reflects a lifetime's exposure to pesticides beginning in childhood. Generally speaking, ingested pesticides, like many other toxins, are stored in fatty tissue and released gradually into the bloodstream, especially during periods of stress. Also in common with many toxic exposures, the early signs and symptoms associated with chronic exposure to pesticides are often labelled 'idiopathic' (of unknown origin) or psychosomatic, a diagnosis that prevents the person from getting the help they need to get well again.

Adult cancers

Throughout the world, studies have shown that the risk of different cancers increases with increasing pesticide exposure. In adults, the use of chlorophenoxy acid herbicides (such as 2,4-D) has been strongly associated with an increased incidence of lung cancer, stomach cancer and leukaemia. Two studies have found a fivefold increased risk of Hodgkin's lymphoma, and other evidence suggests a five- to sixfold increased risk for non-Hodgkin's lymphoma. In addition, many studies have shown a two- to sevenfold increased risk of soft-tissue sarcomas.[78] One showed that farmers in the American state of Kansas using herbicides for as few as 20 days per year have six times the risk of developing lymphoma and soft-tissue sarcomas compared with non-exposed individuals. Those who mixed and applied herbicides and were exposed for 20 or more days per year were eight times as likely to develop non-Hodgkin's lymphoma.[79]

In 1992, a Swedish investigation of 275 confirmed cases of multiple myeloma (cancer that starts in the bone marrow and spreads to various bones, especially the skull) among farmers found that exposure to chlorophenoxy acid herbicides and DDT were primary risk factors.[80]

A review looking at the causes of aplastic anaemia (a serious form of leukaemia resulting from the body's complete failure to produce any type of blood cells) found 280 cases associated with pesticide exposure reported in medical literature. The majority of these cases were in young people (average age 34) with a history of occupational exposure to pesticides. In all of these individuals, the latency period (the time from exposure to development of the disease) was very short – on average, five months.[81]

Neurological disorders

Pesticide exposure is increasingly being linked to a number of neurological disorders now common in old age. While research in this area is still in its infancy, there is a good theoretical basis for the idea that pesticide exposure can lead to degenerative disorders such as Alzheimer's and Parkinson's diseases.

Many pesticides are designed specifically to attack and destroy the nervous systems of insects. Once disabled, the insect is not able to fly or move its legs; paralysed and unable to feed itself, it dies. It is likely that chronic exposure to some pesticides will do much the same to the human nervous system, though research into this area is sparse.

Nevertheless, there is some evidence to suggest that people who are frequently exposed to pesticides, such as farmers and gardeners, have a higher risk of developing mild cognitive dysfunction (MCD). MCD is a somewhat more subtle disorder than dementia, though the two disorders share common symptoms such as memory loss and confusion. In 2000, a study from the Netherlands found that adults exposed to pesticides on a regular basis – for instance, farmers and gardeners – had five or more times the usual risk of developing the subtle neurological impairments or learning problems considered common in MCD.[82]

Osteoporosis

Other deleterious effects of pesticides have increasingly come to light. A recent analysis of bone density in agricultural workers has shown that exposure to pesticides can significantly make bones more porous.

The discovery was made when British researchers assessed agricultural workers seeking litigation for ill health caused by chronic exposure to organophosphates. The men had been exposed to this type of pesticide for between three and 20 years at some point in their lives. Bone biopsies showed significant erosion of the bones in the exposed men as well as much lower bone formation at the tissue and cellular level compared with non-exposed men.

Because of a lack of data, the researchers were unable to say categorically whether the damage to the bone was a direct or indirect result of exposure to organophosphates. While the pesticide can directly enter bone and cause damage, it can also produce other symptoms (such as lethargy, fatigue and depression) that may limit an individual's level of physical activity and, thus, impact on bone health.[83]

Diabetes

Recent research suggests that exposure to herbicides during the Vietnam War, especially Agent Orange (a mixture of the pesticides 2,4-D and 2,4,5-T), may be associated with the development of diabetes later in life.[84]

When published, the results of this study were treated as isolated and relevant only to Vietnam vets. But the use of 2,4-D is particularly widespread even today. It is commonly used by local authorities to inhibit weed growth on roadways and right-of-ways. It can also be purchased at garden stores for home lawn care and is often used by commercial lawn-care companies.

There are, in fact, several studies linking exposure to PCBs and dioxins to insulin effects, changes in glucose metabolism and pancreatic damage.[85] [86] No one understands exactly how pesticides can cause changes in glucose metabolism or lead to diabetes, but it may be the result of the sort of hormonal effects[87] discussed in Chapter 8.

Lowered immunity

It has long been claimed that the present standards for measuring the effects of pesticides on immune function are essentially worthless and do not paint a true picture of the impact of pesticides on immunity. To more fully understand the potential impact, scientists need to begin at the beginning and look at all reports of compromised immunity in terms of how they relate to pesticide exposure.

In the US in 1996, the Washington, DC-based World Resources Institute (WRI) did just that, incorporating data from a number of disparate immunotoxicological studies from around the world into a single report.[88] Its conclusion was that many widely used pesticides are indeed capable of impairing immune function.

Many of the studies reviewed by the WRI scientists came from the former Soviet Union, one of the few places where scientists have examined the impact of pesticides on human immunity. In one investigation of water and soil contamination in Kishinëv, in Moldova, high levels of pesticide residues on many local crops resulted in elevated rates of skin diseases, tuberculosis, tooth decay, ear infections and acute respiratory diseases among children. Infections in adults were also higher than expected and laboratory testing revealed that, as an individual's exposure to pesticides went up, so levels of T cells (infection-fighting cells) went down.

Also noted in the report were data from studies of Inuit children in the northern Hudson Bay area of Canada. The children, nursed on human milk contaminated with organochlorine pollutants, not only suffered an increased risk of infections, but some had immune systems so depressed that they could not receive a standard course of childhood vaccinations.

Pesticides may also interfere with thyroid function and this, in turn, may have a debilitating effect on immunity. The mechanisms by which pesticides might affect human thyroid function are not clear, though some have hypothesised that pesticides may have a chronic mineral-depleting effect that could result in thyroid disorders.[89]

Chronic fatigue

In traditional Indian, or Ayurvedic, medicine, chronic fatigue syndrome (CFS) is the result of accumulated toxins in the body. Western medicine, too, is beginning to acknowledge the link between CFS and chemical poisoning. Pesticide poisoning, for example, can produce symptoms similar to CFS and fibromyalgia,[90] and patients suffering from chronic fatigue have been found to have, on average, twice the levels of pesticides in their blood compared with those not suffering from CFS.[91]

Organophosphate pesticides and insecticides, in particular, are strongly associated with CFS – a condition identical to that suffered by farm workers who regularly work with sheep dips and insecticides.

Looking for more evidence of a connection, scientists in Glasgow studied a small group of individuals who had been experiencing neuro-behavioural symptoms for over a year and who had been exposed to organophosphates – through sheep dip – for between two and five years. Their symptoms included an acute flu-like condition followed by incapacitating fatigue. In all cases, there was a long delay between exposure to the pesticides and the onset of the condition[92] – a problem seen with many toxic exposures and one that, for a doctor who knows nothing about environmental illness, makes diagnosis difficult.

Is Organic a Better Alternative?

The increased demand for organic food has been the result of many shifts in consumer consciousness. Food scares such as BSE and food-borne diseases have affected consumer confidence in conventional farming. Greater awareness of environmental issues has led many people to make the ethical choice of eating organic foods, as has aware-ness of the health hazards of ingesting pesticide-laden foods. Also, the increasing use of alternative therapies that rely on organically grown foods has helped to renew interest in the quality of the food we eat.

In Britain, the sales of organic foods are soaring by 40 percent a year. This is in spite of the fact that customers are still paying more for organic produce than for the conventional variety. In the UK, demand is so great that British farmers are having trouble keeping up with it – with the result that nearly 80 percent of the organic pro-duce in UK shops is imported.

Some critics of organic food have picked up on this issue of organic imports and the possibility that foreign organic produce may not meet British standards – something that many UK consumers are probably not aware of. Organisations such as the Soil Association and the Organic Farmers and Growers, who are responsible for the regulation of organic foods in the UK, admit that monitoring the quality of imported organic produce is notoriously difficult. However, the Soil Association is adamant that the extent of fraud –

that is, non-organic imports masquerading as organic – is very low, in the region of 1 percent.

Where's the proof?

Those looking for research into the nutritional benefits of organic food will find little to help their argument. There have been no human studies on the benefits of organic foods, so we can only guess at how beneficial they may be and whether consumers of organic foods are indeed healthier than those who consume conventionally produced foods. Even if there were research to prove the superior health of organic consumers, the nutrient content of their food may only be one element in the total health picture. Consumers of organic foods may also, for instance, be more active. They may walk or cycle instead of taking the car. They may restrict their use of hazardous chemicals in the home and be non-smokers. They may be better able to manage stress.

In reality, what we know about both conventionally produced and organic food has been gleaned from the jigsaw-puzzle pieces of smallish studies throughout the world. Because of this, both sides of the argument have been able to use the same results in their own way to fight their own corners.

For example, according to the Soil Association, research has shown that organic foods contain more secondary metabolites than conventionally grown plants. Secondary metabolites are substances that form part of a plant's immune system and may also help fight cancer in humans. But even if the theory 'feels right', there is little scientific evidence of the role these secondary metabolites play in human health.

Natural Pesticides?

Conventional growers under pressure from the increasing demands of consumers who want organic foods often point out that the immune systems of organically grown plants contain more 'natural pesticides'. The theory is that, when plants have to rely on their own resources to fight invaders, they step-up production of their inherent pesticides. Phytoestrogens are one type of natural pesticide produced by plants to control the reproduction of their natural predators. But, generally speaking, there is no research on these natural pesticides and how they might affect human health for good or for ill.

The natural-pesticide argument ignores important chemical differences between natural pesticides and synthetic ones; for instance, the latter tend to persist much longer in the environment and in human tissues. In addition, a chemical extracted from a plant may prove to be toxic or carcinogenic in the laboratory, but the whole plant may not be. Indeed, naturally occurring toxins are usually accompanied by naturally occurring antitoxins within the plant to offer a measure of protection that synthetics don't. For example, the natural vitamin C in spinach inhibits the formation of carcinogenic nitrosamines from the nitrates that are also found naturally in spinach.

It is arrogant to assume that, because toxins are found in nature, humans can add to that burden – often with extremely toxic man-made substances – without causing harm to humankind.

In all, approximately 34 studies have compared organic with conventional growing techniques in relation to the nutrient content of plants. While that sounds encouraging, the studies constitute a very mixed bag. Some concentrated only on organic versus conventional fertilisers while others examined combinations of farming practices and farming systems. The crops studied were taken from controlled research plots, working farms, storage facilities and retail outlets.

The result is that few of these studies were truly comparable. Moreover, the findings are difficult to compare because there are many different factors which cannot be controlled for (such as amount of rainfall, light, temperature, maturity at harvest and the variety of the crop itself) and which will affect the nutrient content of plants. Rainfall, light and temperature cannot be controlled in the field and tend to fluctuate from year to year. In addition, depending on the conditions and the length of time involved, there can be changes in nutrient content during storage and distribution.[93]

One review of the scientific literature showed that, in spite of all this, when all the data are taken together, there is a clear trend to support the notion that organic foods are more nutritious.[94] However, the review also noted that, apart from the variables mentioned above, the difference in nutrient content between organic and conventional produce could also be explained by the difference in water content between the two types of produce.

Conventional crops grown with synthetic fertilisers contain a higher proportion of water than organically grown foods. The higher amount of water in conventional produce may 'dilute' vitamins and minerals, resulting in a less nutrient-dense food.[95]

Nevertheless, the claim for the superiority of organic foods is not based on nutrient content alone. In some ways, the nutrient-content argument may even be misleading since it's not what is in organic foods, but what is *not* in them that is probably more important.

Pesticides are harmful to people – no one can reasonably dispute that. When researchers test the amount of pesticide in a single carrot or apple and declare that it is too low to be harmful, they are missing the point. We do not eat foods singly. We eat them in quantity and in combination, day-in and day-out. We have no way of knowing how much pesticide and other toxins we ingest from this quantity of food each day, or who is most at risk from these chemicals.

Government sources continue to insist that pesticide levels in our food are falling. While recent tests by the UK Ministry of Agriculture, Fisheries and Food (MAFF; now subsumed in the Department for Environment, Food and Rural Affairs, or DEFRA) found no pesticide residues in any type of produce, this is inconsistent with many previous reports by MAFF and by other independent groups as well.

There is also a question lingering over the accuracy of such surveys, given that they are largely instigated by complaints from conventional farmers that the organic movement is stealing business away from them. For this reason, it's hard not to view official criticism of the legitimacy of organic foods as more of a sop to conventional farmers, who are undoubtedly feeling the pinch. Unlike other trends in other areas of consumerism, a conventional farmer can't simply jump on the bandwagon and begin producing organics overnight. To go from conventional to organic requires a minimum two-year conversion period for the soil, and many shifts in philosophical outlook and in the day-to-day workings of a farm. Those not willing to make the shift may be looking to government agencies to do what they can to stem the tide of consumer demand for organic food.

Organic food is better for you as eating organically grown produce is still the best way to avoid ingesting pesticides. It may also provide you with more nutrients than conventional produce. However, this is still an expensive option as organic food can be costly. Major supermarkets have recently begun selling selected organic foods at the same price as their conventional counterparts. Should this trend continue, then buying organic food will eventually come within the reach of the average consumer. Until that time, the plain fact is that not everyone can afford to fill their shopping trolley with organic foods. In Chapter 10, however, there are some suggestions to help you make your organic-food budget stretch further.

Lowering Your Pesticide Burden

Though experts argue over just how much danger pesticides pose to human health, few would disagree that less is better. To cut your pesticide exposure, consider the following:

- *Buy organic.* Food and water are our major sources of ingested pesticides. Buying organic food when you can means you are reducing your exposure significantly. Follow the advice in Chapter 10 to help you stretch your organic-food budget.
- *Thoroughly wash all produce* with cool running water. The abrasive effect of running water helps remove some surface chemicals as well as bacteria. Most experts now discourage the use of dishwashing detergent, which can be absorbed into the food. However, if you wish to do so, try the following: for grapes, strawberries, green beans and leafy vegetables, swirl the foods in a dilute solution of dishwashing detergent (look for 'green' or 'eco' brands that don't contain preservatives or colours) and water (about 1 teaspoon per gallon [4.5 litres]) at room temperature for 5–10 seconds, then rinse with slightly warm water. For other fruits and vegetables, use a soft brush to scrub the food with the

solution for about 5–10 seconds, then rinse with slightly warm water. Dry well.

- *Peel fruits and vegetables when appropriate.* This may be especially important when feeding children, and will help reduce their exposure to pesticides concentrated on the surface of foods such as apples, carrots, peaches and potatoes. Likewise, discard the outer leaves of greens, which tend to be more polluted than those nearer the middle.

- *Use a water filter.* Even simple jug filters can remove some chlorine. Reverse-osmosis filters and water purifiers can remove other harmful contaminants and chemicals. See Chapter 10 for advice on which types of filter are best.

- *In the garden,* a simple soap spray is one of the oldest non-toxic pesticides you can use. It can be made by mixing 1–2 tablespoons of mild liquid soap (such as washing-up liquid) to a litre of water. Transfer this mix to a sprayer and use as needed. Similarly, boric acid or borax will kill ants and even cockroaches. Since most ants like sweets, try mixing a bit of honey or other sugar with boric acid to make a paste. Spread this on small cardboard squares and put these in the ant trail so that the ants will eat the mixture and take some back to their nest (you can also find pesticide-free fly and wasp traps at most garden centres). A homemade garden spray can be made from pungent herbs, such as mashed-up garlic combined with cayenne or horseradish. Add a small amount (not more than 1–2 teaspoons) to a gallon (4.5-litre) jug and let it sit for a day or two, shaking it now and then. Test a small amount on a few leaves first to make sure it doesn't burn them. If it does, dilute the mixture with more water. Neem oil is a little less messy and harmless to humans but, diluted in water and sprayed onto garden plants, it discourages all types of fungi, moulds and even ants. Most nurseries sell neem oil products, but you can also buy the oil from healthfood shops and make your own solution.

- *In the house,* opportunist pests can be kept at bay with regular cleaning. Don't leave food out on countertops and, where possible, consider installing screens over windows to keep flying bugs out.

The use of fungicides (for instance, in the bathroom) can be avoided by making sure rooms are well ventilated and humidity levels are kept low. Save common household bug-busters like bleach for when they are really needed as its overuse encourages stronger and more resistant species.

- *Head lice* seem to be a fact of childhood these days. But they don't need to be treated with strong, carcinogenic pesticides. Most lice are immune to conventional formulas anyway. Instead, for quick relief, wash the hair and apply hair conditioner liberally and, before rinsing, comb through the hair using a special nit comb. This will help remove both the lice and their eggs. You should use this procedure several nights running until all the lice and eggs are gone. Neem oil products are also very useful for treating infestations and appears to be non-toxic to humans.

- *Intestinal parasites,* such as threadworms, are also on the rise across all age groups and populations, and are becoming more difficult to treat. Their lifecycle, however, is limited and, if you can prevent reingestion of the eggs, you can avoid using oral pesticides – the side-effects of which include nausea, drowsiness, diarrhoea, loss of muscle control, headache, photosensitivity and skin rashes – to kill them. Keep hands clean and out of the mouth, don't share hand towels with the infested person, and wash sheets and vacuum regularly to prevent eggs being distributed throughout the house. You will need to maintain this kind of scrupulous hygiene for a month or more to beat these bugs.

- *When brushing your teeth,* use only fluoride-free toothpaste and, if your supermarket doesn't sell it, insist that they do. If you still wish to use fluoride toothpastes, use a low-fluoride brand (around 400 ppm). Teach your children to only use a smear of toothpaste on their brushes. Adults should only use a pea-sized amount. This will help avoid excessive ingestion of fluoride – a particular problem with younger children. In fact, not long ago, researchers in Manchester in the UK set out to determine how much fluoride was being retained in children's mouths after brushing with toothpastes containing different quantities of fluoride. They tested toothpaste with 400 ppm and 1450 ppm of fluoride. The average amount ingested per brushing was 0.42 mg when using the 1450-ppm toothpaste and 0.10 mg when using the 400-ppm one. Using the 400-ppm toothpaste twice daily, a child of average weight would not ingest more than 0.05 mg of fluoride per kg of body weight (considered a 'safe' level). But a child using a toothpaste containing 1450 ppm would certainly exceed this level.[96]

- *Watch out for other sources of fluoride.* While water and toothpaste are our major sources of ingested fluoride, there are other sources in our diets and our homes. Those who consume large amounts of tea (independent of whether it is made with fluoridated water) will consume four to 12 times the recommended daily amount of fluoride. Fluoride also comes from foods grown, processed or cooked in fluoridated areas. Teflon cooking utensils also release fluoride. If you are worried, avoid these. Again, choosing a low-ppm toothpaste for your child is essential for limiting the amount of fluoride they ingest.

- *When you bathe*, remember that the longer and hotter the shower, the greater the amount of water contaminants that will pass into your body via your skin and lungs. Baths also produce this effect, but at a much lower level. To lessen your exposure, reduce the water temperature, and keep baths and showers short.

- *Pesticides at school.* Does your child's school have policies in place that emphasise the least use of toxic chemicals, including pesticides? If not, parent involvement can be a catalyst for reassessing the need for using toxic chemicals in school buildings and surrounding play areas. If your school uses wooden play frames, these may have been treated with an arsenic-containing fungicide (*see Chapter 9*). You could reasonably request a policy that children wash their hands after coming in from play, or that the wood be coated with varnish to prevent children from ingesting the heavy-metal pesticide. To protect your child from exposure when pesticides are being used, inform the school that you, as a parent, wish to be notified in advance so that you can make a decision as to whether or not you wish to expose your child to the residues.

- *At work,* employees should be informed of the intention to fumigate premises, and be given the opportunity to work elsewhere during and after. It may be worth speaking to your employer or health and safety officer about the use of pesticides and fungicides in and around the office, and discussing safer alternatives.

7 Turn on, Plug in, Get Sick

WHERE WOULD WE BE WITHOUT ELECTRICITY? IT IS THE INVISIBLE, almost magical, force that powers the many time- and effort-saving gadgets in our homes and offices. It brings us heat, light and sound and, for most people, life without it is frankly unimaginable.

These days, you would have to travel to the furthest and most remote parts of the globe to find anywhere that did not have some form of electrical power to offer its inhabitants. Indeed, today our world is shrouded in an invisible and mostly man-made web of electrical energy. Indoors and out, humans can find little escape from this complex intersection of energy waves in every conceivable frequency range.

Unlike other forms of pollution such as air pollution, which we can see, and toxic chemicals that we can (sometimes) smell, electrical pollution bypasses all of our conscious senses. The only thing that reveals its presence are the end products of its use – computers, TVs, lights, heaters, air conditioners, telephones, microwave ovens, electric shavers, hairdryers, radio alarms and stereos.

Ignored for many years, research into the adverse health effects of electropollution is beginning to show disturbing trends.[1] For instance, the man-made electromagnetic fields (EMFs) that surround us have been linked to higher rates of cancer, depression, suicide and chronic fatigue-like symptoms. They may also cause subtle biological changes that alter the chemical integrity of our bodies, add to the production of cell-damaging free radicals, depress immune function and have reproductive effects. Some authorities suggest that EMFs may also concentrate air pollution and other toxins, especially around high-voltage power lines, causing a range of problems associated with air pollution, including asthma and other respiratory disorders as well as skin cancer. For all these reasons, scientists now believe that our enthusiastic embrace of all things electrical may be doing us more harm than good.

EMFs 101

Most people consider electricity vital because it powers our washing machines, radio/alarm clocks, computers, video games and TVs. But electricity also powers us. The earth is a natural EMF generator, and everything on earth evolved within this dynamic atmosphere. Animals, plants, rocks and the very ground we stand on emanate both electric and magnetic energy.

Humans are also bioelectric beings. Every cell in our body is generating its own EMF as well as contributing to the larger EMF of the whole body. Alternative 'energy' therapies such as acupuncture make good use of these natural electrical fields to produce subtle changes in body chemistry. In many respects, we are like large wet-cell batteries. Our muscle movements are all directed by electrical impulses from the brain through the nervous system. When our brain no longer emits these electrical signals, we are considered clinically dead.

Humans are also natural broadband receivers, picking up signals from the electromagnetic atmosphere around us. Our bodies respond to this natural radiation in unexpected ways. For instance, the incidence of disease, including cancer, and recovery from illness have been found to vary according to geographical region and the relative strength or weakness of the natural magnetic field of that area.

It is inconceivable, then, that electrical life forms such as ourselves – but also other animals such as whales, migrating birds, insects and plants – are not affected by this upsurge in 'man-made' electromagnetic radiation that now shrouds the planet.

Zap!

For 24 hours a day, we are exposed to an alarming array of EMFs.

Inside our homes, we are zapped by:

- Air conditioners/purifiers
- Baby monitors
- Bedside lamps
- Blenders and food processors
- Clocks and clock/radios
- Cordless phones
- Desktop computers
- Dimmer lightswitches
- Dishwashers
- Electric blankets
- Electric fans
- Electric kettles
- Electric ovens and stoves
- Electric radiators
- Electric shavers
- Electric toothbrushes
- Games consoles
- Hairdryers
- Ionisers (if cheaply made)
- Laptop computers
- Lighting
- Microwave ovens
- Power points
- Printers
- Radios
- Reading lamps
- Sewing machines
- Stereos
- Toasters
- TVs
- Vacuum cleaners
- Video recorders/players
- Washing machines
- Water heaters
- Wiring (as well as underground distribution cables)

Inside our offices, we are zapped by:

- Computers
- Electrostatic duplicating machines
- Fax machines
- Fluorescent lighting
- Franking machines
- Heating/air-conditioning units
- Phones
- Photocopiers
- Printers

When we are outside, we are zapped by:

- Airport radar
- Broadcast frequencies from radio and TV
- Communication dishes
- EMFs generated by cars
- High-tension power lines and transformers
- Industrial machines
- Military installations
- Mobile phones and phone towers
- TV transmitters

In addition, when we travel, we are zapped by the EMFs generated by and/or trapped in buses, cars, subways, trains and airplane cabins.

Because utilising electricity often produces instant gratification – hot coffee, cold drinks, a faster Internet connection – it is understandable that many people might want to close their minds to the possible adverse effects it has on human health. Others try to fend off the rapidly accumulating bad news by falling back on the argument that the planet itself is a source of electromagnetic radiation and that humans could not have evolved so successfully if EMFs were a substantial threat to health. This argument, however, misses the point.

While it is true that man-made electromagnetic radiation is not the only source of radiation in our environment, it is equally true that through man-made radiation, our bodies are being exposed – sometimes continuously – to frequencies never encountered before and in a whole different spectrum from those found in the natural world.

Types of Radiation

Man-made electricity is different from the natural electromagnetic emissions from the earth and atmosphere. This difference can be explained in part by the difference between direct currents (DC) and alternating currents (AC). The earth emits a strong electromagnetic current that surrounds us and holds us down; this current is DC, flowing one way – from the earth to us. Man-made electricity is AC – it flows back and forth between objects many times per second, creating a powerful EMF. This cycle of directional changes is measured in hertz (Hz). The fewer changes of direction per second, the lower the frequency and the less energy emitted. The more changes of direction, the higher the frequency and the more energy emitted.

Wherever you have a moving electrical current, you will also have a magnetic field (generally measured in milligauss or mG). Similarly, a moving magnetic field will also produce an electrical field, so the two types of field are really like two sides of the same coin. An electrical field surrounds any appliance that is plugged in, even when it is not switched on. The magnetic field, however, only appears when the appliance is turned on and in use.

Electric and magnetic

Electromagnetic fields are made up of both electrical fields and magnetic fields. The term 'EMFs' generally refers to high-frequency radio waves in which the electrical and magnetic fields are inseparable. However, at low frequencies, including the 50–60 Hz at which electric power is delivered to our homes and offices, electrical and magnetic fields are independent and measured separately.

Scientists tend to worry less about the health effects of electrical fields because we can, to some extent, shield ourselves from these. Solid objects like walls, furniture, fences and trees, for instance, can block them. Magnetic fields, however, can penetrate pretty much anything, with the exception of lead. Because of this, most studies into the health risks of EMFs have focused on the magnetic component.

Many of the documented ill-effects of EMF radiation tend to be linked to increased exposure to the magnetic component of the field, but recent evidence suggests that the long-held assumption that electrical fields are relatively benign may need to be reassessed. In 1996, researchers at the University of Toronto published the results of the first major study into this subject.[2] The participants in the study were electrical utility workers at a Canadian power company, and the results showed a huge increase in their risk of leukaemia.

When the workers' cumulative exposure to magnetic fields alone was considered, the researchers found what they termed a statistically 'non-significant' increased risk of developing leukaemia. In fact, the risk was 60 percent higher in exposed workers than in 'normal' subjects. (It is worth bearing in mind that what research finds statistically significant and what may be significant in human terms is often at variance.)

But when electrical fields were included in the analysis, the cancer risk rose substantially in the exposed workers to more than 10 times more than that of a comparable group of non-electrical workers. The risk of another cancer also increased; exposed workers had an 84 percent higher risk of lung cancer – though, again, this was dismissed as not 'statistically significant'.

In addition, there was also evidence of what is known as a 'dose response' – in other words, the greater an individual's exposure, the higher their risk. This effect was noticeably absent when measuring magnetic fields alone, a finding in common with previous studies in this area.

Thermal and non-thermal effects

Some experts believe that the determining factor for what levels of EMFs constitute a hazard is the difference between thermal and non-thermal effects, and the perception of their harm. All electrical radiation (including ordinary sunlight) generates energy. The higher the frequency, the more likely it is to create what is known as a thermal effect – a heating effect on the body substantial enough to cause tissue and even DNA damage.

Fans of the Marvel comic *The Hulk* will already be familiar with the idea that exposure to gamma rays – super-high-frequency radiation – can cause DNA damage. This is an example of a thermal effect. But we need not be exposed to this kind of extreme high-dose radiation to experience thermal effects. Microwave ovens, for instance, cook food by making use of the thermal effects of high-frequency microwave radiation.

Often, we are given advance warning of thermal effects. When you are out in the sun, you feel heat. When this feeling becomes intense enough, you know that damage to your skin will occur (as sunburn). This warning can help you to take protective action such as going inside or covering up.

The problem is that thermal effects can sometimes occur without any warning signs. The treatment of sports injuries with ultrasound (which makes use of high-frequency radio waves) is a good example of how EMFs can heat tissue without our necessarily being able to feel a strong heating effect. Used in this way, ultrasound is intended to produce controlled tissue changes that are largely perceived to be beneficial. Because tissue temperature is so tightly controlled in the body, it is now believed that even low-frequency electromagnetic energy (for instance, that emitted by mobile phones) can produce a heating effect that is undetectable to our senses, yet strong enough to result in subtle damage to the body's tissues.

In general, thermal effects are easy to recognise and research, and have been the focus of much scientific attention. We know, for instance, that an increase of more than 6° C in the body's core temperature can lead to death. Lesser increases can cause heat stroke, cataracts and localised burns, but also brain damage, infertility in men and birth defects. Now, however, science is turning its attention to non-thermal effects.

Non-thermal effects are those that occur below – in many cases, well below – the level at which tissue heating occurs. A good example of our vulnerability to non-thermal EMF radiation is the way that a flashing light can induce seizures in people with epilepsy. In this circumstance, it is not the light *per se* that causes the seizure, but the electrical information in the form of a coherent signal – in other words, one with a regular pulse, transmitting at around 15 Hz. The brain recognises and is confused by this information because it is similar to a frequency used by the brain itself.

Much of what we know about non-thermal effects comes from animal studies. But human studies have revealed problems as well. For instance, people exposed to mobile-phone frequencies exhibit important changes in their electroencephalogram (EEG; brain wave) patterns that are substantial enough to adversely affect alertness as well as disrupt both deep REM (rapid eye movement) and the lighter dream, or non-REM, sleep.[3] Such frequencies can also adversely affect the memory centres of the brain[4] and increase resting blood pressure.[5]

Measuring EMFs in the Home

You can have the level of EMFs in your home, office or school professionally tested – and this may be a good idea if you live in an area that is near power lines or train tracks. Your local area power company can do this for you. There are disadvantages to doing this, however, since power-company employees generally only work during the day and may turn up at random times when levels of EMF radiation in your particular building may not reflect their true overall values. EMF levels in the home may also change with the seasons – they may, for instance, be higher in winter when we use more lights and heat.

To get a better picture of your EMF environment, you can hire a portable device called a gauss meter, which will allow you to take measurements yourself over a period of days and at various times of the day. This will give you a much better picture of your true EMF exposure.

The gauss meter measures the strength of magnetic fields. These instruments can vary widely in both price and accuracy, but it pays to invest in the best-quality meter you can find because gauss meters can vary in the strength of magnetic field they are capable of measuring.

To get the best out of your meter:

- It should be able to detect levels as low as 0.1 mG
- It should use what is known as a 'triple-axis coil' to calculate EMF levels. Triple-axis gauss meters are considered to be the most accurate, though they are also more expensive
- It should be 'frequency-weighted' – which means that it has the capacity to measure background levels of radiation and incorporate these into its final reading.

Gauss meters can be rented from groups such as Powerwatch and Perspective Scientific (in the UK) and Less EMF Inc (in the US) *(see Chapter 11 Useful Contacts for more details)*.

How EMF Exposure Changes the Body

Several different types of radiation make up the electromagnetic spectrum. These range from extremely low-frequency fields (ELFs), such as those used in radio and TV transmissions, to super-high-frequency fields (SHFs), such as X rays and gamma rays. Microwaves, infrared and the visible-light spectrum occupy a relatively small space somewhere in the middle of these two extremes, but are considered high-frequency fields.

No one disputes the fact that high frequencies can have a deleterious effect on health. High-to-super-high frequencies can have a profound affect on molecules. For example, when microwave energy passes through something containing water (like the human body), it causes the water molecules to vibrate, producing the kinds of thermal effects already discussed. EMFs at frequencies higher than the visual light spectrum are called 'ionising radiation' because they have enough energy to strip electrically charged ions (electrons) from atoms. X rays, which are near the top of the electromagnetic-radiation spectrum, have enough energy to break apart molecules that contain genes. This genetic damage may be what links excessive exposure to super-high frequencies with higher rates of cancer.

The precise mechanism through which exposure to lower-frequency EMFs damages health is not known, though many theories have been put forward.

Electrostress

Most of the concern over EMFs and long-term health has thus far focused upon the possible increased risk of various types of malignancies. However, some scientists now believe that the focus on cancer (which is generally linked with the highest levels of exposure) has become an effective smokescreen to divert attention from the wider range of other effects caused by continuous low-frequency exposures.

We now know that EMF exposure places stress on the body in ways that are not always immediately apparent, but which nonetheless have a profound effect. Studies have shown that when individuals are placed in an induced, artificially made EMF similar to that found in the average home, the body begins to produce stress hormones – the same ones it makes when our fight-or-flight mechanism is triggered.[6] High levels of these hormones have been linked to a huge number of disorders and diseases, including chronic fatigue, asthma, menstrual irregularities, irritable bowel syndrome, depression, heart disease and cancer.

EMFs and Eyes

EMFs can cause eye damage, both directly and indirectly. Low-level microwaves such as those found in everyday communications equipment have been shown to cause direct damage to the retina, iris and macula.[7] Newer studies indicate that radio frequency (RF)-transmitting devices, such as radio sets and mobile phones, may also be a factor in rare types of eye cancer.[8]

Reduced night vision is a further case in point. According to conventional wisdom, it's a condition that comes with age or from wearing certain types of corrective lenses. But it can also be caused by ultraviolet (UV) radiation, and some speculate that sitting in an EMF all day can also be a cause.

The polymers used in the manufacture of contact lenses may also be affected by emissions from visual display units (VDUs) and mobile phones. Ongoing studies have shown that they can be prone to discoloration and, more worryingly, to developing minute holes which, in turn, can irritate and affect the health of the eye. This may be in response to increased retinal temperatures caused by exposure to microwave radiation.[9]

Finally, the metal elements in spectacle frames also constitute a risk. Metal frames can act as antennae, focusing EMFs around your eyes. This effect was first reported by the World Health Organization as early as 1987 and again in 1993, in its report *Electromagnetic Fields 300 Hz–300 GHz*.[10] Both ordinary metallic spectacle frames and certain types of safety spectacles produce this effect.

Conventional science has no explanation for why EMFs should cause this kind of stress. However, practitioners of energy medicine do have a theory. Energy is made up of individual particles – photons and electrons. Many of these are 'coherent' – in other words, they behave in a predictable way (a good analogy might be the way that individual birds in a flock turn together in unison during flight). But some of these particles can behave in a random manner. When there is a lot of EMF radiation circulating around and passing through us, the body may not necessarily be disturbed by the coherent particles. But the random ones are rather like biological snipers, causing random damage that the body must respond to. The body identifies these random particles as foreign, disorganised objects, and responds in a fight-or-flight manner in an attempt to create order again.

This is one reason why some alternative therapists recommend using crystals around computers and other sources of electrical fields. Crystals are forms of coherent energy that exert a stabilising effect on these random particles. This stability is one reason why crystal chips are used in computers and quartz watches – though no one knows for sure if they actually do have a substantial protective effect on humans.

Electrical interference

Because our bodies are electrical, it stands to reason that outside electrical forces may interfere with the organisation of the system in much the same way that running the vacuum cleaner when the TV is on can interfere with the TV signal.

According to one study at Michigan State University in 2000, extremely low-frequency EMFs have the ability to interact with genetic material and damage it, causing the kind of mutations known to lead to cancer. Lab experiments there found that low-frequency EMFs can turn genes on and off at inappropriate times, causing pre-cancerous cells to proliferate when they would normally just remain dormant.[11]

Electromagnetic signals in the microwave- and radio-frequency range (for instance, those used in mobile telecommunications) are also very close to those used by the body to organise cellular activity and metabolism.[12] Some of the frequencies used to power mobile phones correspond to frequencies found in the human brain, specifically, delta waves that relate to sleep, and alpha waves that signify a calm, relaxed, but unfocused state.

In light of this, it is not surprising that neurological complications such as headaches and sleep disturbances are high on the list of adverse effects associated with exposure to mobile-phone use. Such symptoms are consistent with the reported ability of these frequencies to affect the dopamine–opiate system of the brain (that part of the brain that releases pain-relieving chemicals)[13] as well as the permeability of the blood–brain barrier (the protective membrane that prevents toxic substances from reaching the brain).[14] Disruption of either of these systems can act as a trigger for headaches.[15]

Worryingly, emergency services throughout the world are increasingly using a form of mobile telecommunications known as TETRA (terrestrial trunked radio) that mimics frequencies in the human brain. The obvious question is: do we really want our fire fighters and ambulance men and women exposed daily to frequencies that can potentially cause confusion, poor memory and slower response times?

The melatonin hypothesis

The melatonin hypothesis suggests that EMFs can either interfere with the normal function of melatonin or result in such low levels of melatonin that health is compromised.

According to this theory, the pineal gland, which controls hormonal balance throughout the body, can be deeply affected by exposure to EMF radiation. One of the most important hormones it controls is melatonin. Melatonin is important to the synchronisation of our day/night, sleep/wake cycles. When the pineal gland is stressed, melatonin levels go down,[16] resulting in the kind of sleep problems reported by EMF-exposed individuals.[17]

Studies also indicate that people whose jobs expose them to low-level EMFs have lower levels of melatonin than non-exposed individuals.[18] When levels of melatonin are low, the body may also lose its ability to respond to and control abnormal cell growth – a breakdown that has been linked to an increased risk of breast cancer. Laboratory studies show that melatonin can inhibit the proliferation of breast cancer cells, but that this effect is blocked when the cells are exposed to a 60-Hz magnetic field.[19] According to this theory, it may not be that EMFs directly cause cancer. Instead, they cause a breakdown in the efficient running of our bodies, leaving us vulnerable to toxic effects that can lead to cancer.

Reduced levels of melatonin have also been linked to other degenerative disorders such as Parkinson's, Alzheimer's and heart diseases. It is also interesting to note that individuals with multiple chemical sensitivities (a disorder with links to EMF exposure) often have very low levels of melatonin.

Air pollution

A further theory suggests that the high-voltage electricity carried around the country by means of overhead cables suspended between pylons breaks up the air, separating electrons from individual molecules of air (causing the buzzing noise you can hear when you are close to overhead power lines). This process is technically known as ionisation. It results in the production of electrically charged particles, or ions, that have the ability to stick to surfaces (in much the same way that dust particles will stick to a TV or computer screen). In the air, these ions act like magnets attracting microscopic particles of pollution, thus increasing the risk of pollution-related diseases such as skin cancer, lung cancer, respiratory diseases such as asthma, and heart disease.

This theory, put forward by British scientist Professor Denis Henshaw of Bristol University and based on his own research,[20] [21] is not new and is supported by evidence from other scientists.[22] It has long been suspected that the various individual pollutants present in indoor air may combine with indoor EMFs to form a hazard known as 'photochemical smog'. It has been further suggested that UV light from fluorescent tubes provides the energy for reactions to occur between ozone and other pollutants in the air that can, in turn, create a variety of short- and long-term health problems.

Professor Henshaw's work also supports the idea that electrical fields are more harmful than previously thought, and that the combination of magnetic *and* electrical fields may have a greater biological effect than either one on its own.

When it was first published, this work was highly contested by the authorities. But evidence continues to point to the idea that proponents of this theory may be on the right track. For instance, in 2000, British scientists analysed over 10,000 cancer cases in the South West of England. By categorising each case according to where the individual lived – for instance, their proximity to high-voltage power lines – they discovered a significant increase in lung cancer and increases in other pollutant-linked cancers in those living up to more than 500 metres *downwind* of such lines compared with those living upwind of them. Increased rates of skin cancers were also found among those living close to power lines.[23]

Future generations at stake

There are also some still-unanswered questions regarding the passed-on effects of EMF exposure. Some scientists believe EMF exposure can alter DNA, so we must be prepared to address the question of what happens to those future generations whose basic genetic make-up has been subtly altered by EMF exposure.

Swedish studies carried out in the 1980s suggest that the incidence of genetic malformations rises if either the mother or father is exposed to EMF radiation.[24] To date, no UK or US scientists have tried to confirm these findings. However, studies in other fields also show the vulnerability of the developing child to EMF radiation. There is now concern that exposing a developing fetus to ultrasound scans can result in a range of neurological effects, including an increased tendency towards left-handedness[25] and longer-term problems such as learning difficulties,[26] speech delay[27] and dyslexia.[28] Ultrasound has also been linked to immune and neurological damage in animals, the latter resulting in behavioural abnormalities such as social withdrawal,[29] low body weight and poor muscle tone.[30] It also causes thermal effects close to the bone – raising tissue temperature enough to damage brain cells and DNA in the developing child.[31]

Animals and EMF Stress

It is well known that animals have much keener senses of smell and hearing than humans. It seems quite likely that they may also be much more sensitive to weak EMFs and other subtle energy stimuli that may have significant effects on mood and behaviour.

While relatively little attention has been paid to effects on pets and farm animals exposed to EMFs, evidence suggests that they can suffer similar health problems to humans. One study reported that dogs living in apartment buildings where exposure to low-frequency magnetic fields (similar to those found in our homes) was high had an incidence of breast cancer seven times higher than animals in locations with less electropollution.[32] Another found that sheep grazing in close proximity to a high-tension mast had impaired immune-system responses.[33]

Dairy cows with increased exposure to magnetic fields have shown a reduction in milk production and changes in the composition of the milk.[34] Many of these and other effects of EMFs are consistent with the effects of chronic stress in animals such as frequent fertility problems, increased rates of spontaneous abortion and a reduction in milk production.

Scientists have also suggested that the increasing incidence of beached whales may be related to the way in which man-made EMFs interfere with these animals' own radar. Similar problems have been found in migrating birds, which end up miles off their usual migratory paths.[35]

Electrical Sensitivity

The possible adverse effects of man-made electrical forces, like that of all other forms of pollution, are the subject of hot debate. However, many authorities now believe that we are seeing the emergence of a new syndrome related specifically to EMF exposure – 'electro-magnetic hypersensitivity' or, more commonly, 'electrical sensitivity'.

In reality, electrical sensitivity (ES) is not a new concept. Over the years, it has been know by different names, including 'radiowave ill-ness' and 'microwave sickness'.[36] Whatever the name, the symptoms of electrical sensitivity are well documented and most commonly include:

- skin itch/rash/flushing/burning and/or tingling
- confusion/poor concentration and/or memory loss
- fatigue/weakness
- headache
- chest pain/heart problems
- volatile moods.

Less commonly reported symptoms include nausea, panic attacks, insomnia, seizures, ear pain/ringing in the ears, feeling a vibration, paralysis and dizziness. Some ES patients experience only one symp-tom but, more often, a collection of symptoms is present.

Electrical sensitivity is particularly associated with office work, and it appears that EMFs in the office may contribute to the symptoms of sick building syndrome (*see Chapter 5*).

Whether or not individuals succumb to ES may also depend in part on what other stresses they are experiencing in their lives. In a high-stress lifestyle, the extra burden of EMFs may be the straw that breaks the camel's back – bringing on illness that might otherwise have been held in check by the body's own defences.

Some people – for instance, those suffering from multiple chemical sensitivities, chronic fatigue syndrome (CFS) or heavy-metal toxicity from mercury-containing dental fillings – are particularly at risk of

ES.[37] [38] Indeed, ES can occur alongside chemical sensitivity and some believe that one may set the other off.[39] Because the nervous system is a primary target for chemicals and EMFs, those with nervous-system damage (such as multiple sclerosis) appear to be more susceptible to ES as well.[40]

Overexposure to electromagnetic radiation can bring on the symptoms of ES, independent of other illness, but it can also exacerbate any existing health problems. Indeed, if you are already ill, EMF exposure may prevent you from getting better. There is now evidence that patients in intensive care units may be exposed to unacceptable levels of EMFs and that this may slow recovery.[41] In one Italian neonatal ICU, over a period of two working days, peak levels of more than 10 mG were registered – 10 times greater than levels generally accepted as 'safe'.[42] The staff working in such environments may also be affected by these higher levels of EMFs and this, in turn, can bring on ES-like symptoms that affect their health as well as their judgment.

The most electrically sensitive patients need medical help, but simply getting to the doctor's office may prove difficult since a ride in a car can overexpose them to EMFs generated by the vehicle's motor. Once there, they may be surprised to find that the typical doctor's office is a minefield of EMF exposures, with computers, fluorescent and other energy-efficient lights, and medical tests that require exposure to electromagnetic or ultrasound sources.

Once an individual realises that proximity to electrical sources is the triggering event that leads to their symptoms, EMF avoidance will be the most helpful strategy for reducing reactions. Unfortunately, the more we come to rely on wireless technology, such as mobile-phone services and paging systems, the more difficult EMF avoidance becomes. Recent revelations that mobile-phone masts can be hidden in everyday objects in big cities – from church steeples to fake trees, pub and petrol-station signs, and the 'golden arches' outside your local McDonalds[43] – suggest that, in some cases, without a map specifically detailing the locations of these sources of radiation, city dwellers wishing to avoid unnecessary EMFs are at a tremendous disadvantage.

Mobile Phones: Are They Safe?

The World Health Organization (WHO) has called for more research into the potential health hazards of mobile phones and has urged people to limit their use of them. Why? Because nobody can say for sure how dangerous they are. What's more, because most research into adverse effects is funded by major telecommunications companies and others with a vested interest in the widespread use of wireless technologies, we may never see the full and true picture of the health effects of mobiles.

The media, of course, love simple questions like "is it safe?" But when it comes to mobile phones, there is just no simple answer. Indeed, a recent editorial in the medical journal *The Lancet* summed up the problems eloquently in its title: 'Mobile phones and the illusory pursuit of safety'.[44] The editorial was commenting on two papers in that particular edition of the journal, one of which suggested that it was too soon to come to any conclusions about the safety of mobile-phone use[45] while the other suggested that, as the human body is an electrochemical instrument of exquisite sensitivity, the possibility of EMFs not interfering with its orderly function was quite ridiculous.[46]

Mobile phones make use of microwave technology – the same technology that heats your food to a high degree in such a short amount of time. Cellular phones emit a mixture of high (microwave)- and low (radio wave)-frequency radiation. For instance, cell-phone lines use microwaves in the 900–1800 MHz frequencies. But the phones themselves emit pulsed bursts of low-frequency radiation at up to 217 Hz, which peaks when talking and troughs when listening. In addition, when you use a mobile phone, its battery also emits low-frequency 'harmonic' energy pulses at 2.4 and 8 Hz.

As with all types of EMFs, no one is sure whether it is thermal effects caused by the microwaves or non-thermal effects caused by the radio waves that have the most significant effect on health.

It has been estimated that the temperature in the head rises 0.5–2° C over 30 minutes when exposed to a mobile phone. However, once the blood flow through the head is taken into account, this rise in temperature drops to 0.01–0.1° C – too low to be considered a risk. Nevertheless, the amount of radiation absorbed into the head can be increased considerably by the enhancing effect of metal in and around the head   for instance, amalgam and other metal tooth fillings, earrings and eyeglasses (especially the metal-rimmed variety). The results are 'hot spots' in the head, with temperatures easily above accepted thermal guidelines. To date, this enhancement effect has been all but ignored by researchers.

Others believe that it is non-thermal effects that will ultimately prove to be the biggest threat from mobile phones. The low-frequency 'harmonic' pulses emitted by the phone's battery that direct energy into the brain are thought to be one of the principal ways that mobile-phone radiation can affect brain function[47] and sympathetic nervous system activity (for instance, control of blood pressure).[48]

Indeed, some authorities believe that the headaches associated with extended mobile use, while debilitating in themselves, are also a foretoken of much more significant effects yet to be revealed.[49]

Given this uncertainty, it is not surprising that a report by the UK Independent Expert Group on Mobile Phones noted recently that the lack of conclusive data so far does not put mobile phones in the clear, that no evidence of harm should not be confused with evidence of no harm, and that a precautionary approach is warranted, especially where children are concerned.[50] Such is the weight of evidence that, if mobile phones were food, the chances are they would simply not be licensed for sale.

The picture of mobile-phone safety has been further complicated recently by concerns that the cordless phones used in our homes may be as dangerous, if not more dangerous, than mobiles. Such phones are popular because they give the user the freedom to wander as far as 100 metres away from the phone's base unit while talking.

But newer cordless phones using DECT technology operate in a similar manner to mobile phones, using microwave radiation at around 1900 MHz. Both the phone and the base station emit pulses of microwave energy so, if you are using the phone close to its base, you are getting a double dose of radiation. Furthermore, unlike mobile phones which 'power down' when talking, the DECT system gives off continuous pulses of both electrical and magnetic radiation directly into the head.[51]

Scientists say radiation emitted by the handsets, which are found in many modern homes, could interfere with the brain to cause memory loss, headaches, dizziness and even cancer. Cordless phones may even turn out to be more risky than mobile handsets because they are used more frequently and for longer periods.

Longer-Term Risks

Both adults and children can be affected by chronic low-level as well as high-level exposure to EMFs. Of most concern to the general public is the association between EMFs and cancer. But EMF exposure is also linked to a range of other disorders, including memory loss, behavioural changes and depression. It is up to each individual to make up his/her mind about the relative risk of EMF exposure in their life. Nevertheless, the stockpile of evidence suggesting harm continues to grow and simply ignoring the bad news won't make it go away, however comforting it may be in the short-term.

Children's health

Children are particularly susceptible to the effects of radiation.[52] Children's thinner skulls make it easier for radiation to penetrate the normally protective skull. In addition, the synchronisation of alpha and delta brain-wave activity in children under 12 is not stable, and is more easily disrupted by outside forces. Immunity, too, is not as robust in children and is therefore more vulnerable to the disrupting effects of microwave radiation.

Childhood cancer

Childhood leukaemia is perhaps the most well-proven effect of exposure to EMFs. Denied for many years by the authorities, who claimed that older studies were poorly conducted and proved nothing, newer and better studies have only served to strengthen the evidence.[53] Nevertheless, a recent 'definitive' report from the UK's National Radiological Protection Board (NRPB) still hedged its bets.[54] Their official conclusion was that, overall, there was no proof that EMFs caused cancer. Yet, tucked away in the body of the report was the admission that current evidence suggests roughly a doubling of the risk of leukaemia in children (from one in every 1400 to one in every 700) with heavy exposure to very-low-frequency EMFs – a conclusion in line with those of previous studies done in the US, Canada and the UK.[55]

Evidence is also accumulating to show that living near even relatively low levels of magnetic radiation from mains electricity or power lines can significantly raise a child's chance of developing leukaemia. In 1979, the first major study linking EMFs from power lines and domestic wiring to childhood cancer was published.[56] Other studies followed, including a Swedish study, involving around a half-million children under the age of 16, which showed that children exposed to varying levels of household EMFs had up to a fourfold greater risk of developing leukaemia.[57]

Other studies have reached mixed conclusions.

The United Kingdom Childhood Cancer Study (UKCCS) – an 18-year study of EMFs in 2226 cancer-stricken children and an equal number of healthy children – did not support a definite link between EMF exposure and risk of childhood cancer.[58] And because this study was conducted by an 'official' body, it was greeted with open arms in the press.

This conclusion was, however, at odds with previous studies and even the authors admitted that the study design may have been flawed (an admission that was omitted from most of the reporting). For instance, only a few children – 2.3 percent – in the study fell into the higher-exposure category. Also, the study, which began in 1991, used a criterion known as the 'time-weighted average' (TWA) – where the amount of EMF exposure was averaged out over a period of years and which, some scientists believe, does not give a true picture of EMF exposure, particularly periods of high exposure. By employing TWA, a researcher effectively removes the periods of short but intense exposure that may damage human tissue or alter DNA irrevocably.

At around the same time, a smaller study from New Zealand also failed to find an association between leukaemia and EMF exposure. Similarly, this study suffered from the same design problems as the UKCCS study.[59]

In Britain, it is believed that less than 1 percent of children are exposed to EMF levels high enough to cause leukaemia. This is why the possibility is dismissed as small and not warranting any regulatory action by the authorities. However, it is cold comfort to the parents of a child dying of cancer to know that their child only had a 'small' risk of developing the disease in the first place.

Sudden infant death syndrome

Some scientists have observed that cases of sudden infant death syndrome (SIDS) seem to cluster around places with abnormal geo-magnetic fields (GMFs; where there is strong natural radiation from the earth) and/or EMFs.[60]

In the UK, scientist Roger Coghill is one of the few investigators who has put time and effort into studying the effects of EMFs on infants.[61] In one study, he examined the location of all SIDS cases in four North London boroughs between January 1986 and July 1988 in relation to obvious sources of EMFs. He found that not only were SIDS infants living significantly closer to EMF sources than healthy babies, but also that the nearer the EMF sources, the younger the age at which the infants died.[62] To date, few other researchers have investigated this possibility, even though SIDS is the single most important cause of infant mortality in industrial countries.

Adult health

Links with adult leukaemia and other cancers have proven more elusive in adults. In many ways, this is to be expected since a developing child is particularly sensitive to the effects of EMF exposure. Nevertheless, there is growing evidence that adults are not immune to the adverse health effects of EMFs.

Adult cancers

Evidence from Sweden, Norway and Finland, which have the most mobile phones per person in the world and where they have been in use for longer than elsewhere, has shown that adults who regularly use mobile phones have two to three times the risk of developing a brain tumour.[63] [64] In these studies, the risk was related to the use of older-style analogue phones, which cause two to three times greater exposure than the digital system, which is now more common – at least in Europe.[65] Whether this means that digital phones are safer or whether it will simply take longer for them to induce a tumour remains to be seen.

Several studies suggest that exposure to EMFs is associated with breast cancer in both men[66] and women,[67–69] possibly because exposure to magnetic fields inhibits the nightly synthesis of melatonin by the pineal gland.[70] This, in turn, can result in higher levels of circulating oestrogens – a known risk factor for the development of breast cancer. While it is true that not all studies have found this association,[71] and no one knows exactly how EMFs influence melatonin,[72] research continues to receive funding in this area because here at least scientists have what they consider a 'plausible' theory as to how EMF exposure could lead to breast cancer.

Other studies have suggested a link between EMFs and increased skin cancer risk. In one, undertaken in Devon and Cornwall, persons living within 20 metres of a power line had an overall increase of 62 percent in skin cancer over those in low-exposure areas. This increased to 99 percent if the properties had high radon levels in addition to high EMF levels.[73] Other researchers have also noted this effect.[74] One reason for this phenomenon may be the presence of a greater number of carcinogens concentrated in and around areas of high EMF radiation. In such circumstances, a higher number of toxic particles and gases, including radon decay products, may be landing on the skin.

Increased risk of lung cancer in EMF-exposed adults may be due to inhaling the same type of carcinogens implicated in skin cancer. Several studies have shown increased risks of anywhere from 13 percent for those in average-exposure groups to 600 percent for those in the highest-exposure groups.[75] Five major studies in this area have showed a statistically significant excess of lung cancers in those exposed to the highest levels of EMF radiation.[76] One of the studies reviewed was carried out in East Anglia in the UK, where it was discovered that women living under high-voltage power lines had a 75 percent increased risk of developing lung cancer.[77]

There is also research to suggest that exposure to EMFs may also lead to a risk for more rare cancers such as non-Hodgkin's lymphoma (NHL). According to available data, those exposed to EMFs on a regular basis may have one-and-a-half to more than twice the risk of non-exposed individuals.[78]

Chronic fatigue

Fatigue and mood swings are well-documented symptoms of electrical sensitivity. Left untreated, these problems can grow in intensity, occasionally leading to severe depression and suicide. In one study, the risk of severe depression was increased by nearly fivefold among subjects living within 100 metres of a high-voltage power line.[79]

Further evidence suggests that people may be more likely to commit suicide if they are regularly exposed to low-frequency EMFs. In one US study of nearly 6000 workers employed by five electric-power companies, suicide deaths were twice as high among those whose work regularly exposed them to electromagnetic radiation.[80] Once again, disruptions in melatonin, the hormone that maintains the normal daily rhythms of the body, including the sleep and wake cycle, as well as serotonin, the neurotransmitter that has a calming effect on the nervous system and emotions, were put forth as a possible cause.

Reduced immunity

Several reports show that EMF exposure can adversely affect the human immune system.[81] This reduced immunity associated with EMF exposure has also been linked to the melatonin hypothesis. One of melatonin's functions is to support the immune process and, when levels are low, the immune system becomes less effective at dealing with toxic chemicals, losing its ability to metabolise them or transport them out of the body. In one study in New Zealand, adults living near power lines had significantly increased risks for asthma, arthritis and type II diabetes as well as a range of other chronic health problems.[82]

In another, scientists found that chronic human exposure to low-frequency EMFs can cause disorders of the nervous, circulatory and immune systems. More specifically, they found that electrical workers exposed to low-level magnetic fields had significantly lower lymphocyte counts than a similar control group which was not exposed to such levels.[83] Lymphocytes are among the body's most powerful toxin- and infection-fighting cells.

Miscarriage

For women who have trouble getting pregnant or a history of miscarriage, it may be prudent to take steps to avoid excessive EMF exposure. Evidence of a possible link between EMF exposure and miscarriage first emerged in the 1980s and 1990s when researchers discovered that using an electric blanket could increase the risk of miscarriage.[84] The results of more recent studies have been mixed probably, say experts, because such studies fail to take into account brief but significant periods of high exposure.

One study that did take these brief periods of high exposure into account showed just how significant this kind of exposure can be. In this case, researchers followed nearly 1000 women from early pregnancy. The women were asked to wear devices that would monitor EMF-exposure levels during a single day of their pregnancy. What the researchers found was that women exposed to the highest levels of EMFs were more likely to miscarry than women whose daily exposure was low.

In this investigation, single high exposures appeared to have the most devastating effects. For instance, exposure to a magnetic field of more than 16 mG (16 times higher than recognised 'safe' levels) increased a woman's risk of miscarriage sixfold in the first 10 weeks of pregnancy, and this effect was most pronounced in women with a history of miscarriage or problems becoming pregnant. To put this figure into perspective, the researchers noted that standing next to a microwave while heating a cup of coffee in the morning can expose a person to 100–300 mG, and appliances such as electric blankets, commonly used electrical appliances such as vacuum cleaners or hairdryers, and electrically powered vehicles all emitted similarly high levels of EMFs.[85]

How Much is Too Much?

Given these findings, what most of us would like to know about EMFs is very simple – at what level does exposure become harmful? It is the one question that scientists have failed to adequately address. Perhaps they are afraid of the answer.

It is, for instance, unclear whether it is your cumulative exposure or intermittent high frequency exposures that cause the most harm. Chances are, it is a combination of both. Electric razors and hairdryers emit alarmingly high EMFs in the short time we use them. However, these levels are generally highest close to their energy source and drop off rapidly with distance. Thus, levels may register very high close to an appliance, but virtually disappear at distances of no more than three to five feet. For this reason, it is possible to be exposed to higher levels of EMFs from certain home appliances than from nearby power lines.

Nevertheless, your background level of exposure also appears to be important. Scientists now believe that weak EMFs may be able to produce debilitating 'low-dose' effects in the same way that weak oestrogens and low doses of other environmental toxins can.

Different people, different risks

Since there is no longer any large group of people in the world who have not been exposed to EMFs at some time or at some level, scientists have no healthy unexposed individuals to make comparisons against. This makes research into this area a difficult proposition. However, in trying to sort out the electrochaos, researchers have divided exposure into three significant levels.

Continuous high exposure
People in this group tend to work in jobs that expose them day after day to high-frequency EMFs. Indeed, the earliest studies into the effects of EMFs were done with high-risk groups such as power-industry workers. However, these are not the only people with this sort of exposure. Other risky occupations include industries that use electricity, including smelting, electrical workers (such as electrical engineering technicians, electrical engineers, electricians, power-line and cable workers), power-station operators, telephone line workers, TV and radio repairmen, welders and flame cutters, dressmakers, data-entry workers, radio- and TV-station employees and those working in sound-recording studios, radio operators (such as in army communications), scientists working with microwave technology, and hospital workers, especially doctors and nurses in intensive-care departments.

Single or intermittent high exposure

Individuals in this category regularly use appliances that produce high-energy EMFs, but are generally exposed for only short periods of time. Such appliances include those in the home such as hair-dryers, microwaves, washing machines and dryers, electric shavers, electric blankets, blenders, electric can openers, power saws and drills, electric cookers and vacuum cleaners, as well as office equipment such as photocopiers and franking machines. EMF radiation tends to drop off sharply with greater distance from such appliances, and people can protect themselves from exposure by simply putting space between themselves and their appliances.

Continuous low exposure

This group includes the entire population. Examples of things that generate more or less continuous low-frequency fields include the wiring in your home and pretty much anything you plug into an electric socket. Even when the appliance is switched off, it will be generating an electrical field. Some of these appliances – for instance, microwave ovens, mobile phones, and all wireless forms of communication including the TV and radio – can also generate higher-frequency fields once they are switched on. Other appliances and machines that emit low-frequency EMFs include radio alarm clocks, battery chargers, baby monitors, telephones and fax machines, desk and bedside lamps, video and DVD players, and VDU screens. Because of the technology required to produce a picture on a screen, TVs and VDUs are particularly complex and produce both a low- and a high-frequency field at the same time.

Even if you are generally surrounded only by low-frequency fields, this does not mean they will have no effect on your health. Low-frequency energy fields from different sources may even combine to produce a synergistic effect. So, switching on the light in one room may push EMF levels much higher elsewhere in the home or office.

While many scientific studies do indicate that exposure to EMFs can result in statistically significant adverse health effects, there is also research to suggest no harmful effects. Official bodies cling to such research as proof that their position is sound. However, there are other hurdles in the way of sensible regulation of EMF exposure.

Wielding Power

Power companies don't just hold sway over our electricity supply, they also wield considerable political power. In March 1990, when the US Environmental Protection Agency first drafted tough guidelines on EMF exposure, these were swiftly vetoed by the power industry in favour of weaker ones that still stand today.

The original report recommended that EMF radiation be classified as a "probable human carcinogen". This recommendation meant that EMFs would join the ranks of formaldehyde, DDT, dioxins and PCBs.

Utility, military and computer lobbyists were outraged, and extreme political pressure was applied. When the final revision of the report was released, it was clear that the power industry had won – the EPA had revoked its original recommendations on the basis that "the interaction between EMFs and biological processes leading to cancer is not understood".

Scientists and government authorities continue to hold the line that, until they fully understand how EMFs affect health, they should not be setting limits for human exposure nor should they be issuing warnings that might alarm the public. Nevertheless, official levels of 'safe' exposure have been silently and without fanfare dropping lower in the last few decades.

Those experts, public officials and governments that have bothered to make any effort to devise guidelines have proposed that a safe ambient level of a 60-Hz magnetic field is 3 mG. However, opinions vary. The EPA has proposed a safety standard of 1 mG, and other scientists such as Robert Becker, author of the book *Cross Currents* and a doctor who has been studying EMFs for 20 years, concur.[86] There is some logic behind this belief. When electricians try to solve a magnetic-field problem, they do their best to drop the level to 1 mG or below. For safety purposes, you should consider that anything higher than 0.5–1 mG is unusual and may be unsafe.

Such information, however, is useless unless you can find out whether the levels of EMFs you are exposed to at home or at work fall within these safer boundaries. The only way to do this is to have your home or office levels measured either by the local power company or with a hired gauss meter (*see pages 136–137*).

Governments' continued inaction on the EMF question exposes a frustrating double standard. The excuse that regulation is not reasonable until we understand how EMFs damage health greatly contradicts the relatively swift action taken when CJD was first linked to beef consumption. Even now, we still do not fully understand the connection between eating beef and developing CJD. No one can say for certain, for instance, if the prions found in contaminated meat really do cause this debilitating and ultimately fatal condition. There is good evidence linking CJD with pesticides and deficiencies in modern animal feeds (*see Chapter 6*). Nevertheless, governments were forced to bring in regulations – mostly because of consumer pressure.

If we were dealing with this much evidence against a carcinogen of any other kind, the scientific and medical community would be calling for immediate government action. Consumers, too, would be outraged – and consumer outrage is the only thing stronger than the political power of the utility companies.

Consumer outrage, however, has been slow to emerge. Either through ignorance or a lack of motivation, consumers have done little to stem the tide of electropollution in their homes or on the streets. Yet, every time you use your computer on the train or phone a friend while grocery shopping, you are adding to the growing problem of second-hand EMF pollution.

A good example of the risks involved was recently discovered by a Japanese physicist working at the Curie Institute in Paris. He calculated that trains, because of their largely metal construction, trap the microwave radiation emitted from mobile phones in the carriages. According to his calculations, the average EMF in a train carriage greatly exceeds the recognised safe exposure levels. Similar problems can arise in other metal vehicles, such as buses, tube trains and lifts, where every time someone gets out their mobile phone, the other occupants are caught in the crossfire of EMFs bouncing off the walls.[87]

As with all forms of pollution, the full picture of the toxic effects of electropollution may take years, even decades, to develop. However, based on the evidence at hand, there is good reason to believe that, one day, second-hand electropollution will be acknowledged as having as great an impact on health as second-hand smoke.

Switching Off

You can't avoid EMFs completely but, if you believe that it is best to limit your own exposure and that of your family, there are several easy and inexpensive methods of doing so. With regard to electrical appliances, simply turn them off and preferably unplug them when not in use. Because EMF levels drop off rapidly with distance, exposure can be reduced by not staying any closer to a working appliance than is necessary. Consider increasing your distance from electric or microwave ovens while they're cooking, and avoid electric heaters, washing machines and dryers when they're operating.

In addition:

- *Cut down on unnecessary electrical gadgets.* Most of us have far more than we need. Be especially wary of cordless appliances such as electric toothbrushes, razors and cordless phones as well as plug-in devices such as hairdryers and electric can openers.
- *Consider removing the microwave from your kitchen.* If you only use it to heat coffee, or cook potatoes or prepackaged meals, you probably don't need it. Getting rid of your microwave will also vastly improve the quality of the food you eat since food that has been microwaved has fewer nutrients in it. In addition, proteins, such as those found as meats, are significantly altered during the microwave process. Eating food directly from the microwave may also mean ingesting food that is still giving off radiation; this is why users are advised to let food 'sit' for a few minutes afterwards – to let all this radiation disperse.

- *Ground yourself and your home.* Modern synthetic materials such as nylon can spark electricity (as anyone walking across a nylon carpet towards a metal doorknob will know). Being surrounded by synthetics (acrylics, nylons) can help conduct electricity into your body whereas natural fibres like wool, linen and cotton, on the other hand, are neutral. Replace man-made shoe soles with leather ones. Similarly, plastics and synthetics in the home and office can attract static charges (as well as emit toxic gases). Replace these with natural wood and ceramics where possible.

- *Before buying a home.* Assess prospective new neighbourhoods from an electromagnetic point of view. Do any power lines run directly under the property? Does the property back onto power lines or train tracks? Is there a power station nearby? If so, you may wish to consider another location.

- *Do you really need to be in touch all the time?* Is it really important to chat to your friends while doing the shopping or to talk business at the bus stop? Try keeping your mobile phone for emergencies only. Switch to a pay-as-you-go plan and keep calls to an absolute minimum. In addition, don't let your kids have mobile phones. They are more vulnerable to the adverse health effects and sociological evidence suggests that mobiles are now officially an addiction with youngsters.[88] Don't feed the fire.

- *Put your cordless phone somewhere safe.* DECT phones use microwave radiation similar to mobile phones. To avoid being blasted with radiation, put the base unit somewhere away from people, like in a hallway or passage. Since microwaves can travel through walls, be aware of what furniture lies on the other side of the wall. Keep the unit away from where you sit or sleep and always away from children.

- *Rearrange your office and living spaces* so that you are not exposed to EMFs from the sides/backs of electric appliances and computers. In the home, all major electrical appliances, such as computers, TVs and refrigerators, should ideally be placed up against outside walls. That way, you avoid creating an EMF in the adjoining room. Try to not put sofas, chairs and beds near significant sources of EMFs such as electricity metres and TV sets. As a rule of thumb, allow at least six to eight feet from such sources, especially for beds. Also, try not to run electrical wires under beds or chairs.

- *Make the bedroom an EMF-free zone.* You spend eight or more hours there – time that your body uses to repair and recover. Make sure you have as few electrical gadgets as you feel comfortable with in the bedroom. Put stereos, computers and TVs somewhere else; consider a battery-powered alarm clock. Don't sleep under an electric blanket or on a waterbed. If you insist on using these, unplug them before going to bed (don't just turn them off). Even though there is no magnetic field when they are turned off, there may still be a high electrical field. Brass and metal bedsteads are beautiful, but they can also concentrate EMFs around you; wood is a better alternative. Similarly, consider replacing metal bedside lamps or make sure they are three feet away from your head. Wires in mattresses can also concentrate EMFs; if you are at all concerned about this, consider switching to a latex-rubber mattress such as a Tempur mattress or use a *futon*.
- *Don't forget the kids' room.* EMF avoidance is especially important for children whose growing bodies may be more sensitive to the damaging effects of EMFs. Get rid of electrical gadgets that produce light shows or purport to 'lull babies to sleep'. They are expensive, unnecessary and may up the EMFs in your baby's room to above safe levels. Be wary, also, of baby monitors. Some newer models use ultrasound and microwave technology, which babies should never be exposed to. Instead, keep your baby by your side (the way other animals do) and/or let the baby sleep with you at night.
- *Plant trees.* If your garden backs onto a railway line, trees as well as high fencing can provide some shelter from electrical fields.
- *Don't sit too close to your computer.* Computer monitors vary greatly in the strength of their EMFs, so you should check yours with a meter. When you are working within 10–12 inches of a VDU, the highly positive electrical field can change the polarity

of your skin from negative to positive. This effectively turns you into a magnet for bacteria and viruses, which are easily drawn to exposed skin. Place a radiation shield on the front of your computer screen – and make sure that it really is a radiation shield and not just a glare-reducing screen. But remember that these will only shield you from the radiation emitted from the front of the machine. The back and sides of the machine also emit radiation. If you work in an office where you are sitting near the back of someone else's computer screen, you will not be protected. In this case, rearranging the seating plan in the office may be called for.

- *Eyeglass frames* should ideally be made from plastic with no wires in them; otherwise, they can serve as an antenna to focus the radio and mobile-phone waves directly into your brain. If you work on computers all day, consider having a pair of computer glasses made with plastic frames to minimise eye damage. Many opticians offer 'two for the price of one' deals these days, so this need not be an expensive option.

- *Bras with metal underwires* can act like mini-antennas on your body, directing EMFs into your breasts. If you are sitting in an EMF field all day, consider wearing a different kind of bra.

- *Quartz analogue watches* radiate pulsating EMFs along the acupuncture meridians on your wrist. An older or second-hand mechanical wind-up watch may be an acceptable alternative for the very electrically sensitive. Kinetic watches – which work by using the energy generated from your hand movements – are also becoming more widely available and (a little) cheaper. Also, try wearing as little jewellery as possible when working near EMFs as they will concentrate EMFs around your body. Always take jewellery off at night and when working on computers, photo-copiers or franking machines.

- *Keep your laptop off your lap.* Laptop computers use liquid-crystal displays (LCDs) that do not give off hazardous magnetic fields. Nevertheless, when you use them on your lap, they will be emitting electrical impulses into sensitive parts of your body. In addition, evidence from Australia suggests that the use of laptops among children on places other than desk tops encourages poor posture and raises the risk of repetitive strain injury.[89]

- *Watch out for transformers.* To adjust the voltage down from a power station to the home, a transformer is needed. Each neighbourhood power supply will have a series of transformers which step down the voltage from the power station to the lower voltage required by most household equipment. Transformers are also used to boost electrical power. For example, fluorescent lights usually have a transformer attached since they require more energy to function. Halogen lights, on the other hand, require a lower voltage to operate and so require a transformer to step voltage down. The same is true for dimmer switches. Transformers can create powerful electrical fields around us, and those who wish to avoid powerful EMFs in their homes and offices should reconsider the use of lighting that requires a transformer.

- *Redecorating?* Consider using an EMF-shielding paint in rooms that may be close to outside sources of EMFs. This may be particularly useful for children's rooms and bedrooms, and will help block EMFs from the outside. But this will not protect against magnetic radiation nor will it reduce indoor EMFs. EMF-shielding paint can be used as a base coat under normal (preferably low- or zero-VOC) paints.

- *Your diet is important.* A poorly nourished body will be less able to fight off the effects of increased free-radical production caused by EMF exposure. A diet high in fresh fruits and vegetables will help the body fight the increased level of free radicals. Increasing your intake of antioxidant vitamins such as A, C and E may also be useful. Babies should be breastfed for as long as possible to build up a strong immune system, and the less junk food your kids eat, the more they will be able to deal with the effects of EMF exposure.

- *Lobby your local council* to make locations of mobile telephone masts public so that you can avoid these areas. Don't let your children play near power lines, transformers, radar domes or microwave towers.

8 Fooling the Body

A WOMAN'S UNCONTROLLABLE EMOTIONS, A TEENAGER'S UNREASON-able behaviour, a man's serial infidelities, a disgraced athlete on steroids. Think of 'hormones' and these are the images that come to mind.

With a little help from the media, hormones have become the easy excuse for every kind of unfathomable and objectionable human behaviour; and it's the kind of bad press that obscures the real truth about hormones: we simply can't survive without them.

The endocrine or hormonal system is composed of many different organs and glands – such as the pituitary, hypothalamus, thyroid, adrenals, pancreas, thymus, ovaries and testes – that produce and secrete a variety of unique hormones directly into the bloodstream.

Once in the bloodstream, they travel to special receptors throughout the body. Each type of hormone has a specific target, or 'receptor', that it must connect with to transmit its information. Hormones are essentially chemical messengers transmitting information between cells. The interaction between hormone and receptor is vital to maintaining optimal hormone levels as well as controlling normal physiological processes and maintaining the body's natural state of balance.

This balance, however, can be thrown out by the presence of chemical interlopers – synthetic hormones that can interfere with the normal interplay between hormones and target organs and cells within the body.

Once in the body, these hormonally active agents can mimic or interfere with the actions of almost any hormone-producing gland in the body. Because of this, these toxic substances may have a role to play in a range of common disorders such as hypothyroidism, diabetes mellitus, hypoglycaemia, reproductive disorders and cancer. But without a doubt, the greatest amount of attention in this field has centred around oestrogen mimics and their effect on the body.

Environmental oestrogens (known as xenoestrogens – literally oestrogens produced outside the body) can produce powerful oestrogenic activity within the human body by mimicking an oestrogen called oestradiol, the strongest of the body's oestrogens and one produced naturally in women.

Because the endocrine system is so complex, xenoestrogens can interfere with the normal function of the body at any of a number of points along a hormone's pathway of production, regulation and action.

Oestrogen is, of course, primarily a female sex hormone, so it is often assumed that this form of pollution mainly affects women's health. Certainly, many of these synthetic toxins are believed to raise the risk of breast and reproductive cancers in women. But the problem of xenoestrogens affects us all.[1] They can, for instance, increase the rate of abnormalities in sexual development and reproduction in both men and women, and have also been associated with a range of male problems, including prostate and testicular cancer.[2]

Scientists also speculate that even those who do not experience immediate and noticeable health effects from exposure to environmental oestrogens may be affected in more subtle ways over the longer term. For instance, a man exposed to synthetic oestrogens may not perceive any obvious health problems or symptoms. But looked at under a microscope, his seminal fluid may contain fewer and less motile sperm. Such a man may have a reduced chance of producing a son and/or he may even be in danger of passing on endocrine damage to his children in the form of genital abnormalities (in boys) and higher risk of cancer in later life (in both girls and boys).

Everyday Encounters With Hormone Disrupters

Most of us believe we are safe from the industrial chemicals that cause hormone disruption. After all, how could an average person living an average life be exposed to relevant levels of such damaging substances? Yet, these days, we live in a world awash with synthetic hormones. We eat them, drink them, breathe them and absorb them through our skin. We use them at work, at home and in the garden. They are present in soil, water, air and food.

Below is a list of 15 common ways in which we all encounter hormone disrupters. Women taking the Pill or hormone replacement therapy (HRT) should be aware that they are already significantly hormone-disrupted even *before* they encounter these other synthetic oestrogens and hormone mimics.

1. Tapwater

The endocrine-disrupting chemicals most commonly found in water include: alkyl phenols and alkylphenol ethoxylates; bisphenol-A; cadmium; dioxins; pharmaceutical hormones (the Pill, HRT) and their metabolites (breakdown products); lead; organochlorine pesticides (such as endosulfan, lindane, methoxychlor, atrazine, DDT); phthalates and polychlorinated biphenyls (PCBs). You drink and cook with this water, but you also wash yourself with it and many industrial contaminants, including oestrogen mimics, can easily pass through the skin into the body during showers, baths and dishwashing.

2. Bottled water

Worries about harmful chemicals in tapwater have led many people to use bottled water instead. But the plastic bottles used for bottled water may leach the endocrine-disrupter bisphenol-A into your water.[3] Similarly, there is concern that milk and juice cartons may also leach this chemical into their contents.

3. Tinned food

Metal cans are lined with a plastic to prevent metal contamination. Ironically, this coating contains bisphenol-A, a powerful endocrine disrupter that can easily leach into food.[4] Fatty foods (such as tinned meats and fish in oil) may contain the highest concentrations, though studies have shown that bisphenol-A can migrate into tinned fruits and vegetables as well.[5]

4. Soya-based infant formula

Infants fed soya formula are at the highest end of human phytoestrogen exposure because all of their calories are derived from soya. In a typical day, such an infant will receive 11 mg of phytoestrogens per kg of body weight compared with just 1 mg/kg in the average-sized adult.[6] At best, research into potential harmful effects is sketchy and, for the moment, has only revealed subtle changes in menstrual patterns in offspring.[7] This may change over the next few years. Soya-based infant formulas may also contain high levels of thyroid-disrupting cadmium.[8] Heating formula in plastic bottles may release bisphenol-A and phthalates into the liquid. This risk is higher with older bottles that have been repeatedly scrubbed clean and sterilised.[9]

5. 'Natural' plant-oestrogen supplements

We take far too many and they are not magic bullets (*see pages 194–200*).

6. Car exhausts

Emissions from car engines contain several unhealthy chemicals. In terms of endocrine disruption, polycyclic aromatic hydrocarbons (PAHs), in particular benzo(a)pyrene, in car exhaust may be the most significant.[10] PAHs are also generated by burning incense and candles (*see Chapter 5*). Burning petrol may also release cadmium into the atmosphere.

7. Cigarettes

Cigarette smoke is a source of hormone-disrupting cadmium and PAHs. There is also extensive documentation of the presence of multiple pesticides in tobacco products, some of which have confirmed or suspected endocrine-disrupting effects.

8. Paper products

Including paper towels, coffee filters and tampons, most paper products that are chlorine-bleached can contain dioxins. Tampons are of particular concern because they are worn inside the body. While levels of dioxins in tampons are probably low, they can accumulate, helped along by the way that women are encouraged to use tampons – for hours, sometimes whole days at a time, for several days each month, over the course of approximately half a woman's lifetime.

9. Toiletries and cosmetics

Including body lotions, hairstyling products, makeup and sunscreens, these products contain oestrogenic preservatives known as parabens[11] (ethyl-, methyl-, butyl- and propylparabens). Hairsprays and nail varnishes can contain phthalates. Many sunscreening agents (such as benzophenone-3, homosalate, 4-methylbenzylidene camphor (4-MBC), octylmethoxycinnamate and octyldimethyl-PABA) are oestrogenic[12] – and even more so when combined in one product.

10. Disposable nappies

The bleach used on both outer and inner materials can produce detectable levels of carcinogenic and endocrine-disrupting dioxins. The gel used in the 'super-absorbent' core of disposables has been associated with a number of risks to health, including hormone disruption. It has also been linked to lower sperm counts. Recent studies have detected another endocrine-disrupting compound, tributyltin (TBT), an industrial-strength antifungal, in disposable nappies.

11. Flea collars

Of particular concern are the oestrogen-disrupting organophosphates such as diazinon, and carbamates such as carbaryl used in these products. Many flea collars are also made of PVC, another endocrine disrupter, creating an oestrogen-disrupting double whammy for pets and those who love them.

12. Air fresheners

These completely unnecessary products (and related products such as perfumes) contain a variety of endocrine disrupters. For example, the fragrance ingredient musk ambrette has been found to cause atrophy of the testicles in animal studies.[13] Citral, a common substance used in both fragrances and flavours, causes enlargement of the prostate gland and is oestrogenic.[14] This has been put forward as one reason why men working in perfume and soap manufacturing have an increased risk of developing prostate cancer.[15] Phthalates are also common in scented products, where they are used as solvents.[16] [17] In an analysis of the popular perfume Calvin Klein's *Eternity*, diethyl phthalate (DEP) made up over 10 percent of the fragrance portion of the product.[18]

13. Animal fat

Most of the endocrine-disrupting pesticides used on farms make their way into our livestock. These substances prefer to be surrounded by fat and so are stored in the animal's fat. When we eat animal fats, we ingest these harmful substances as well.

14. Non-organic foods

Similarly, when we eat conventionally produced foods such as vegetables and grains, we are ingesting the whole range of pesticides currently used on our foods during their growth and storage. These substances cannot be effectively washed off; traces will always remain.

15. Sitting at home watching TV

Wall coverings, carpets, furnishings and TVs are treated with hormone-disrupting brominated flame retardants. In the home environment, these chemicals can rub off onto your hands and face, or off-gas into the atmosphere. Many flame-retardant chemicals are hormone disrupters. In particular, polybrominated diphenyl ethers (PBDEs), pentabromophenol (PBP) and tetrabromobisphenol-A (TBBPA) are known to interfere with thyroid function.[19]

The origins of endocrine disrupters

Widespread industrialisation creates a range of dangerous and un-intended byproducts, among them, endocrine disrupters. Pesticides, emissions from incinerators and other combustion processes, and the production and disposal of plastics and heavy metals can all be sources of environmental oestrogens as well as other hormone disrupters.[20]

In addition to pesticides and industrial chemicals, women taking the Pill or HRT as well as those taking 'natural' oestrogen supplements, all in quantities much larger than their bodies could ever produce and metabolise on its own, are also adding to the worldwide problem of environmental oestrogen pollution.

The greater your exposure to oestrogenic substances, the more your body will collect and store. However, there comes a point at which the body can no longer process or store unneeded oestrogens. During times of stress, when losing weight as well as during pregnancy or breastfeeding, these chemicals are released from fat and redistributed in the body, passed on to offspring and/or excreted in the urine. Oestrogen from the Pill and HRT also enters our waterways via human urine and eventually reenters the human and animal food chain.

The list of recognised xenoestrogens is growing all the time and, clearly, it is getting harder to avoid them. The box below provides an overview of the most common xenoestrogens in the environment, listed in broad categories.

In reviewing this list, it is important to remember that it is the *total* exposure to oestrogens *from any source* that ultimately influences health for good or ill.[21][22] In his book *The Breast Cancer Prevention Programme*,[23] Dr Samuel Epstein, a leading light in the war against environmental toxins in everyday products, confirms that among the most influential factors in the development of breast cancer is the total amount of oestrogen to which a woman is exposed – whether natural, synthetic, pseudo and phytoestrogens – and the length of time for which she is exposed.

Major Sources of Hormone Disrupters	
Toxin	**What you should know**
Pesticides	
Insecticides e.g. carbaryl, chlordane, o,p-DDT (short for o,p´-dichlorodiphenyltrichloro-ethane), dieldrin, dicofol (a version of DDT), endosulfan, kepone, lindane, methoxychlor, synthetic pyrethroids, toxaphene	Widely used in agriculture to kill plant-eating pests; agricultural and some factory workers have highest exposures. Ingested mostly from food, but also in air and water, and on textiles, particularly cotton, beds, sofas, carpets and other household furnishings.
	Used in ant, roach, fly and wasp sprays, no-pest strips, flea collars and powders, tick and lice treatments, mosquito repellents, and oral treatments for intestinal parasites.
	DDT is still the top insecticide toxin. Even though its agricultural use in the West was stopped years ago, it remains in our soil. DDT is used in agriculture and to kill

Toxin	What you should know

Pesticides *contd.*

	mosquitoes in many developing countries. In the body, DDT is converted to DDE. While DDT is only weakly oestrogenic, DDE is a powerful antiandrogen (blocks the action of male sex hormones). Another commonly used insecticide, endosulfan, is an oestrogen mimic. In tests, found on almost all produce samples. Other widely used insecticides include carbaryl, dicofol (a version DDT) and synthetic pyrethroids.
Herbicides e.g. alachlor, amitrol, atrazine, nitrofen	Used on crops, but also in garden weedkillers; have a range of hormonal effects; some are oestrogenic, some also affect the thyroid.
Fungicides e.g. benomyl, mancozeb, tributyltin, vinclozolin, EBDC fungicides (used on fruits and vegetables, but rarely tested for by the FDA)	Used widely in agriculture, but also in supermarkets to preserve food in storage. In the home, fungicides are found in bathroom and kitchen cleaners, and wallpaper paste.

Industrial Chemicals

Alkylphenols	Used to make detergents and surfactants for the home (in the US) and industry (in Europe), though this use is being scaled down (*see listing below*). Also added to some plastics and pesticides. Exposure is by inhalation or ingestion of pesticide sprays, and contaminated food and water from fields spread with sewage sludge.
	Alkylphenols prevent oestrogen from binding with receptors. They are reproductive toxins and toxic to breast cells, causing them to multiply in lab conditions at very low concentrations.

Toxin	What you should know

Brominated flame retardants e.g. polybrominated biphenyls (PBBs)	Similar to PCBs and added to many products including computers, TVs and household textiles to reduce fire risk. Also found in baby mattresses, foam mattresses, car seats and PVC products. Office workers who use computers, hospital cleaners and workers in electronics-dismantling plants are at particular risk from these chemicals.
	PBBs are oestrogen mimics (similar in action to bisphenol-A – *see below*) and can also affect the thyroid.
Nonylphenol, octylphenol	Related to alkylphenols (*see above*) and used widely as a surfactant (e.g. in pesticides and detergents) and added to certain plastics; often used to soften plastics such as polystyrene and polyvinyl chloride (PVC). Found in paints, lubricating oils and farm chemicals. The breakdown of certain chemicals in industrial detergents, pesticides and personal-care products give rise to nonylphenol in the environment. In the body, they have a similar action to alkylphenols.
Polychlorinated biphenols (PCBs)	Related to DDT and dioxins, PCBs were once used extensively in transformers, insulating cooling equipment, hydraulic fluids, lubricants and other electrical components. Banned since the 1970s, they are still present in many older electrical installations. PCBs resist biodegradation, are fat-soluble and tend to accumulate in animals higher up in the food chain.
	Found in plastics, dyes, inks, older types of carbonless copy paper, adhesives, wood treatments and pesticides; detected in foods such as meat and fish, water fowl, poultry, eggs and milk.

Toxin	What you should know

Industrial Chemicals *contd.*

	PCBs are both antioestrogens and anti-androgens. Exposure to PCBs in food linked to delayed brain development and reduced IQ in children.
Polychlorinated dibenzofurans (PCDFs or furans)	Byproducts of incineration of organochlorine chemicals; also used as intermediates in the preparation of pharmaceuticals, insecticides and other chemicals, and as solvents for the resins used in lacquers.
	Effects on human health are broadly similar to those of dioxins.
Polychlorinated dibenzo-*p*-dioxins (PCDDs or dioxins)	Tetrachlorodibenzo-*p*-dioxin (TCDD) is the most well-researched dioxin and arguably the most toxic. When scientists refer to the toxic effects of dioxins, they usually mean TCDD.
	Dioxins are the toxic byproducts of several types of industry: during incineration of organic waste containing chlorine (i.e. plastics); and during manufacture of paper, wood preservatives and chlorinated aromatics such as 2,4,5-trichlorophenol (an intermediate in the manufacture of the herbicide 2,4,5-T). Found in paper products, including disposable nappies, pants liners, tampons, toilet paper, milk and juice cartons, and paper containers for microwaveable food; also found in some pesticides and herbicides.
	However, more than 90 percent of human exposure to dioxins comes from food, mainly animal fat.
	Many PCDDs are known to be toxic and carcinogenic. They are also antioestrogens.

Toxin	What you should know

Industrial Chemicals *contd.*

Polycyclic aromatic hydrocarbons (PAHs) e.g. phenanthrene, fluoranthene, benzo(a)pyrene, benzo(ghi)perylene, coronene	Created by incineration of plastic waste such as polyvinyl chloride (PVC), high-density polyethylene (HDPE) and polypropylene (PP) as well as other industrial waste; large quantities released during natural events such as volcanic eruptions and forest fires, but also by many human activities, such as burning coal, oil and wood for heat, smoking cigarettes, frying food and gas-powered motor travel. Found in asphalt, creosote, coal-tar pitch, roofing tar, coal and crude oil. A few are used in medicines, plastics, dyes and pesticides.
	Many, including benzo(a)pyrene, are known to cause cancer or genetic damage and are oestrogen mimics.[24]

Plastics

Bisphenol-A	A major endocrine disrupter used to make clear, hard, reusable plastic products; also used in the manufacture of polymers, fungicides, antioxidants, dyes, phenoxy, polysulphone and certain polyester resins, flame retardants and rubber chemicals. Some (but not all) dental resins contain this. Also an ingredient in pesticides.
	Found in food and drink packaging, soft-drink bottles, milk and juice cartons, baby bottles, microwaveable dishes and water-supply pipes; also an ingredient in epoxy resins commonly used to coat metal products such as food cans and bottle tops. It easily leaches into food at room temperature, but the effect is even more pronounced when heated (i.e. babies' bottles).
	Acts like an oestrogen mimic and binds to hormone-receptor cells. Implicated in increased risk of breast cancer, is a testicular

Toxin	What you should know

Plastics *contd.*

	toxin and a factor in low sperm counts, and may be linked to diseases of the prostate and uterus.
Phthalates e.g. diethylhexylphthalate (DEHP), monoethylhexylphthalate (MEHP), dimethylphthalate(DMP), butylbenzylphthalate (BBP), dibutylphthalate (DBP), dioctylphthalate (DOP)	Found in our groundwater, rivers and drinking water. Around 95 percent of its production over the last few decades tied to the PVC industry. Also used in the inks used to print on plastic, board and foil-packed products, and in some of the adhesives used in packaging, in vinyl flooring, emulsion paint, PVC baby toys and some cosmetics (*see separate listing below*).
	Foods stored in plastic-coated containers such as baby-milk formula, cheese, margarine and crisps may contain measurable levels. Many of the bags and tubes used in hospitals are made of phthalate-containing PVC and the US FDA now recommends against using DEHP in medical equipment. Phthalates are fat-soluble, so tend to concentrate in foods such as meat, fish, eggs, milk and milk products;[25] also likely to accumulate in body fat.
	Stop oestrogen and androgen from binding to receptors. Toxic to the breast and testicles, high levels are reported to lead to miscarriage and other complications of pregnancy.
Polyvinyl chloride (PVC)	Commonly known as vinyl, this is one of the most toxic plastics on the market. While no longer used in Europe in toys for children under age three or in food packaging (where the food comes into direct contact with it), PVC is still widely used in plastic pipes, cables and wire insulation, flooring, wallpaper, shower curtains, moulded furniture, Venetian blinds, toys and food containers.

Toxin	What you should know

Plastics *contd.*

Not recyclable and a major pollutant throughout its entire lifecycle – from manufacture to incineration (which releases dioxins). In the body, it blocks oestrogen and androgen from binding to receptors.

Food Additives

Butylated hydroxyanisole (BHA)

An antioxidant in fat-containing foods and in edible fats and oils, it prevents food from becoming rancid. Also a preservative and antioxidant in cosmetics.

High levels found in chewing gum, active dried yeast, prepared snacks, processed foods, cereal products and fatty foods. Generally added to packaging rather than food but, during storage, it vaporises and can leach into food.

In the body, it is an antioestrogen, preventing oestrogen from binding to receptors.

Drugs and Supplements

Hormone replacement drugs

Birth-control pills, diethylstilboestrol (DES), cimetidine and HRT are all hormone disrupters that we take as medicines. They are also excreted in urine, where they contaminate waterways and work their way back into the food chain.

Phytoestrogens

Found in 'natural' plant-oestrogen supplements for treating menopause and other 'women's problems'. Of the several types, it is primarily isoflavones (found mainly in legumes, particularly soya beans), lignans (found in whole grains, flaxseed, berries and nuts) and coumestans (found in forages, clovers and legumes) used in such supplements.

Toxin	What you should know

Drugs and Supplements *contd.*

	Taken in quantity, they are oestrogen mimics that can cause many of the same problems associated with less 'acceptable' xenoestrogens.
Spermicides	Condoms, and spermicidal foams, jellies and films contain the spermicidal lubricant nonoxynol-9, an alkyphenol (*see above*) that blocks oestrogens from binding to receptors.

Household Detergents

Alkylphenols e.g. nonylphenol, octylphenol	Mainly used to make alkylphenol ethoxylate (APE) surfactants (detergents). In the US, found in many liquid clothes detergents; in the UK, not used for this, but present in industrial-strength detergents and surfactants. Break down into oestrogenic nonylphenol and octylphenol, which get into our water supply and are re-ingested every time we drink water. Their use has been scaled down in Europe over the last decade via voluntary industrial measures, though Norway instigated the first outright ban of endocrine-disrupting industrial detergents in 2001 on the basis that they are harmful to health (*see listing under Industrial Chemicals for more*).

Toiletries and Cosmetics

Alkanolamines	DEA, MEA and TEA are found most often in foaming toiletries such as shampoos and bodywashes. Easily absorbed through the skin and, once in the system, act as oestrogen mimics.
Benzophenone	Fixative for heavy perfumes, especially in soaps. Also used in the manufacture of antihistamines, hypnotics and insecticides. A weak oestrogen mimic.

Toxin	What you should know

Toiletries and Cosmetics *contd.*

Citral	A perfume ingredient found to cause enlargement of the prostate gland in animals; has oestrogenic effects.[26]
Parabens (alkylhydroxy benzoates)	These preservatives are in almost all toiletries and also in foods. Identified as oestrogen mimics in late 1988.[11] Each type has a different oestrogenic potency. Methylparaben is the least potent followed by ethylparaben, propylparaben and finally butylparaben.
Phthalates	Found in nail varnish, hairspray, some conditioning shampoos and hair conditioners, deodorants and in large quantities as fixatives in perfumes. Also in PVC products (*see listing above for more details*).[27]
Resorcinol (carbolic acid)	Fixative in hair dyes.
Sunscreens e.g. benzophenone-3, homosalate, 4-methylbenzylidene camphor (4-MBC), octylmethoxycinnamate, octyldimethyl-PABA	Researchers in Switzerland and Japan have found that the most common UV-screening chemicals are adding to the xenoestrogen burden.[28][29] Generally these are oestrogen mimics.

Heavy Metals

Arsenic	Common in soil and in rock, particularly ores. Most are water-soluble, so may occur in groundwater. Also released into the air as dust from soil or from the ore smelting or waste burning (e.g. arsenic-treated lumber). Principal commercial use is as a wood preservative, and also as a component of agricultural pesticides.
	A glucocorticoid disrupter.

Toxin	What you should know
Heavy Metals *contd.*	
Cadmium	Cadmium is used in batteries, metal plating, fungicides, as an absorbent in nuclear reactors, and in the production of plastics and pigments. Present in air as a result of burning of fossil fuels or municipal waste. Metal-smelting operations or soldering may release it into the air. Used as a pigment dye in cosmetics. A thyroid-hormone disrupter.

What are the Risks?

To understand how environmental oestrogens can disrupt the body, it is useful to think of the relationship between hormone and receptor in terms of a key (the hormone) and a lock (the receptor). When the key fits, it opens the pathway for a variety of bodily functions. Natural hormones fit their receptor sites perfectly; synthetic hormones do not. Some synthetic hormones are structurally similar to natural ones but, once in the receptor, they transmit confusing or wrong messages that not only disrupt hormonal actions at the target organ, but also have a knock-on adverse effect in other parts of the body.

Xenoestrogens can fool the body in several ways. Some can *mimic* the actions of natural oestrogens – though their effect may be weaker or stronger than the real thing. Using the lock and key metaphor, mimics could be said to be the right kind of key, but they open the door at the wrong time, or for too short or too long a time, thereby causing a general imbalance in hormone levels.

Other xenoestrogens *block* normal hormonal actions and are called antioestrogens (or, if they block the effects of male hormones, antiandrogens). These, too, can cause a disruption in normal hormone levels. For instance, when an antiandrogen blocks the effects of male hormones, the man will experience a relative rise in oestrogen that can affect his sexual and reproductive health.

Just to complicate things, some xenoestrogens act as both mimics and blockers.

Still others, known as *disrupters*, can affect how natural hormones are produced and eliminated, or they can alter the number of receptors available to specific hormones or damage target organs, making them either less or more receptive to the actions of hormones. Other disrupters work by stimulating the release of other hormones or other natural substances that can upset the normal balance of hormones in our bodies.

In contrast to oestrogens made in the body, which are short-lived and have a specific purpose in the body, xenoestrogens are thought to pose a particularly high risk because:

- They are not easily or readily broken down by the body or in the environment
- They remain intact and active in living organisms and in the environment for many years
- They are lipophilic – in other words, they prefer to be surrounded by fat molecules. Because of this, they accumulate (are stored) in the fat and tissue of animals and humans. In addition, endocrine disrupters present in pesticides cannot be washed away by water and so cling to crops and foodstuffs. In this way, they are passed up the food chain to humans.

Hormonally active chemicals also defy much of what we know about toxicology since minute quantities appear to cause biological havoc that is out of all proportion to the dose.

One reason for this is that the hormones in our bodies are tightly controlled and present only in small amounts. It has been estimated, for example, that the total amount of oestrogen in a woman's body at any given time is less than a teaspoon. Yet, this tiny amount is responsible for orchestrating myriad functions. For instance, in addition to maintaining our reproductive cycles, reproductive hormones such as oestrogen regulate growth, metabolism and immunity, helping to maintain hormonal balance in a variety of systems in both sexes.

Although no one knows exactly how or to what extent environmental oestrogens affect us, there is growing concern because reproductive hormones are so important to our wellbeing. This concern is heightened by evidence that, to a greater or lesser extent, we all carry these environmental oestrogens in our bodies. No one is free of them, and most babies born today are born with them already in their bodies.

Children at risk

Many factors affect the potential toxicity of xenoestrogens, including length of exposure, dose, age and individual differences. Of these factors, timing – that is, when the individual is exposed – appears to be more important than dose. In all children, hormones are what orchestrate the body's normal development. This is why a developing fetus or infant exposed to xenoestrogens may be more obviously and immediately harmed than an adult. Adolescents, of course, are also more sensitive to the effects of environmental oestrogens because they, too, are still developing.

Reproductive abnormalities

The number of male babies born with reproductive abnormalities such as cryptorchidism (undescended testes) and hypospadias (where the urethra opens on the underside of the penis) appears to be increasing.[30] Data on these two disorders are, however, increasingly difficult to collect. In some places, hypospadias has become so commonplace that physicians are no longer required to report it as an abnormality. Factoring out abnormalities in this way is becoming more and more common, and is one way in which statisticians perform the medical magic of making disturbing trends disappear overnight.

Nevertheless, studies in England and other countries that have attempted to track the incidence of these reproductive abnormalities conclude that the trend is towards higher rates of both.

Are environmental oestrogens to blame? At the moment, we have only the adverse effects of medically prescribed synthetic oestrogens to guide us. The synthetic oestrogen diethylstilboestrol, or DES, was used in the US between 1938 and 1971 to prevent miscarriage. Over time, it was found that not only did DES not prevent miscarriage, it also caused cancers of the vagina and cervix. In addition, women exposed to DES had a higher incidence of male children with hypospadias[31] and, because of this, scientists have theorised that male babies exposed to other types of oestrogens in the womb may be similarly affected.

Fewer male babies

Throughout the world, fewer male babies are being born than would normally be expected. This phenomenon has been noted over the last 20–40 years in a number of countries, including Denmark, the Netherlands, Sweden, Germany, Norway, Finland, Canada and the US. It is not clear why this is happening, though environmental pollution and hormone-disrupting chemicals have been suggested as possible causes.

This hypothesis is supported by data from Seveso, Italy, where an industrial accident in 1976 resulted in the highest known human exposure to the dioxin 2,3,7,8-tetrachlorodibenzo-*p*-dioxin (TCDD). The population was followed for several years to determine what the effect might be on reproduction. While mothers' exposure to dioxin was not influential in determining the sex of their offspring, fathers exposed when they were less than 19 years of age sired significantly more girls than boys. In the eight years after the accident, 12 daughters and no sons were born to nine couples who had the highest dioxin exposure, thus supporting the theory that the time before and during puberty may be a very sensitive period for dioxin toxicity in men.[32 33]

Early puberty

Hormone-disrupting chemicals may be robbing children, especially girls, of a normal childhood and normal sexual development.[34] In 1997, researchers from the University of North Carolina first reported that American girls were entering puberty at earlier ages than in the past. The study involved 17,000 girls and revealed that, between their eighth and ninth birthdays, 48 percent of black girls and about

15 percent of white girls had begun breast or secondary hair development, or both. Exposure to oestrogenic chemicals in the environment was put forward as one reason for this phenomenon.[35]

The potential role of chemicals in early puberty was supported by a further study that examined the onset of puberty in children exposed to the polybrominated biphenyls (PBBs), which are used in flame-retardants. Accidental contamination of the Michigan food chain with PBBs led to the exposure of more than 4000 individuals in 1973. By following the girls through puberty, scientists discovered that exposed girls began menstruating around 11 months earlier than non-exposed girls.[36] Such findings have implications for adult health since studies have shown that girls who enter puberty earlier are at increased risk of breast cancer.

In Puerto Rico, girls now have the highest rates of early puberty in the world.[37] Phthalate exposure is believed to be one cause;[38] pesticide exposure (which is high in that country) and hormones in meats are another.

Women at risk

In women, oestrogens (mainly the hormone oestradiol) are responsible for the development of female characteristics (such as breasts and light facial hair) as well as regulating mood and behaviour. They also protect bone strength and the cardiovascular system, regulate liver metabolism, influence ovarian and menstrual cycles, stimulate uterine growth and maintain pregnancies.

Pesticides and other chemicals collect in body fat and may affect women's health in a variety of ways. For instance, in the short-term, exposure to environmental oestrogens may be associated with disorders such as:

- Endometriosis
- Premenstrual symptoms
- Irregular menstrual cycles
- Pelvic inflammatory disease

- Fibrocystic disease of the breast
- Polycystic ovarian syndrome
- Uterine fibroids.

The longer-term outlook is even more grim.

Once again, data from Seveso have proved instructive. When researchers looked at the health of exposed women 20 years after the accident, they found that the women had a 20–110 percent higher risk of developing endometriosis. Those with the highest risk also had the highest blood concentrations of the dioxin TCDD.[39] Among girls who had not started their periods at the time of the accident, exposure was associated with longer menstrual cycles and scantier periods.[40] Elsewhere in the world, Taiwanese women exposed to PCBs through contaminated rice were found to have double the rate of abnormal menstrual bleeding and nearly three times the risk of delivering a stillborn baby.[41] Exposure to DDE and PCBs has also been suggested as a cause of early menopause.[42]

Breast cancer and more

Breast cancer rates are on the rise throughout the world and no one seems to know why. Recent studies have implicated exposure to organochlorines such as DDT, but also other industrial chemicals as risk factors for breast cancer in the US, Finland, Mexico and Canada. Several investigations have discovered associations between breast cancer risk and exposures to endocrine disrupters in the environment as well as in the workplace.[43]

Breast tissue, it seems, acts rather like a sponge when it comes to organochlorines. Not only are levels of these compounds higher in the blood and fatty tissue of breast cancer patients, they are also higher in the cancerous tissue than in nearby healthy tissue.[44]

While studies in this area have been far from conclusive, disturbing trends have emerged. Seveso survivors, for instance, have a greatly increased breast cancer risk.[45] Similarly, a 1998 study from Denmark found that, even after taking into account all other known risk factors for breast cancer, women who had the highest concentrations of the organochlorine pesticide dieldrin in their blood were twice as likely to develop breast cancer as those with the lowest concentrations.[46] Dieldrin was banned from use in the late 1980s but, because it lingers in the environment for years, it continues to influence the rate of breast cancer development.

Women exposed to the organochlorine DDE (a close relative of DDT) have also been found to have more than twice the risk of developing breast cancer,[47] [48] with postmenopausal women being most at risk.[49]

Prolonged breastfeeding has been shown to slightly decrease the risk of breast cancer, independently of a woman's level of DDE exposure. Unfortunately, DDE has been shown in several studies to decrease the length of time that breastfeeding mothers can produce milk for their babies[50] – a finding that has serious implications for the health of both mothers and babies.

Biological Warfare

Gaseous (or elemental) chlorine was first produced in the 19th century by breaking the chemical bond between sodium and chlorine in sodium chloride (ordinary salt). It soon became widely used as a bleaching agent and disinfectant. During World War I, the chlorine derivative mustard gas became a potent chemical weapon.

During World War II, scientists on both sides began combining chlorine with other organic (carbon-containing) substances to create even more destructive chemical weapons. Many of these were first tested on insects and, when the war ended, they found their way into agriculture as pesticides. DDT is an example of this kind of WWII experimentation.

Post-WWII, chlorine combined with organic substances (now known as 'organochlorines'), often petrochemicals, was used to produce plastics, paints, dyes, deodorants, bleaching agents, refrigerants and wood preservers, and in paper milling and the production of synthetic materials such as rayon, cleaning solvents and even more pesticides.

Some natural organisms produce organochlorines in minute quantities, though these tend to have very precise functions (for instance, they might act as a natural antibiotic). Industrially produced organochlorines, on the other hand, are freaks of nature, but are nevertheless similar enough to naturally produced organochlorines as to trick living organisms into using them – a process illustrated by the hormone-disrupting effects of many organochlorines such as dioxins and PCBs.

Once in the body organochlorines accumulate in fat. However, while they are in the environment they are highly mobile, and are easily carried around the globe by atmospheric winds, river systems and ocean currents.

The damage they can do is considerable. For instance:

- **Chlorofluorocarbons (CFCs)** are largely responsible for destruction of the ozone layer
- **Polychlorinated biphenyls (PCBs),** widely used as electrical insulators until the 1970s, are no longer in production, yet they continue to wreak havoc on human and other animals, interfering with reproduction, causing birth defects and depressing immunity
- **Dioxins and furans** are chlorinated chemical 'accidents' that have no useful function in the natural world. They result from a variety of processes, including the bleaching of wood pulp (to create bright white paper products), copper smelting, and the burning of municipal and toxic waste, and leaded petrol. The dioxin 2,3,7,8-TCDD (tetrachlorodibenzo-*p*-dioxin) is thousands of times more toxic than thalidomide or cyanide, and is considered by scientists to be the most potent synthetic poison ever created
- **Household chlorine bleach** – a dilute solution of sodium hypochlorite – produces trace amounts of chloroform, a known animal carcinogen and a suspected human carcinogen.

Miscarriage and stillbirth

Studies in this area are not plentiful but, given the fact that pesticides are both endocrine disrupting and capable of causing reproductive abnormalities, their link to miscarriage and stillbirth cannot be entirely discounted.

Known risk factors for miscarriage include smoking, being an older mother and a previous history of miscarriage. However, a recent study of women living close to farmland where pesticides are sprayed found that the women had an increased risk of miscarriage due to birth defects, especially if they were exposed during the first trimester of pregnancy.[51] Specifically, the researchers found that if the woman was exposed during the third to eighth weeks of pregnancy – a sensitive time as the internal organs are being formed – the fetus seemed to be especially vulnerable to developing birth defects.

This study was particularly important because it illustrated the devastation of close proximity to pesticides during pregnancy, but also because it was able to measure pesticide exposures objectively rather than simply relying on guesswork or a person's memory of what they might have been exposed to.

Another, earlier study of pregnant women's exposure to workplace or household pesticides in early pregnancy also found an increase in the risk of stillbirth.[52] The researchers discovered that just one month of maternal exposure to workplace pesticides during the first two months of pregnancy resulted in a nearly two-and-a-half-fold greater risk of having a stillbirth, again due to congenital defects, compared with women with no pesticide exposure.

In this study, the home environment was by far the most common source of pesticide exposure. Even though these types of pesticides are considered weaker than those used in occupational settings, women exposed during early pregnancy to insecticides such as cockroach and ant sprays in the home environment were also found to have a 70 percent raised risk of stillbirth due to congenital defects.

Macho women?

While much of the focus on endocrine disrupters has been on the feminisation of men, very new research, mostly based on observations of animals in the wild, suggests that the opposite effect can also occur in women. Observations of the mosquito fish in Florida have shown that female fish living in polluted rivers are developing male characteristics. The cause is a chemical called androstenedione. Known among weightlifters as andro, this anabolic steroid is widely available over the counter, and widely used by sportsmen and weightlifters. In humans, andro triggers the production of testosterone, the body's primary androgen (masculine hormone).

The andro in the Florida river, however, was not from a bottle. It was the result of the biotransformation of industrial pollutants. This was the first environmental androgen ever discovered, and the researchers believed it was responsible for giving the female mosquito fish their masculine fins.[53] Similar studies with rats have shown that exposure to diesel fumes *in utero* can masculinise pups through accumulation of testosterone in their mothers.[54] Can women look forward to the same effects? Watch this space.

Men at risk

In men, oestrogens play a secondary role to androgens (male hormones like testosterone), which define male characteristics (for example, more body hair and greater strength) and aid sperm production. Male sexual development is critically dependent on the normal levels and action of androgens, and unbalanced androgen/oestrogen ratios can easily disturb this process. Again, studies of men's health over the past 20 years show worrying trends.[55]

In men, hormone disrupters that mimic oestrogens – pesticides such as DDT, kepone, dieldrin, PCBs, plasticisers and polystyrenes – as well as those that block the action of androgens – pesticides such as linuron, vinclozolin and DDE as well as combustion byproducts such as polycyclic aromatic hydrocarbons (PAHs) – are associated with poor semen quality (low sperm counts, low ejaculate volume, high number of abnormal sperm, low number of motile sperm), testicular cancer, reproductive abnormalities (undescended testes, small penis size), prostate disease and other recognised abnormalities of male reproductive tissues.[56]

Sperm counts

Concern over the effect of environmental changes on male reproductive health has now become a major preoccupation in developed countries. In the early 1970s, a number of studies suggested that sperm concentration was declining. However, it wasn't until the early 1990s that the true extent of the problem was revealed. In 1992, the British Medical Journal published an analysis of 61 studies in this area. The authors concluded that the average sperm count in healthy men had declined by 1 percent each year over the previous 50 years.[57] The suggestion caused a furore, and much rebuttal, but a reanalysis of the same data by another group of scientists five years later suggested that the original researchers had got it right.[58] Since that time, different studies have come to different conclusions regarding this issue. However, taken as a whole, the evidence does suggest a decline in sperm counts worldwide.[59]

Environmental pollutants and pesticides may have a role to play in this decline.[60][61] A 1999 study of couples seeking in-vitro fertilisation (IVF) therapy concluded that sperm from men with either high or moderate on-the-job exposure to pesticides was associated with a 78 percent and 48 percent decline, respectively, in IVF success rates compared with sperm from unexposed men. The men with the highest levels of pesticide exposure tended to work in jobs such as fruit or flower harvesting, livestock, poultry or dairy farming and gardening.[62]

After studying the children of Taiwanese mothers who were poisoned in 1979 by the large-scale ingestion of rice oil contaminated with polychlorinated biphenyls (PCBs) and dibenzofurans, Chinese researchers found that the sperm of the teenagers exposed prenatally to these substances showed abnormalities such as reduced motility and an inability to penetrate eggs. The researchers also found that, on average, the exposed youths were 2.7 cm shorter than controls and also more sexually mature.[63]

Testicular cancer

According to a Cancer Research Campaign report published in January 1998, testicular cancer has increased in incidence by 55 percent between 1979 and 1991 in England and Wales. Rates of increase found in other countries include a 300 percent increase between 1945 and 1990 in Denmark, and an annual increase of 2.3 percent in the Baltic countries. While rates of increase appear to be less dramatic in the US, the trend is still towards an increase, rather than decrease, in this cancer.

Since testicular cancer is mainly a disease of young men, the increased age of the population is not a reason for the increase of this form of cancer (as it is assumed to be with many other cancers). Instead, the influence of environmental factors is now widely acknowledged.[64][65]

It is now believed that testicular cancer is initiated during the development of testes while the fetus is still in the womb, and hormone-disrupting chemicals are thought to be a cause of the increase.[66–68]

Even so, adult males are also vulnerable to these toxic exposures. There is, for example, evidence that plastic workers exposed to PVC occupationally have a sixfold higher risk of testicular cancer.[69]

Prostate cancer

Around the world, the incidence of prostate cancer is increasing annually by 2–3 percent. Small amounts of oestrogens from, for instance, dietary intake of phytoestrogens may protect men against this disease.[70] But higher exposures to synthetic oestrogens, particularly while in the womb, may tip the scales in the direction of harm.

Once again, the extensive human data on DES-exposed men provides a useful basis for assessing the effects of other xenoestrogens.[71] At the moment, we only have laboratory studies to go on, though one recent study found that bisphenol-A – an endocrine disrupter found in plastics – stimulates the growth and proliferation of prostate cells.[72]

While not all authorities agree,[73] it still remains possible that real-world exposure to sufficient quantities of xenoestrogens other than (and maybe even weaker than) DES in the womb can alter sexual development[74] and lead to an increased incidence of disorders of the male reproductive tract.

Other Hormone Systems

Because the endocrine system is composed of so many different types of hormones, each with specific functions and each connected to the others through complex pathways, exposure to hormonally active agents in the environment can have an impact on the body that goes well beyond the reproductive system.

Several scientists, including Dr Theo Colbin and colleagues (authors of the book *Our Stolen Future*), and Dr Michael Warhurst, an environmental chemist working for the World Wildlife Fund in Brussels, Belgium, have dedicated themselves to the study of the bigger picture of endocrine disruption.[75] [76]

Their work suggests that, with over 70,000 chemicals in commercial use today, the fact that synthetic hormone disruptors have not been identified for every hormone system is probably due to the lack of proper evaluation and testing rather than the inherent safety of these chemicals. This is very much work in its early stages, although trend-watchers suggest that a wide range of other hormone systems can and are being disrupted by environmental endocrine disrupters.

The thyroid gland

Thyroid hormones are essential to metabolism, brain development, and the ability to learn and memorise. They also regulate our auditory (hearing) function and behaviour. The thyroid gland is also an important component of the immune system. Since the nervous, immune and endocrine (hormone) systems are all closely related and in constant communication with each other, it stands to reason that if any one of the three systems is damaged or degraded, the other two may be adversely affected.

For some time, we have only had animal studies to guide us. Animals living in polluted areas, for instance, are increasingly showing signs of thyroid disruption and humans may eventually suffer the same fate.[77] [78] In addition, studies have shown altered thyroid-hormone activity and an increased tendency toward aggression in animals exposed to pesticides and, again, some researchers believe that this tendency may surface in humans as well. The effect may be even more devastating when mixtures of different pesticides and industrial chemicals are combined.[79]

Human data, however, are now also emerging. The fungicides maneb and zineb have been found to inhibit the production of thyroid-stimulating hormone (TSH) – which is responsible for regulating the release of thyroid hormones controlling our metabolism. When this happens, the body experiences a drop in thyroid-hormone levels. In an attempt to regain hormonal balance, the body responds by producing excessive and largely uncontrolled quantities of thyroid hormones. Researchers have speculated that, because of this, exposure to fungicides may be one cause of the overactive thyroid (hyperthyroid) condition known as Graves' disease.[80]

More recently, drinking water contaminated with small amounts of perchlorate – an industrial chemical used in the manufacture of rockets, missiles and fireworks, but also, and some would say inexplicably, found in fertilisers – has been identified as the reason behind the higher-than-normal thyroid-hormone levels identified in some newborns in Arizona.[81]

Progesterone

Progesterone is another reproductive hormone important to both women and men. In women, progesterone is involved in maintaining the menstrual cycle. It is the '*yang*' to oestrogen's '*yin*', switching off the activity that oestrogen switches on. Pesticide exposure may interrupt this cycle by damaging the follicles of the ovaries, reducing their capacity to release an egg, or ovulate, every month like they're supposed to.

During pregnancy, progesterone relaxes the uterine muscle, allowing it to expand to accommodate a growing baby. If the level of progesterone (which is vital in early pregnancy) is too low, there is an increased risk of miscarriage in the first 10 weeks. Exposure to PCBs is thought to increase the risk of miscarriage by accelerating the breakdown of progesterone in the liver, thus making less available to the body.

Progesterone is also involved in the synthesis of testosterone. In males, a relative imbalance of oestrogen-to-progesterone while still in the womb may have serious consequences later in life. Again, we only have animal data to go on, but a study carried out in the US revealed that exposing fetal mice to either natural oestradiol (the most potent of the oestrogens and the one which pesticides mimic) or synthetic oestrogen caused the prostate to become hypersensitive to male sex hormones for the rest of the animal's life.[82] In humans, this same type of hypersensitivity is a risk factor for prostate cancer.

Polychlorinated biphenyls (PCBs) have also been reported to interfere with the production of progesterone-supported testosterone. While testosterone is primarily a male reproductive hormone, women's bodies also require small amounts of it to function properly.

Retinoids

Retinoids (the basis of vitamin A) have a powerful effect on fetal development and, if a growing animal is exposed to them in the wrong amounts at the wrong time or in the wrong place, they can cause deformities. This is one reason why, for instance, pregnant women are advised to limit their intake of vitamin A (retinol) and avoid the use of skin medicines (for instance, acne creams) that contain retinoids.

'Sensitive' Plants Damaged by Waterborne Hormones

All the pesticides we use in agriculture and those from household waste ultimately end up in our water supply and, although water companies tell us that levels of these are low, their effects on other living things are already becoming apparent.

For instance, in New Zealand in 1995, farmers took their local water company to court, claiming that high levels of the hormone-disrupting pesticide tridopyr – a component of the herbicide Grazon, which the water company had used in the area around their reservoir – had damaged tomatoes that were being grown hydroponically (in water and without soil). The farmers lost the case on the basis that: a) the water company only had a duty to supply water fit for human consumption and not for horticultural use; and b) current water-testing standards in New Zealand (as in the rest of the world) did not require the water company to specifically test its supply for the presence of hormone-containing pesticides.

The farmers were also let down by a lack of scientific evidence on the effects of hormone-containing weedkillers on crops such as tomatoes. However, it is important to understand that lack of evidence of harm cannot be taken as evidence of safety. Crops such as tomatoes have a shorter lifespan than humans and may therefore react more swiftly to the presence of hormone disrupters in the water. Hydroponically grown crops are more sensitive still since they do not have the buffer of soil to 'dilute' the contaminants commonly found in the water. Nevertheless, these 'sensitive' plants may eventually prove to be a forewarning of the risks for humans of ingesting hormone-disrupting water.[83]

Some pesticides have been found to bind to retinoid receptors in mammals and amphibians. In parts of North America, frogs with gross deformities – missing backs, or with legs protruding from their stomachs or no legs at all, or eyes on their backs and/or suction-cup fingers growing from their sides – are turning up with alarming frequency.[84] Amphibians are often sensitive predictors of what can happen to humans and this has led scientists to speculate that retinoid mimics might have a similar effect on human health.

Many factors could contribute to these frog deformities, including parasites and fungal infections. But pesticide poisoning is now believed to be a major contributor. One explanation is that exposure to retinoids may alter the frogs' immunity in some way, making them more susceptible to infectious diseases. The pesticide most likely to initiate such deformities is methoprene, a retinoid mimic that is a popular anti-mosquito insecticide and a common ingredient in flea powder.[85]

Glucocorticoids

Glucocorticoids are steroid hormones in the same class as oestrogen, progesterone and testosterone. Glucocorticoids help regulate embryo development, stress responses, immune function, bone metabolism and central nervous system activity, blood glucose levels, blood vessel function, and lung and skin development. They are also responsible for 'switching-on' genes that may suppress cancer.

PCB metabolites (breakdown products in the body) have been reported to bind to glucocorticoid receptors. Similarly, laboratory studies have shown that, even at extremely low levels, arsenic (still used as a pesticide) appears to suppress the ability of glucocortoid receptors to respond to their normal hormone signals.[86]

How Safe are Plant Oestrogens?

In the midst of all this information about the damage caused by synthetic oestrogens, many readers may be surprised to find an examination of so-called 'natural' plant oestrogens. And yet, looking at the whole of the endocrine system, it is interesting to note that scientists specialising in environmental oestrogens make only a small distinction between synthetic oestrogens such as the Pill, oestrogen mimics such as those found in pesticides, and what have been dubbed 'phytoestrogens,' oestrogens which occur naturally in plants. Each, they say, is a potential endocrine disrupter.[87] It is for this reason that the US Centers for Disease Control (CDC) has now added phytoestrogens to the list of potential human toxins it is currently monitoring. Likewise, concern over the phytoestrogen content of soya has led, in March 2003, the UK government's Committee on Toxicity of Chemicals in Food to conclude that there is cause for concern regarding the widespread use of soya-based infant formulas.

Many different plants produce compounds that may mimic or interact with oestrogen hormones in animals. Most of us are exposed to small quantities of phytoestrogens through our food. They can be found, for instance, in herbs and seasonings (garlic, parsley), grains (soybeans, wheat, rice), vegetables (beans, carrots, potatoes), fruits (dates, pomegranates, cherries, apples) and drinks (coffee and wine).

Unlike their man-made counterparts, these relatively weak, naturally occurring, endocrine disrupters do not appear to be stored in the body for long periods of time. Some, when taken as nutrients in the diet, may exert beneficial effects and may even protect the body against certain cancers (breast, uterus and prostate) in humans.

But several questions remain unanswered. For instance, what happens when we begin to deliberately bombard the body with phytoestrogens, either through increased dietary intake or in supplement form?

Phytotherapy versus Phytonutrition

To support the use of phytoestrogens, many alternative practitioners cite the example of Oriental women who have a higher intake of phytoestrogens and who, research tells us, are longer-lived, have lower rates of heart disease and breast cancer, and do not suffer from menopausal symptoms to the same degree that Western women do.[88]

But women in Far Eastern cultures take in plant oestrogens through their food as phytonutrients whereas, in the West, they are taken primarily as supplements, or phytotherapy. Phytonutrition differs from phytotherapy in several important ways. Natural foods contain literally hundreds of different phytochemicals in delicate synergy. Many of these may work through as yet unknown, non-hormonal pathways to promote good health. In contrast, purified concentrates are designed to increase the dose of a specific, known active ingredient while downgrading or eliminating others. Long-term use of such supplements may deprive women of the full spectrum of beneficial phytonutrients.

Even when we in the West try to include more phytoestrogens in our diet, we generally get it wrong. For instance, our overenthusiasm for the use of soya protein in everyday processed foods such as bread and other bakery items as well as many prepared meals means that both men and women are getting a potentially dangerous daily dose of xenoestrogens without knowing it, all the while being sold the idea that soya is the healthy alternative.

In spite of all this, it is the unbridled use of phytoestrogen supplements especially among women that is the most worrying, since it is likely that the influence of concentrated phytoestrogens in the body may be quite different from those observed at the lower levels available through food. A typical phytoestrogen supplement may contain as much as 250 mg of phytoestrogens. Compare this to Germany, where the recommended dose is 40 mg, and women are advised not to take it for more than six months because of the lack of long-term safety studies.

Do phytoestrogen supplements protect women's health?

If phytoestrogen supplements were really providing unequivocal health benefits, then such worries would seem miserly and unfounded. But, in reality, they provide only marginal benefits.

Phytoestrogens are primarily 'prescribed' to women going through menopause, this in spite of the fact that they have shown, at best, mixed results in relieving menopausal symptoms.[89–91] Indeed, several recent trials have concluded that a placebo works as well as red clover and better than soya isoflavones at relieving hot flashes.[92]

Some studies have shown positive effects on cholesterol.[93] [94] Though most of what we know about the heart-protective attributes of isoflavones is based on animal and laboratory studies,[95] small-scale human studies continue to show some positive effects.[96]

There is evidence that isoflavones can lower cholesterol levels, but so can many other things, such as regular exercise and low-fat, plant-based diets. What's more, the benefits of isoflavones only seem to work in persons suffering from high cholesterol. Supplementation does not appear to lower cholesterol in healthy individuals[97] and, therefore, is unlikely to be a useful preventative.

Small benefits have also been noted in cases of osteoporosis,[98] [99] though again, much of the evidence is from animal studies.[100]

While phytoestrogens are generally promoted as being anticancer, test-tube studies – the only controlled studies ever done – show mixed results, with some concluding that soya isoflavones can inhibit tumour growth,[101] [102] while others show that they actually promote it. In a recent study of the effects of different phytoestrogens on breast cancer cells in the lab, red clover caused cells to multiply to the same degree as oestradiol.[103] Similarly, there is some evidence that a high intake of dietary soya for just 14 days can significantly stimulate the proliferation rate of healthy breast cells.[104] This is why phytoestrogen supplements are now being offered as a means of 'natural' breast enhancement, though whether this kind of hyperstimulation could, in some vulnerable women, lead to cancer is not yet known.

Once again, the majority of the evidence for cancer protection comes from animal and laboratory studies,[105] which cannot necessarily be applied to humans.

Before You Take Phytoestrogen Supplements . . .

It would be wonderful if plant oestrogens were the answer to all women's health problems. But they are not. Before you start adding lots of pills to your daily regime, take a moment to consider how inconclusive most studies into supplementation are. Consider also that problems experienced in menopause may be the result of other aspects of your life – stress, lack of exercise, smoking and alcohol consumption – and not related to menopause at all. In addition:

Eat a variety of plant-based foods. This increases the number of different phytochemicals you ingest, and decreases the likelihood that any one type will be ingested in unbalanced and overly large amounts. Such foods also provide fibre that binds to hormone disrupters and can aid their excretion from the body.

Supplement with fish oil and vitamin B12. This can alleviate some of the more common perimenopausal problems, including dysmenorrhoea, bloating, headaches, nervousness and irritability.[106] However, fish-oil supplements can sometimes be contaminated with the heavy metal mercury, so choose carefully. Alternatively, get your oil from dietary fish sources such as salmon, mackerel and herring.

Support your adrenals. Healthy adrenal glands will continue to supply your postmenopausal body with a form of oestrogen. Keep them working well by reducing stress as adrenals under stress are too busy producing the stress hormone cortisone to produce any other useful substances. Adequate levels of vitamins C, B5 and B6, and the minerals zinc, potassium and magnesium are all necessary for the manufacture of hormones by the adrenal gland. Increasing levels of brightly coloured fruits and vegetables will help you obtain these nutrients.

Is it your thyroid? New data suggest that hypothyroidism (an underactive thyroid) is twice as common as previously thought in women over 60.[107] The complications of low thyroid function – osteoporosis, high cholesterol, tiredness, weight gain, constipation, dry skin and brittle hair – may be confused with the 'symptoms' of menopause.

Hot flashes can be triggered by dietary factors such as hot cups of tea and coffee, and alcohol and spicy foods. Removing these 'thermogenic insults' from the diet can decrease the number of hot flashes by as much as 50 percent.[108]

Surround yourself with supporters. The social context in which a woman ages has a great deal to do with her perceptions.[109] It is likely that Eastern women do not experience disruptive menopausal symptoms because their society accepts ageing as a natural progression.[110]

Quit smoking and limit alcohol. Smoking increases your risk of developing brittle bones by 400 percent. High alcohol intake is associated with an increased risk of many diseases, including heart disease, cancer and brittle bones.

Consider boron. This element may help the body make better use of circulating oestrogen[111] and is useful in the prevention of postmenopausal osteoporosis.[112] Useful levels can be found in fruit (especially apples, pears, grapes, dates, raisins and peaches), legumes (especially soybeans), nuts (including almonds, peanuts and hazelnuts) and honey.

'Weak' oestrogens?

Depending on whose research you read, phytoestrogens either have no oestrogenic effect or only a weak one.[113] However, the emerging view is that phytoestrogens are not really 'weak' at all and that they can, in sufficient quantities, evoke all the same responses as physiological oestrogens.[114]

What is not disputed is that oestrogen is toxic to the system in high doses. A look at the accumulating evidence on HRT will prove this.[115] There is also the issue of how to define a 'weak' oestrogen. The example of diethylstilboestrol (DES), an oestrogen given to women to prevent miscarriage, may be instructive. DES was considered a weak oestrogen in that it did not compete with natural oestrogens by binding to oestrogen receptors. Today, we are only just beginning to understand the devastating generational effects of taking DES; even the granddaughters of women who took this 'weak' hormone have a higher risk of ovarian cancer.

The generational effects of plant oestrogens have also been studied, albeit in animals. In one study, high levels of soya during pregnancy increased the risk of breast cancer in female offspring.[116] The study suggested that the risk is dose–dependent – the more the mother ate, the greater the risk – and that genistein, a phytoestrogen present in soya, was responsible.

Oestriol (an oestrogen metabolised in the body from plant sources) is also considered a weak oestrogen yet, in large enough doses, it can produce quite profound oestrogenic effects.[117] There is even evidence that oestriol binds more strongly to receptors than DES. In one study, when oestriol was added to a long-term culture of human breast-cancer cells, it not only stimulated their growth, but was powerful enough to negate the antioestrogenic effect of tamoxifen.[118]

Likewise, coumoestrol, a plant isoflavone found in high doses in red clover, is unique among phytoestrogens in that it has been shown to have powerful oestrogenic effects[119] – six times that of regular isoflavones.[120] Years ago, agricultural research showed that red clover caused permanent sterility in the sheep that consumed it[121] as well as their offspring.[122] Some argue that these effects have only been demonstrated in sheep and that such data cannot be extrapolated to humans. And yet, a significant proportion of the 'evidence' for the benefits of phytoestrogens in humans is also based on data from animals. Proponents can't have it both ways.

Much of what women are told about the actions of phytoestrogens is intelligent guesswork. In reality, we have no idea what will happen when we begin to deliberately and dramatically change the ratios of naturally produced to synthetic hormones in the body. These unknowns have led some observers to postulate that the unbridled consumption of plant oestrogens may yet prove to be one of the greatest uncontrolled experiments in human health to date.

Standing up to the hype

Phrases like 'perimenopause' and 'oestrogen deficiency' are marketing tools, not medical diagnoses. Australian evidence culled from studies of women aged 15 to 69, for instance, has shown that as many as 32 percent of young women between the ages of 15 and 19 had signs of 'oestrogen deficiency' (as defined by marketeers and medical men). Nearly half of all the women sampled also showed these signs. It is clearly ludicrous that so many otherwise healthy women should be considered oestrogen-deficient. Don't buy into it.

Menopause is not a 'disease' of 'oestrogen deficiency' – it is an age-appropriate decline in oestrogen levels. Equally, the problem of environmental oestrogens cannot be fixed, as some have suggested, by simply adding progesterone (or, more correctly, progestin) to the female body. Whatever the marketeers tell you, there is no such thing as natural progesterone – all progestins, whether they come from wild yams or any other source, are synthesised in the lab. This typically hamfisted way of dealing with potential oestrogen excesses has *never* been scientifically proven to be effective.[123] Since both oestrogen and progesterone are recognised carcinogens when present in the body in amounts higher than needed, it may even be dangerous.

Indeed, as of December 2002, the synthetic oestrogens used in HRT and oral contraceptives have been added to the federal list of known human carcinogens compiled by the US National Toxicology Program.[124]

Minimising Hormone Disruption

There are a number of things you can do to protect you and your family from the short- and long-term threats of endocrine disrupters.

- *Use a water filter.* Pesticides, fertilisers, industrial chemicals and other debris have contributed to dangerously high levels of toxic chemicals in our water. Toxic metals from household pipes and plumbing can be an added concern. This means that a good-quality water filter is becoming one of life's necessities. Your best choice is probably a reverse-osmosis water filter. However, if installing one is too expensive, buy a jug-type filter and make sure the filter is changed regularly.
- *Use safe, natural household supplies.* Reconsider your use of garden chemicals and fertilisers, mothballs and strong household cleaners which can all contain a range of endocrine disrupters. These days, they are almost totally unnecessary since good natural alternatives are plentiful and easily obtainable.
- *Avoid plastic wrap.* You'll find this on a wide range of foods, from cheese to meat to precut vegetables. It may contain endocrine disrupters that have the potential to interfere with hormones in the body. For instance, the chemical di-(2-ethyl-hexyl)adipate (DEHA), which gives the 'cling' to plastic wrap, is still used in some brands of household wrap and in grocery-store wrap for cheese and meat. DEHA has been proven to interfere with male fertility in most animal species.

- *Avoid microwaving foods in plastic containers*, even those marked safe for microwave use. Plastic contains oestrogenic compounds that can be released when heated. Use a glass container instead or, better yet, get rid of the microwave and prepare your food yourself and in good-quality cookware.

- *What price beauty?* Many of the preservatives and other chemicals used in cosmetics have an oestrogenic effect on the body. Watch out for preservatives such as parabens (butylparabens, propylparabens, methylparabens and ethylparabens). These are found in both men's and women's toiletries and cosmetics. Sunscreen agents, too, are oestrogenic, so consider covering up with clothes instead of creams during the hottest part of the day.

- *Buy organic fruits and vegetables* and buy locally whenever you can. If you can't purchase organic produce, be sure to wash your produce carefully and peel thin-skinned produce such as apples and carrots. Choosing produce carefully may also help limit your exposure. For instance, the following fruits and vegetables have been found by the US Environmental Working Group to contain the most pesticides: spinach, strawberries, apricots, cantaloupe, green beans, peaches, bell peppers, celery, cucumbers, cherries and grapes (*see Chapter 10 for more information*).

- *Eat organic meats whenever possible.* Environmental pesticides and chemicals accumulate in animal products, especially in animal fat. If you eat meat, it is especially important to purchase organic. With conventionally produced meats, trim fat, and discard poultry and fish skins. Cook in a grill-type pan that allows fat to drip away from the food.

- *Increase good fats* such as flaxseed oil and fish oils. Because pesticides are fat-soluble, you should supplement each day. Flaxseed oil can be included in your diet as a dressing and can help to leach out fat-soluble chemicals from the body. Use freshly pressed flaxseed oil in salads or drizzled on food (*see Chapter 10 for more information*).

- *Think functional foods.* Include the following foods for protection against pollution: turmeric, milk-thistle extract, sea vegetables, rosemary, broccoli and other cruciferous vegetables. Glutathione-rich foods like asparagus, raw spinach, parsley, avocados, watermelon, cauliflower, broccoli, pears, squash and potatoes help the liver to remove environmental waste. Allyl sulphide-containing foods like garlic, shallots, onions and chives stimulate glutathione production. Finally, consider using *miso* (a fermented soya paste that can be added to soups, stir-frys, etc.) which contains a range of helpful enzymes and friendly bacteria that are reputed to help expel pollutants and protect the body from radiation.

- *Protect your children.* Unless there is a sound medical reason why you can't, you should breastfeed your child for as long as possible. Similarly, if you have no good reason to give your child soya formula, don't. Consider also the use of reusable nappies made from natural fabrics, and choose pacifiers and children's teething toys made from materials other than PVC. Buy toys that are clearly PVC-free, such as those made from wood, metal or hard plastics without additives.

- *Exercise* can help reduce your body's load of a whole range of chemicals. By working up a sweat two or three times a week or, even better, every day, you are supporting your body's natural eliminatory channels. The most recent evidence suggests that women who exercise just half-an-hour daily cut their risk of developing breast cancer by 10 percent; an hour a day will cut the risk by 20 percent.[125]

- *Menopausal women* should consider options other than HRT and phytoestrogens. See pages 197–199 for tips on how to get started.

9 Metallica

IMMUNE DEFICIENCY, LOWERED INTELLIGENCE, AGGRESSION, VIOLENCE and birth defects – this is the legacy left to us after years of exposure to toxic metals such as lead, mercury, cadmium, aluminium, arsenic and copper in our environment.

You can encounter these metals almost anywhere, but the most common sources include tapwater, air pollution particularly in areas of heavy traffic, old paint, tobacco smoke, fish and shellfish, pesticides, medications such as antacids, and also children's vaccines, intrauterine devices, enamelled and aluminium cookware, dental fillings, copper pipes, the disinfectant used in public swimming pools, processed foods, cosmetics and toiletries. Unlike the beneficial trace metals we get from our diet (and with the exception of copper), these metals have no function in the body and can be highly toxic if ingested in high-enough quantities.[1]

Traditionally, where metals are concerned, scientists have believed that "the dose makes the poison" – in other words, the higher the dose, the more toxic the metal becomes. But dose is only one facet of metal toxicity.

Indeed, because toxic metals are bioaccumulative – that is, stored in body tissues – it is now believed that they do not need to be present in your day-to-day environment in high concentrations to produce adverse health effects. All you need to produce a state of toxicity is for your body to accumulate these elements faster than it can dispose of them.[2]

Although these metals are commonly referred to as 'heavy' metals, in reality, they are not all heavy and some, like arsenic, are only semi-metallic. But these elements possess other properties that make them dangerous to humans: they do not dissolve, evaporate, or decompose; and in general, they stay put in the environment until someone becomes concerned enough (or sick enough) to do something about them.

While all of these 'heavy' metals can be poisonous, the degree to which they damage human health depends to a large extent on the form the metal takes. Metals come in inorganic and organic forms. An inorganic metal is in its raw elemental state – the same stuff you find in the ground. Generally speaking, these elements are poorly absorbed by the body but, through ingestion and metabolism, they can sometimes be converted in the body to more potent and poisonous forms.

In chemistry, 'organic' does not mean the same thing as in a grocery store. Organic metals are those that have been combined (either in nature or in the lab) with some other carbon-containing substance, such as a petroleum derivative. Complexes of toxic metals with carbon compounds can greatly increase the health risks associated with the metal itself. This is, in part, because the carbon molecule gives the metal more power to interact with other substances. In the body, this interaction is known as oxidation and involves the production of free radicals. The higher the level of free radicals in the body, the greater the likelihood of illness (*see Chapter 3 for more details*).

Toxic metals are particularly harmful to the reproductive system. They can also interfere with detoxification pathways, including the colon, liver, kidneys and skin. Some are also endocrine disrupters. The immune system's function is also compromised by the presence of toxic metals,[3] and they can weaken our energy production pathways. Because of this, they are believed to be involved in disorders such as chronic fatigue syndrome.

Toxic metals also appear to increase the acidity of the blood. When this happens, the body responds by drawing alkaline, in the form of calcium, from the bones to help restore the proper pH (alkaline-to-acid balance) of blood. In the presence of toxic metals, calcium may also be drawn to areas of damage and inflammation (for instance, joints and arterial walls). While this process acts like a bandage, patching up one problem area, it can create other problems such as hardening of the artery walls and arthritis. In addition, without the replenishment of calcium, the constant removal of this important mineral from the bones can result in brittle bones (osteoporosis).

However, it is damage to the neurological system, particularly the brain, which is the most well researched. In addition to generating harmful free radicals, toxic metals also interfere with the body's uptake of essential nutrients such as magnesium, lithium, zinc, iron and several of the B vitamins. The resulting deficiencies have been linked to increased neurological damage.[4]

Evidence also implicates toxic metals in a range of emotional and behavioural problems in children such as autism, dyslexia and attention-deficit and hyperactivity disorder (ADHD),[5] as well as learning difficulties, including decreased concentration and organisational skills; speech, language and comprehension difficulties, and lowered intelligence. Adults are affected, too, as studies show higher rates of violence,[6] dementia[7] and depression among exposed individuals.

This means that metal toxicity is as much a social problem as it is an environmental one. While toxic metals may not be the whole answer to the problem of learning difficulties in children and increasing levels of violence in our society, they certainly appear to be an important piece of the puzzle. Equally, while some would argue that small decreases in intelligence are unlikely to be important, consider the knock-on effect of a general lowering of IQs by just five points.[8] Extrapolated to the entire population, this would mean that millions of people would drop below the threshold of average intelligence and be labelled 'learning impaired'.[9] The changes in social policy needed to meet such a decline should not be underestimated.

Short-Term Effects

Current studies indicate that even minute levels of toxic elements can have negative health consequences, though these vary from person to person.

Over the short term, they can cause a variety of symptoms, most of which are linked to neurological dysfunction. In general, these include:

- mental confusion
- headaches
- short-term memory loss
- vision problems
- numbness or tingling in the extremities
- joint pain and/or swelling
- drowsiness.

Other common symptoms are:

- pain in muscles and joints
- gastrointestinal upsets
- food intolerances/allergies
- chronic fatigue
- skin rashes
- hypoglycaemia
- depression
- fatigue
- nervousness and irritability
- aggressive behaviour in children.

Aiding Metal Absorption

Toxic metals can be absorbed through inhalation, ingestion and through the skin. They do not need to bioaccumulate to disrupt the body. Several factors make us more vulnerable to exposure and absorption of heavy metals. These include:

- *Your genetic inheritance* – inherited 'weak spots' may make you vulnerable to specific types of toxic metal damage.
- *The 'window of exposure'* – in other words, how long you were exposed for, at what levels and, crucially, at what age. Children and the elderly, whose immune systems are either underdeveloped or age-compromised, are more vulnerable to toxicity. Exposure while in the womb or in early infancy is considered particularly devastating.
- *Nutritional status* – those on a poor diet are more vulnerable.

- *Decreased function of the body's detoxification pathways* – in other words, your body's ability to metabolise, neutralise and excrete toxic substances.
- *The mode and degree of toxic metal exposure* – for instance, occupational exposures can be particularly devastating, though poor housing conditions are also relevant.
- *Relative levels of poverty or affluence* – the poorest families may be particularly vulnerable because their economic status may affect other risk factors, such as diet and housing.

Exposure to hidden sources of metals may also be important to our overall absorption of these substances. For instance, 90 percent of the fluoride used to fluoridate water systems (particularly in the US) is industrial waste produced by the phosphate-fertiliser industry. The chemical hydrofluorosilicic acid is an industrial-grade (as opposed to pharmaceutical-grade) product that contains trace amounts of lead, mercury and arsenic.

Proponents claim that these toxic metals, when poured into the water supply, are diluted to the point that they pose no threat to human health. Once again, this misses the point. Anything that adds to the total exposure to these substances is a threat to health. What's more, toxic metals in the water supply are particularly insidious since they can be taken into the body via numerous pathways. For instance, when we take hot showers, they are inhaled as minute droplets in the steamy air or absorbed through the skin. When we cook with or drink water, or brush our teeth, they are ingested directly.

Lead and arsenic are both human carcinogens (and so is fluoride) and, while levels required to produce health effects vary from one individual to another, the question remains: *Do we really want these things in our water?*

Mind, Body, Metals

Some scientists speculate that there may even be an emotional element to how we absorb heavy metals and where they eventually accumulate in our bodies. It's an intriguing possibility that goes some way to answering why individuals exposed to toxic metals end up storing them in various, seemingly random, areas of the body.

Mercury is a good example. With chronic exposure, some individuals deposit this metal in the hypothalamus of the brain (and develop multiple hormone problems) or in the limbic system (where it can lead to depression). Others deposit mercury in the adrenals (leading to fatigue) or in the long bones (a risk factor for osteoporosis and leukaemia). Drawn to the pelvic area, it can lead to interstitial cystitis and, deposited in the autonomic and sensory ganglia, it is linked with chronic pain syndromes. In the connective tissues, it is related to scleroderma and lupus; in the cranial nerves, it may lead to tinnitus (constant ringing in the ears), cataracts, temporomandibular joint (TMJ, or alignment of the jaw) problems and loss of the sense of smell and, in the muscles, fibromyalgia.

According to Dietrich Klinghardt, MD, PhD, who has spent many years researching the effects of heavy metals and their behaviour in the body, the subject is complex. Patients usually consult their practitioners when they are feeling out of sorts – for instance, with the kinds of symptoms associated with metal toxicity and other forms of environmental pollution.

However, a symptom is rather like the outer layer of an onion. Peel it back and you usually find other problems that have made the person vulnerable to metal toxicity. In Klinghardt's view, underlying our symptoms may be, for instance, a chronic infection and underlying that may be the presence of toxic metals and, underneath that, the reason (other than the obvious one of exposure) why the person is so ill. Klinghardt believes, somewhat controversially, that the type of metal and where it eventually is stored in the body are largely guided by the subconscious mind and determined by the emotional state of the individual as well as aspects of their lifestyle.[10]

Those aspects of our life and personality that he believes can 'direct' metals to different parts of the body include:

- **Past physical trauma** (such as a head injury), which can turn the brain into a storage site for lead, aluminium and mercury.

- **Food allergies**, which can often cause a low-grade encephalitis or joint inflammation, setting up those areas to become reservoirs for toxic deposits.
- **Geopathic stress** as a result of sleeping above underground waterlines or too close to electrical equipment, or living in an area of unusually high natural magnetic radiation, which can weaken the entire system, thus allowing metals to concentrate in vulnerable areas of the body.
- **Scars and sites of inflammation**, which can create abnormal electrical signals that can alter the function of the autonomic nervous system. These abnormal impulses can create areas of decreased blood flow that can encourage metal accumulation in specific areas.
- **Structural abnormalities**, such as jaw or spinal misalignments, which can also be responsible for impaired blood flow as well as poor lymphatic drainage in specific areas and, thus, encourage metal deposition.
- **Nutritional deficiencies**, such as a chronic zinc deficiency, which can cause organs like the prostate, which has a large turnover of zinc, to incorporate other reactive metals such as mercury and lead instead.
- **Environmental toxicity**, such as from solvents, pesticides, wood preservatives and industrial chemicals, which can act in synergy with most toxic metals. Metals will often accumulate in body parts that have been chemically injured.
- **Unresolved psychoemotional trauma** and other unresolved familial problems, which can also be a factor in determining where a metal will be stored in the body and which infectious agent will thrive in what part of the body.

The evidence for this is anecdotal, but nevertheless intriguing. Indeed, the theory may not be as farfetched as it appears to be. There is already a considerable body of evidence on the way that loneliness, for instance, can damage the heart.[11] There is also evidence of a 'cancer personality' – a chronic emotional state that predisposes certain people to the development of cancer.[12] Similar studies are emerging for diabetics[13] and those suffering from other autoimmune disorders.

Interestingly, American naturopath Hulda Clark has hypothesised much the same idea about parasites – suggesting that the areas in the body that are most vulnerable to infestation differ from person to person according to their toxic exposures. Different toxic substances have affinities with different organs and, once damaged, these organs become weakened and, thus, more accommodating for parasitic infestation.[14] Taking these theories to their logical conclusion, it may be that whenever an organ is weakened – whether through toxic environmental exposures, toxic emotions or straightforward genetic inheritance – it then becomes vulnerable to further damage from other sources. Put more simply, each of us has a weak spot that needs acknowledging and protecting.

Metal Poisoning Through the Ages

Throughout history, there have been many famous cases of metal toxicity.

- Lead has been implicated in the downfall of the Roman Empire. During that era, the ruling classes had lead piping installed in their homes and drank from goblets made from a lead alloy.
- The film *Erin Brockovitch* is based on a true case of environmental poisoning from a highly reactive form of chromium called hexavalent chromium. This resulted in a highly publicised and successful lawsuit for damages against the company which discharged the waste that had contaminated the local water supply.
- Tests carried out recently on strands of Beethoven's hair have found very high concentrations of lead. This may have accounted for his deafness and distressing abdominal pain as well as his reputed irritability and depression.
- In Naples, Italy, during the late 1600s and early 1700s, Madame Giulia Toffana provided a unique service for women. Her main business was the production of fine cosmetics. But she was also renowned for her open-minded attitude towards women who wished to 'dispose' of their unwanted husbands, unfaithful boyfriends and troublesome ex-lovers. To these women, she would provide poisonous potions, usually arsenic trioxide, disguised as cosmetics. During her long and successful career in 'cosmetics', she contributed to the demise of more than 600 unfortunate individuals.

- During the 1800s, mercury was used in hat making. The phrase 'mad as a hatter' was coined because of the way chronic mercury exposure altered the emotional stability of felters.
- The violinist and composer Paganini suffered an early death due to chronic mercury poisoning. The reason? He was receiving mercury-containing treatment for suspected syphilis as well as abusing laxatives containing calomel (mercuric chloride).
- The famous neo-Baroque Spanish painter Francisco Goya (1746–1828) became lead-intoxicated through the mixing of his white paint pigments. His depression and mood swings, often reflected in his paintings, have been attributed to lead encephalopathy (lead in the brain).
- King George III suffered violent episodes of nervous breakdown, paralysis and delirium, which appeared to be madness to his ministers. Recent conjecture suggests that he suffered from chronic lead poisoning from tainted wine – the lead having leached into his preferred tipple from the original royal casks.

The Heavy Hitters

Metal toxicity has been with us for a very long time. Greek and Roman physicians were diagnosing symptoms of acute lead poisoning long before the science of toxicology was founded. Today, much more is known about the health effects of these metals. Research into acute, usually occupational, exposures is relatively plentiful and forms the basis of much of our knowledge. However, as more and more scientists accept the idea of low-dose effects, it's becoming clear that you don't need to have acute exposures to develop symptoms of metal toxicity. Over the years, many of these metals can accumulate in body tissues, where they slowly but steadily reach toxic levels, and it is now believed that metal toxicity represents an uncommon, yet clinically significant, medical condition. If unrecognised or inappropriately treated, this toxicity can result in significant illness and even death.

In spite of this, our exposure to toxic metals continues largely unabated and may increase further still in the absence of any directed effort to protect human health by restricting their use. While most metals are toxic at some level, those that we come into contact with on an everyday basis are of greatest concern.

Lead

Lead is the most significant of all these metals because it is both toxic and very common. Professions that put their employees at risk of lead exposure include lead-smelting, -refining and -manufacturing industries, brass/bronze foundries, the rubber and plastics industries, steel-welding and -cutting operations, and battery manufacturing plants. Construction workers and people who work in municipal waste incinerators, in the pottery and ceramics industries, radiator-repair shops and other industries that use lead solder may also be among the high-exposure groups.

But we are all exposed to lead to some extent. Since the advent of unleaded petrol, emission from cars has ceased to be the major source of lead for the majority of us. Nevertheless, lead still enters our atmosphere as toxic emissions from factories and from cigarette smoke.

Lead has been used as a plumbing material since Roman times, and it can still be found in the solder joints on older copper pipes, and in fittings and faucets made from brass. As these plumbing materials corrode, they leach lead into the water.

Older lead-based paints, which may be anywhere from 5–40 percent lead, also contribute to lead pollution. Lead-containing dust is tracked in from outdoors and airborne particles are created when this type of paint is improperly removed from surfaces by dry scraping, sanding or open-flame burning. Lead-containing dust is particularly risky in households where there are young children who play on the floor and who put things found on the floor into their mouths.

Women should be aware that some cosmetics and hair dyes also contain lead compounds. In addition, if their partners work in jobs where they are exposed to high levels of lead (plumbers, painters and motor mechanics, for example), women may become contaminated with lead through her partner's semen. Once pregnant, such women might consider having their husbands use a condom to prevent lead being absorbed into their bodies (and into their babies) from their partner's seminal fluid.

Foods such as fruits, vegetables, meats, grains, seafood, soft drinks and wine can be contaminated by lead in the soil and air during growth, storage and transport. They may also absorb lead from water used in cooking and processing. Lead may leach into foods if they are stored in improperly glazed pottery or ceramic dishes, or in leaded-crystal glassware, and can be released from the soldered joints in kettles. Since lead can be stored in the liver of animals, it is also found in foods that contain organ meats such as processed liverwurst, sausage and some sandwich spreads.

Lead in the body

Lead exposure at any level can affect numerous body systems. For instance, low levels can adversely affect the central nervous system (brain and spinal cord), heart, red blood cells and kidneys. Chronic exposure in adults is associated with endocrine and reproductive dysfunction — specifically, deformed and dead sperm, infertility, repeated miscarriage, stillbirth, fetal abnormalities and low birthweights. It is also associated with hypertension, headaches, confusion, irritability, motor dysfunction and insomnia. Higher levels cause drowsiness, loss of muscle coordination, kidney damage, fatigue, apathy, susceptibility to infections, gouty arthritis and anaemia.

Most lead in the body is stored in the bones,[15] and some can stay in the bones for decades. However, under certain circumstances – for example, during periods of stress, during pregnancy and breastfeeding, after a bone is broken or with advancing age – some lead is liberated from the bones and can reenter the bloodstream and organs.

Lead also interacts and competes with several essential elements in the body – principally, calcium, iron, and zinc – and high body loads can cause deficiency in these nutrients. Conversely, dietary deficiencies of both calcium and iron are known to enhance the absorption of lead. It has also been suggested that lead can affect bone growth in children by interfering with vitamin D metabolism.[16]

Even though studies show that blood lead levels in humans have dropped significantly in the last 30–40 years, lead is still with us. Children are particularly at risk from lead exposure because, compared with adults, more of the lead they ingest stays in their bodies. While about 99 percent of the lead ingested by an adult will be excreted within a couple of weeks, over the same time period, only around 32 percent of the lead ingested by a child will be excreted.

Children, like adults, are prone to neurological damage from lead ingestion, and it has been found to lower intelligence and cause behavioural problems in some youngsters.[17][18] In one 1996 UK study, researchers took blood samples from 69 children (average age 5.7 years) with behavioural and/or developmental problems and compared concentrations of lead in their blood with children who were behaviourally normal. The children with behavioural problems were more than 12 times more likely to have toxic lead concentrations in their blood.[19]

The same year, Australian researchers reported that exposure to environmental lead during the first seven years of life was associated with learning difficulties – including poor verbal skills and test performances, and a decline in IQ. Indeed, those with the highest lead concentrations in their blood had IQs that were, on average, three points lower than those who had the lowest lead concentrations. All these difficulties persisted into early teenage years.[20]

In the US, studies by lead expert Dr Herbert Needleman have uncovered similarly disturbing trends.[21] In 1996, Needleman published a study showing that those with relatively high levels of lead in their bones were more likely to engage in antisocial activities like bullying, vandalism, truancy and shoplifting.[22] Later, he showed that children with high lead levels in their teeth, but no outward signs of lead poisoning, had lower IQ scores, poorer attention spans and poorer language skills.[23] Needleman's research in this area was, in fact, instrumental in getting lead banned from paint, petrol, and food and beverage cans in the US and elsewhere.

Protect yourself

The most important way families can lower exposure to lead is to know about the sources of lead in their homes and, as far as possible, avoid or eliminate these. To reduce your exposure to and intake of lead:

- *Do not bring lead dust into the home.* Remove your shoes and use doormats to wipe your feet before entering the home. If you work in any of the professions mentioned on page 213, or your hobby involves lead (such as some types of model-making or using oil paints), you may unknowingly bring lead into your home on your hands or clothes. Consider changing clothes and, if possible, showering before leaving work. Bag up work clothes securely before bringing them into the home for cleaning, and wash these clothes separately.

- *The soil in your garden* and other outdoor areas may be contaminated from lead paint on the outside of the building or from years of exposure to exhaust fumes from cars and trucks using leaded gas. Planting grass and shrubs over bare soil areas in the garden can reduce the contact that children and pets may have with soil and the tracking of soil into the home.

- *How old is your home?* Adding lead to paint is no longer allowed. But if your house was built before 1978, it may have been painted with lead-based paint and this lead may still be on walls, floors, ceilings and windowsills or on the outside walls of the house. The paint may have been scraped off by a previous owner, and paint chips and dust may still be in the garden soil. Lead paint in good condition is usually not a problem except in places where painted surfaces rub against each other and create dust (for example, when opening a window). If potentially lead-based paint in your home is in good condition, leave it alone – do not sand or burn it off. If you must strip it, use a solvent-free paint stripper and dispose of the residues carefully.

- *Eat right.* A healthy diet will help combat the effects of lead. Make sure your diet includes plenty of antioxidant foods, such as fresh fruits and vegetables that are rich in vitamins A, C and E. Maintaining adequate levels of the minerals iron, calcium, magnesium, manganese, selenium, chromium and zinc as well as getting adequate protein and fibre is also important. In particular, calcium and iron can block the absorption of lead. Foods rich in iron include eggs, red meats and beans. Dairy products and dark-green vegetables are high in calcium. Eating lots of fresh garlic can also help combat the effects of excessive lead.

- *Consider having a water filter installed.* Older homes that have plumbing with lead or pipes with lead solder may leach higher amounts of lead into drinking water, particularly in soft water areas. You cannot see, taste or smell lead in water, and boiling the water will not get rid of it. What's more, lead taken in from water and other beverages tends to be absorbed to a greater degree than lead taken in food.[24] If you are concerned about lead in your water, contact your local health department or water supplier to find out how to get your water tested. If levels are high (more than 10 microgrammes per litre), consider installing a good-quality water filter (*see Chapter 10 for advice on water filters*). If this proves too costly, run your water for 15–30 seconds before drinking or cooking with it. This will help to flush out lead that may leach out from the pipes, especially if you have not used your water for a while – for example, overnight or when you've been away.

- *Do not store food or liquid in lead-crystal glassware, or imported or old pottery.* Lead can leach out of these and into the food.

- *Some types of paints and pigments* that are used as facial make-up or hair dyes contain lead. Cosmetics that contain lead include surma and kohl, popular in certain Asian countries. Lead acetate is approved for use in progressive hair dyes (most often used by men), despite it being a known carcinogen and endocrine disrupter. Read the labels on hair-colouring products and avoid those that contain this substance. If you must use such products, keep them stored where children cannot be exposed to them.

- *Keep areas where children play as dust-free and clean as possible.* Most multipurpose cleaners will not remove lead in ordinary dust. Instead, mop floors, and wipe window ledges and chewable surfaces such as cribs with a solution of powdered automatic dishwasher detergent in warm water. (Dishwasher detergents are recommended because of their high content of phosphate, which binds with lead.) Launder soft toys and stuffed animals regularly.

- *Make sure that all members of the family*, especially children, wash their hands before eating or preparing meals and before naptime and bedtime.

Candle, Candle, Burning Bright

Research by the US Environmental Protection Agency has shown that burning a candle with multiple wicks or multiple candles can lead to high levels of pollutants called particulates – tiny droplets or particles of soot plus a variety of toxic chemicals – indoors. According to the report, scented candles, so popular for the romantic ambience they lend to a room, are more likely to give off black soot than unscented candles.

Most of us are also unaware that candlewicks can contain lead,[25] even though they are not supposed to. Indeed, in the US 25 years ago, the candle-making industry vowed to remove lead from their products. Nevertheless, lead is still used by some manufacturers to stiffen candlewicks. Every time you burn one of these lead-containing candles, you release significant amounts of neurotoxic lead into the atmosphere.

In one recent US study, different types of candles were purchased from 12 different stores. Testing revealed that 30 percent had metallic wicks and 10 percent of these (3 percent of all the candles purchased) contained lead.[26] Burning these lead-containing candles for just three hours, said the researchers, would result in air levels of lead 36 times over the safe limit. Breathing this air would certainly result in lead poisoning.

In April 2003, the US Consumer Product Safety Commission finally banned the sale and import of candles with lead wicks in the US. Other countries have yet to follow suit. There is no way to distinguish lead-containing wicks from safe ones nor are candle manufacturers obliged to state on product labels what their wicks contain. However, there is some evidence that candles from the US and China are among those with the highest lead content.

Mercury

For centuries, mercury was an essential ingredient in many different medicines, such as diuretics, antibacterial agents, antiseptics and laxatives. As evidence of mercury's toxicity grew, these uses were phased out. Nevertheless, our exposure to mercury continues to rise due to the increased use of fossil fuels and agricultural products that contain this toxic metal. This fact was highlighted in March 2001, in the *National Report on Human Exposure to Environmental Chemicals*,[27] compiled by the US Centers for Disease Control. The report noted that, while levels of lead in human tissues appear to be slowly declining, there has been a rise in, among other things, levels of mercury.

There are three basic forms of mercury in the environment: metallic, inorganic and methylmercury.

There are many different uses for liquid metallic mercury. It is used in the production of chlorine gas and caustic soda, and in the extraction of gold from ore or articles that contain gold. It is also used in paper-pulp production, photography, thermometers, barometers, batteries and electrical switches as well as in fluorescent, mercury and neon lighting. Amalgam dental fillings are typically about 50 percent metallic mercury.

Some inorganic mercury compounds are used as fungicides. Mercuric sulphide and mercuric oxide may be used to colour paints, and mercuric sulphide is one of the red colouring agents used in tattoo dyes and other inks. Mercuric chloride is a topical antiseptic or disinfectant. Other chemicals containing mercury (such as thimerosal and phenylmercuric nitrate) are still used as antibacterials and can be found in cosmetics such as skin-lightening creams, mascara and perfumes, and in over-the-counter medicines such as spermicidal jellies. Most controversially, it is also used in common vaccines such as the ones for diphtheria–tetanus–whole cell pertussis (DTP), *Haemophilus influenzae* (HIb) and hepatitis B.

Methylmercury, however, is the form most easily absorbed through the gastrointestinal tract – studies show that around 95 percent of it reaches the bloodstream in this way. Once there, it quickly finds its way to vital organs. Indeed, approximately 98 percent of the total mercury found in the brain is in the form of methylmercury. Methylmercury is also lipophilic, which means that it tends to be stored in the body fat of humans and other animals.

Methylmercury can be synthesised in the lab or in nature. Microorganisms such as bacteria, phytoplankton in the ocean and fungi can convert inorganic mercury to methylmercury. Until the 1970s, methylmercury and ethylmercury compounds were used to protect seed grains from fungal infections. Once the adverse health effects of methylmercury were known, this use was banned. Up until 1991, however, a related compound phenylmercury was used as an antifungal agent in both interior and exterior paints. Again, this use was banned when it was confirmed that dangerous mercury vapours were being released from these paints.

Occupations that have a greater potential for mercury exposure include manufacturers of mercury-containing electrical equipment or automotive parts; chemical-processing plants that use mercury; metal processing; construction industries where building parts contain mercury (such as electrical switches and thermometers); and the medical profession where equipment such as thermometers and devices that measure blood pressure contain liquid mercury. Dentists and their assistants may be exposed to particularly high levels of mercury vapour in their day-to-day work (*see below*).

Some people may also be exposed to higher levels of methylmercury if they have a diet high in fish, shellfish or other marine mammals (for instance, whales, seals, dolphins and walruses) harvested in mercury-contaminated waters.

Mercury in Your Mouth

The 'silver' fillings that most of us have in our mouths are known as amalgam fillings. Not everyone realises that dental amalgam is made of equal parts of mercury and a 'carrier' powder made from other toxic metals. The composition of amalgams varies with each manufacturer; however, a typical formula includes: 48–60 percent mercury, 15–37 percent silver, 12–13 percent tin, 0–26 percent copper and 0–1 percent zinc. Some also contain small amounts of nickel and cadmium.[28]

Studies show that, for the average individual, the mercury from dental amalgam may contribute anywhere from 50–75 percent of their total daily mercury ingestion,[29][30] depending on the total number and size of fillings in the mouth, and the chewing and eating habits of the person as well as other environmental factors.

Almost anything you put in your mouth can cause mercury to be released from amalgam fillings. Brushing your teeth can release mercury, as can hot or acidic drinks or foods. Chewing anything, including gum, can also cause mercury vapour to be released.[31] People who frequently grind their teeth increase the amount of mercury normally released from amalgam fillings over time.

In addition, metal fillings can act like small electrical conductors when they come into contact with saliva. Dr Jack Levenson, President of the British Society for Mercury Free Dentistry, maintains a large file of case histories illustrating how mercury fillings can exert a distorting effect on the normal electromagnetic field of the body. Sitting in a strong EMF all day, your fillings may well be conducting electricity directly into your head.[32] While evidence is still anecdotal, it is entirely possible that some of the symptoms of amalgam poisoning can be related to the mild but continual electrical current they produce.

Mercury in the body

Like lead, mercury toxicity is associated with a wide range of non-specific health problems such as poor digestion and absorption of nutrients, chronic enterocolitis, food allergies, depression, dementia, fatigue, headaches and memory impairment, nausea, stomach pains, weakness, eczema, travel sickness, infections, headache, dizziness, dulling of the senses and gingivitis. The combination of vague symptoms and lack of knowledge within the medical profession means that, very often, mercury poisoning is misdiagnosed and remains untreated.

The US EPA has determined that mercury chloride and methyl-mercury are possible human carcinogens. In addition, all forms of mercury can cause kidney damage if large enough amounts enter the body. Mercury is also known to cause reproductive abnormalities.

However, it is mercury's effect on the nervous system that is most widely acknowledged. The nervous system is very sensitive to mercury, and toxicity can result in a variety of symptoms, including personality changes (irritability, shyness, nervousness), tremors, changes in vision (constriction, or narrowing, of the visual field), deafness, muscle incoordination, loss of sensation and difficulties with memory.

At the extreme end of the scale, studies conducted at the University of Kentucky have found abnormally high mercury levels in the brain of people with Alzheimer's disease.[33] Likewise, excessive mercury in children has been linked to learning disabilities and hyperactivity.[34]

During critical periods of development before they are born and in the early months after birth, children are particularly sensitive to the harmful effects of mercury on the nervous system. Mercury easily crosses the placenta, and there is evidence that a mother who is herself carrying a large body load of mercury can pass this on to her child. In one study, women with 10 or more amalgam fillings gave birth to babies who had twice the level of mercury in their bodies as mothers with two or fewer fillings.[35]

In some cases, this heavy body load of mercury may interfere with the child's development. The child may be slow to reach developmental milestones, such as the age of first walking and talking. More severe effects such as incoordination or brain damage with mental retardation may also surface over time.

A Slap in the Face

Think of the days when it was considered fashionable to paint the face white with lead paint. Many of us now laugh at such obviously dangerous practices, and believe that today's cosmetics represent a huge step forward in both beauty and safety. But how safe is modern makeup really?

Recently, concern has been escalating over the use of mercury preservatives in children's vaccines. Many parents are rightly concerned since exposure to mercury is associated with a range of long-term, often irreversible, health problems. So great has been the concern that mercury-containing vaccines have now been recalled in the US, UK and elsewhere.

This concern, however, has not yet extended to the mercury-containing ingredients, such as phenylmercuric acetate, still commonly used in cosmetics. Indeed, the same preservative used in vaccines, thimerosal, can also be found in a wide range of toiletries including soap-free cleansers, antiseptic sprays, makeup remover, eye moisturisers and mascara. In these products, it is not usually called thimerosal, but one of its many synonyms, including mercurochrome, merthiolate, sodium ethylmercurithiosalicylate, thimerosalate, thiomerosalan, merzonin, mertorgan, ethyl (2-mercaptobenzoato-S), mercury sodium salt, merfamin or [(o-carboxyphenyl)thi] ethylmercury sodium salt.[36] A glance at this list and its easy to see how the use of mercury in products used on the eyes has escaped the attention of the vast majority of us.

A surprising percentage of cosmetics (75 percent in one study[37]) also contain a range of other toxic metals such as lead, cobalt, nickel and chromium and arsenic, most commonly as contaminants in pigments and talc. These metals can be absorbed through the skin or inhaled during application and as they degrade throughout the day.

Protect yourself

Both metallic and inorganic mercury can be brought into the home on clothes and shoes, so if you work with mercury on a regular basis, make sure you don't bring your work clothes home. If you do, bag and store them securely away from children and launder them separately from other clothes, making sure to rinse the washing machine afterwards. In addition, get into the habit of removing your shoes before entering your home to minimise tracked-in mercury dust. In addition:

- *Have your amalgam fillings replaced with composite fillings.*
  Metals in the mouth are released during everyday activities such as toothbrushing, drinking fruit juice or eating. Having mercury-containing fillings removed can be expensive – although there is no rule that says you have to do it all at one time. If you are planning on having a baby and want to have your mercury fillings removed, it is best to do this before conception. Don't attempt to have them removed during pregnancy since airborne particles of the drilled mercury can be inhaled and reenter your system. Instead, do what you can to reduce your mercury intake by, for instance, avoiding high-risk fish and mercury-containing cosmetics. Where possible, choose a dentist who runs a mercury-free practice. Every time you enter a conventional dentist's office – even if it's just for a clean – you are inhaling mercury vapour.
- *Limit your fish consumption*, and especially if you are pregnant. In the US, the Food and Drug Administration currently advises that pregnant women and women of childbearing age who may become pregnant should limit their consumption of high-risk fish such as shark and swordfish to no more that one meal per month. Other popular types of fish and seafood – shrimp, pollock, salmon, cod, catfish, clams, flatfish, crabs and scallops – are less polluted and may even contribute to overall levels of health (*see box on page 229 for more details*).
- *Foods high in selenium* or selenium supplements will afford some protection against mercury. Try including more Brazil nuts, tuna,

oysters, turkey, chicken, sole or flounder, wheatgerm, brown rice and oatmeal in your diet.

- *Check the wiring in your home.* Damaged electrical switches in the home may result in exposure to mercury vapours in indoor air.

- *Educate your children* about the dangers of playing with mercury (for instance, from a broken thermometer). Keep metallic mercury items in a safe and secured area (such as in a closed container in a locked storage area) so that children do not have access to them without the supervision of an adult.

- *Check your medicine cabinet.* Chemicals containing mercury, such as mercurochrome and thimerosal (sold as Merthiolate and other brands), are still used as antiseptics or as preservatives in eyedrops, eye ointments and nasal sprays. Some skin-lightening creams contain ammoniated mercuric chloride and mercuric iodide. Some traditional Chinese and Hispanic remedies for stomach disorders (for example, herbal balls) contain mercury and giving these remedies to your children may harm them. If you are pregnant or breastfeeding and use mercury-containing ethnic or herbal remedies, you could pass some of the mercury on to your unborn child or nursing infant.

- *Is that vaccination necessary?* The decision to vaccinate or not is a difficult one and can only be made with a full consideration of the facts. However, many parents throughout the world are beginning to question the effectiveness and necessity of routine childhood vaccinations. Certainly, you have a right to protect your child from vaccines that contain mercury. Indeed, throughout the world, mercury-containing vaccines are being recalled because they are not safe. If you are in doubt about the ingredients of any proposed vaccine, get your doctor to make a thorough check before your child is jabbed. In addition, parents may also wish to consider how necessary vaccines are for mild childhood illnesses such as measles and mumps and, where possible, refuse these. Many adult vaccines such as the flu jab are also of limited effectiveness. Don't take them without full consideration of the benefits and risks.

- *Dispose of mercury-containing items carefully.* Metallic mercury is used in a variety of household products and industrial items, including thermostats, fluorescent light bulbs, barometers, glass thermometers and some blood pressure-measuring devices. You must be careful when you handle and dispose of all items in the home that contain metallic mercury. Metallic mercury and its vapours are extremely difficult to remove from clothes, furniture, carpet, floors, walls and other such items. If these items are not properly cleaned, the mercury can remain for months or years and continue to be a source of exposure.

- *Be careful with spills.* If small amounts of mercury are spilled, be very careful during clean up. Do not try to vacuum spilled metallic mercury as this causes the mercury to evaporate into the air, creating a bigger health risk. On carpeted and uncarpeted floors, clean up the beads of metallic mercury by using one sheet of paper to carefully roll them onto a second sheet of paper, or using an eyedropper to suck up very small beads of mercury. After picking up the metallic mercury in this manner, put it into a plastic bag or airtight container. The paper and eyedropper should also be bagged in the same container. All plastic bags used in the clean up should then be taken outside and disposed of properly, according to instructions provided by your local health department or environmental officials. Try to ventilate the room with outside air, and close the room off from the rest of the home. Use fans to direct the air to the outside and away from the inside of the house for at least one hour to speed up the ventilation.

Cadmium

In everyday life, the most common source of cadmium is cigarette smoke. On average, smokers have four to five times higher blood cadmium concentrations and two to three times higher kidney cadmium concentrations than non-smokers. Despite this, exposure from passive smoke appears to only contribute minimally to cadmium exposure.

Nevertheless, cadmium can build up in our water and air (and consequently our food) from a number of other sources. Workers can be exposed to cadmium in air from the smelting and refining of metals, or from the air in plants that make cadmium products such as batteries, coatings or plastics, or when soldering or welding metal that contains cadmium.

Cadmium also has a number of uses in consumer and industrial products. Its principal uses include as a protective plating for steel, in electrode material in nickel–cadmium batteries and as a component of various alloys.[38] It is also present in phosphate fertilisers, fungicides and pesticides.

It can enter the air from burning fossil fuels, including automobile exhaust, and the incineration of household waste. Cadmium is also used as a stabiliser for polyvinyl chloride (PVC) and in the pigments (especially reds and oranges) used in plastics and paints. Our overuse and consequent incineration of plastics is thought to contribute significantly to increasing levels of cadmium in the environment.

In addition, there may be cadmium in refined cereal products such as white flour and bread, alcohol, oysters, gelatine, some canned foods, pigs' kidneys from animals treated with a wormkiller containing cadmium, and caffeinated drinks such as cola, tea and coffee.[39] Cadmium in the soil is taken up through the roots of plants and distributed to edible leaves, fruits and seeds,[40] and eventually passed on to humans and animals, where it can build up in milk and fatty tissues.[41]

Cadmium in the body

As with many metals, the route of exposure determines just how toxic cadmium is. Both the US Environmental Protection Agency and the International Agency for Research on Cancer (IARC) have concluded that cadmium, especially when inhaled, is carcinogenic to humans.

Some cooking implements such as enamelled pans and ceramics also contain cadmium and, if the products are poorly made, it can leach into food during cooking and storage. Many non-fatal cases of 'food poisoning' have followed ingestion of food kept for brief periods in these types of containers. Even so, ingestion is still considered the least risky type of exposure because cadmium is absorbed poorly through the gastrointestinal tract.

Inhalation is toxic because inhaled cadmium tends to bioaccumulate. When taken in via this route, cadmium can take anywhere from 10–30 years to clear from the body,[42] even after sources of exposure have been eliminated.

The traditional signs of cadmium overload in the body are yellow teeth, dry skin, chronic bronchitis and fatigue. Over time, it can also have a debilitating effect on the liver, kidneys,[43] bones and testes as well as on the immune and cardiovascular systems.[44]

Cadmium is also considered an endocrine disrupter. It has been shown to cause birth defects in mammals, and has been linked with both stillbirths and low birthweights. Cadmium has also been implicated in the increase in prostate cancer in men exposed to high levels such as welders, battery manufacturers and rubber workers.

Protect yourself

To avoid cadmium overload, take an inventory of items in and around your home that might contain cadmium. This may include fungicides (cadmium chloride), batteries (nickel–cadmium, or Ni-Cad batteries) and hobbies that use materials containing cadmium (electroplating or welding, fabric dyes, and ceramic and glass glazes). If you or your family members have a hobby where metals or materials that contain cadmium are being heated or welded, you should seek advice on proper ventilation of your workspace and the proper use of a safety respirator. In addition, consider the following measures:

- *Is your work polluting your home?* It is sometimes possible to carry cadmium-containing dust from work on your clothing, skin, hair, tools or other objects removed from the workplace. Without due care, you may contaminate your car, home or other locations outside work that children have access to. As with other toxic metals, try not to bring it home (*see advice under Lead*).

- *Think zinc.* Cadmium competes with zinc in the body and this may be one reason why men who work with cadmium have a higher rate of prostate cancer.[45] The prostate naturally concentrates zinc and, when levels are low, prostate health can be compromised. But it's not just men who should consider their zinc status. Studies show that most of us don't get enough zinc and this can have an adverse effect on immunity as well as make us vulnerable to cadmium overload. Natural sources of zinc include eggs, leafy green vegetables, nuts and seeds, seafood (especially shellfish), red meat and whole grains.
- *A balanced diet* that includes enough calcium, iron and protein will also help reduce the amount of cadmium that may be absorbed into the body from food or drink. Keep your diet low in refined, prepackaged and convenience foods that may also contain traces of cadmium.
- *Avoid cigarette smoke*, even the passive kind.
- *Consider changing your enamelled pans* since cadmium can be released during cooking.
- *Keep nickel–cadmium (Ni-Cad) batteries out of the reach of small children*, and teach your older children that the contents in Ni-Cad batteries can be harmful to their health if swallowed or burned. To prevent cadmium from being liberated into the environment, take advice from your local council on the safe and ecologically sound ways to dispose of these batteries. Better yet, consider using rechargeable batteries.
- *If you are using fungicides or fertilisers* that contain cadmium on your lawn or garden, read the instructions to learn the safe way to use these materials. It is very easy to inhale small particles of cadmium-containing dusts when using cadmium-containing fungicides or fertilisers. Wear protective safety gear, including dust masks, which can be bought at most hardware and building-supply stores. Remember not to track these products into your home after use, and keep children and pets away from treated lawns.
- *Water filters* – even simple, inexpensive jug types – can remove some cadmium as well as other metals from drinking water.

Thou Shalt Have a Fishy . . .

Fish is undeniably good food. Not only is it low in artery-clogging saturated fats, but it is rich in artery-friendly omega-3 oils. All fish contains these heart-healthy oils, though fatty, cold-water varieties are the richest sources – a good reason not to shun high-fat fish such as salmon. Research suggests eating fish regularly can reduce the risk of sudden cardiac death, improve blood pressure and blood fat levels. It can also reduce some of the symptoms of rheumatoid arthritis.

But as our oceans become more polluted, so have our fish and, these days, a high fish intake comes with a caution because of the threat of mercury contamination.

Almost all fish contain some mercury, but it's only a significant problem in large predators like shark, swordfish and large species of tuna (used mostly for fresh steaks or sushi). Much less mercury is found in the smaller species of tuna typically used for canning. Nevertheless, there is evidence that eating more than 30 g of high-mercury fish daily may double the risk of coronary heart disease.[46]

Fish, even those from the deepest, coldest parts of the ocean, also harbour dioxins and other industrial contaminants like polychlorinated biphenyls (PCBs). These substances can promote cancer, damage the immune system and interfere with hormone function.

So which fish are safe to eat? Since fish is such an excellent food, some scientists consider that any risk posed by mercury and other industrial contamination is outweighed by the nutritional benefits.[47] Nevertheless, to be on the safe side, choose small fish – those lower down in the aquatic food chain – to limit mercury exposure.

Consume no more than seven ounces a week of large fish like shark, swordfish and fresh tuna (pregnant women should limit their intake to once a month). Remove visible fat (and skin, when possible) from fish before cooking to limit exposure to dioxin and PCBs. Bake or broil on a rack or grill to let the fat drip away. Varying your fish choices will also help to limit your exposure to any one chemical contaminant.

Eating up to 2.2 pounds (1 kg) of less-polluted fish – shrimp, pollock, salmon, cod, catfish, clams, flatfish, crabs and scallops – per week is considered both safe and healthful.

Aluminium

A certain amount of aluminium is naturally present in our food and drinking water. But these days, pollution-induced acid rain is causing more aluminium than normal to be dissolved in groundwater. In addition, water treatment plants use aluminium sulphate as an antibiotic, and to remove suspended clays and silts from drinking water. This use can increase the level of aluminium in water and on our land by up to five times.

Some people are exposed to aluminium when they ingest medicinal products like antacids and buffered aspirins. The amount of aluminium in some antacids can be as much as 200 mg per tablet. Aluminium compounds are also added to vaccines (both childhood and adult) to boost their effectiveness.

Some cosmetics and toiletries contain aluminium-based preservatives or, in the case of antiperspirants, active aluminium ingredients. Many processed foods – such as processed cheese – and cakes contain aluminium-based preservatives and additives (like baking powder). Aluminium is also used as an anticaking or bleaching agent in foods you use every day such as salt, milk substitutes and flour. Soy-based infant formula may also contain moderate amounts of aluminium, and food stored in aluminium containers or wrapped in aluminium foil (especially if it is fatty or acid) will absorb some of this metal.

Your Daily Cuppa

Moderate consumption of any kind of tea can be part of a healthy lifestyle. But as with any food, the quality of the product you consume and your ability to moderate your intake seems to hold the key to maximising its benefits.

More urgent than caffeine content is the problem of heavy metals and pollution in both black and green teas. According to estimates from the Ministry of Agriculture, Fisheries and Food (MAFF), the average adult aluminium intake in Britain is around 5–6 mg per day. Around half of this comes from drinking tea.[48] Levels are particularly high in teas from Assam, Darjeeling, Ceylon and some supermarket blends, which contain more aluminium in their leaves than do other teas. Aluminium can also be present in tapwater.

British scientists have concluded that there is between 2–6 mg of aluminium per litre in brewed teas[49] and, because of the way aluminium molecules bind to organic matter in tea, they can in theory become highly bioavailable.[50] Water quality also has some effect on the release of aluminium during infusion. For instance, tea samples brewed using soft tapwater tend to have higher levels of aluminium than those brewed in hard water.

The good news, however, is that the tannins in tea appear to mitigate the effect of the high aluminium content of tea.[51] Drinking tea with milk rather than lemon also reduces aluminium absorption.[52]

Tea drinkers should also consider what else they are getting when the brew up. Conventional tea production means that tea plants are sprayed liberally with pesticides and that their soil is treated with a range of chemical fertilisers. The first brew off any teabag or handful of leaves may produce nothing more than a cup full of toxic sludge. For this reason, those wishing to get the best out of any kind of tea should consider switching to organic brands.

Aluminium in the body

Although aluminium is generally lumped in with the 'heavy' metals such as lead and mercury, it is, in fact, one of the lightest metals on the planet. Equally, although it is present in high concentrations in the earth's crust, no biological role for this metal in the human body has been recognised. For years, scientists considered aluminium non-toxic except at extremely high levels. Recent evidence, however, suggests that it may be implicated in a wide range of conditions from dementia to cancer.[53]

Many body systems can also be affected by high aluminium exposure. Common symptoms of toxicity include respiratory disorders, cough, weakness, fatigue, aching muscles, rickets, osteoporosis, skin reactions (from aluminium antiperspirants), liver and gastrointestinal complaints, and hyperactivity and other emotional disturbances in children.

Aluminium phosphate and aluminium hydroxide are added to vaccines such as the DPT (diphtheria–pertussis–tetanus) to improve their effectiveness. Studies show that some people are extremely sensitive and may experience allergic-type reactions to these vaccines.[54]

However, it is the recent link made between Alzheimer's disease and aluminium that has grabbed most of our attention. Aluminium is a potent neurotoxin that can penetrate the blood–brain barrier and accumulate in the central nervous system (brain and spinal cord). Studies of workers who inhale aluminium dusts or aluminium fumes show measurable decreases in neurological function.[55]

There is now evidence that people with Alzheimer's disease have significantly higher (in some cases, double) blood aluminium levels than healthy people of similar ages or, indeed, those with other types of dementia.[56] [57] What's more, as the levels of aluminium in the body go up, so does the level of central nervous system degeneration. For instance, in areas with higher aluminium content in the drinking water, the incidence of Alzheimer's also goes up – in some cases, by as much as 46 percent.[58]

A lifetime's use of aluminium-containing antiperspirants – but not the use of antiperspirants and deodorants in general – has also been associated with a risk of Alzheimer's dementia and, once again, the greater the exposure, the more the risk rises.[59] This relationship, however, does not appear to extend to aluminium-containing antacids, although these have been shown to induce calcium loss by increasing urinary excretion of this mineral.[60] Calcium loss is, of course, a risk factor for osteoporosis.

Similarly, patients receiving dialysis and whose tapwater contains significant levels of aluminium have been found to develop osteomalacia, a weakening of the bones. This effect has been observed in North America, Australia and Europe.[61] These patients also have a greater tendency to develop dialysis encephalopathy, a disease resembling Alzheimer's.

Protect yourself

It can be difficult to minimise the exposure to aluminium no matter how careful you are. Nevertheless, there are certain things you can do to help.

- *Avoid ingesting large quantities of aluminium* such as aluminium hydroxide-containing antacids (Maalox) and buffered aspirin. In addition, these products should have childproof caps so that children will not accidentally ingest them. Families should also be aware that soya-based infant formulas may contain high levels of aluminium and may want to consult their physician on an alternative choice of formula.
- *Steer clear of cooking utensils made from this metal.* Every time you cook in an aluminium saucepan, you expose yourself to this

toxic metal. If the food you are cooking is acidic (such as apples, spinach or rhubarb), it can release more metal into the food. Many pressure cookers are made with aluminium and this cooking method can also concentrate the metal in your food. Try using stainless-steel cookware instead.

- *If you use aluminium foil or containers*, make sure the foil coverings are not touching fatty foods during cooking. Keep your use of foods heated in tin foil or served up in freezer-to-oven foil trays to a minimum. If you do use them, transfer their contents to glass containers before cooking.

- *Avoid foods with added aluminium.* These include bleached white-flour products and foods containing the additives E556 (aluminium calcium silicate), E173 (aluminium; CI77000) or E554 (aluminium sodium silicate).

- *Foods rich in manganese* such as whole grains, green vegetables, nuts, peas and eggs will help counteract the harmful effects of aluminium.

- *Avoid aluminium-containing antiperspirants.* If you don't tend to sweat heavily anyway, consider using a deodorant rather than an antiperspirant. Healthfood shops stock a wide range of aluminium-free deodorants. Beware, however, of rock-crystal deodorants, some of which contain ammonium alum (aluminium sulphate). Labels on these products are rarely instructive so, if in doubt, check with the manufacturer.

- *Check bottled-water labels.* Aluminium levels should be low. Some bottled-water companies provide an analysis of the aluminium content of their water. You might also find out from your public water company what the aluminium level is in the local drinking water. If levels are high (over 200 ppb, or parts per billion), consider using a jug-type water filter or installing an under-sink filter (*see Chapter 10 for more details*).

- *Silica might help.* High levels of silicic acid in drinking water do appear to protect against the adverse effects of aluminium ingestion.[62] Whether silica supplements such as gels that you rub into your gums can protect against the development of dementia, however, has yet to be determined.

- *Use minerals.* Ensuring adequate levels of calcium, magnesium and zinc – either in your diet or through supplementation – should help protect against aluminium accumulation.[63] Deficiencies of these important minerals are common among the elderly[64] and in low-income populations,[65] and supplementation may protect these individuals.

Arsenic

Arsenic is not a true metal, but a semi-metallic compound that can enter the atmosphere as a consequence of arsenic, tin and copper mining and smelting. Indeed, a thousand-year history of mining and smelting has left a legacy of arsenic pollution in Devon and Cornwall in the UK. During the last half of the nineteenth century, Cornwall was the world's largest producer of arsenic,[66] and the soil in some parts of Cornwall has the world's highest concentrations of arsenic.

Similarly, the largest mass poisoning in history involved arsenic. It occurred in Bangladesh as a result of arsenic that had leached into deep wells dug by well-meaning aid agencies in the 1970s and 1980s. Arsenic poisoning now affects more than 77 million people and causes 3000 deaths a year.

Throughout the rest of the world, arsenic is used as an alloy in the lead-acid batteries used in automobiles; it is also used in semiconductors and light-emitting diodes. Some pesticides also contain arsenic. Long before organochlorine and organophosphate pesticides became widespread, arsenic-based pesticides were the most common type used in agriculture. Organic arsenicals – namely, cacodylic acid, disodium methylarsenate (DSMA), and monosodium methylarsenate (MSMA) – are still used as pesticides, mostly on cotton. Arsenic in the form of lead arsenate is no longer used in vineyards and orchards. However, its legacy is a lasting one; significant lead arsenate residues can still be found in older orchards.[67]

However, it is through pressure-treated woods that we now get our biggest exposure to this toxic substance. At present, about 90 percent of all arsenic produced is used as a wood preservative – namely, chromated copper arsenate (CCA).

CCA is poisonous to humans, and manufacturers admit that it easily leaches out of treated wood. Very young children, who are always putting their hands into their mouths, can ingest up to 2016 microgrammes of arsenic per day from just playing on treated wood. To put this into perspective, the maximum safe amount of arsenic for a 25-pound child is 3.4 microgrammes per day. CCA also leaches into the surrounding soil, where it eventually gets into the groundwater.

Arsenic in the body

Inorganic arsenic (the same stuff now found in pesticides and wood preservatives) has been recognised as a human poison since ancient times, with large oral doses capable of causing death. Particularly high levels can accumulate in the body when the kidneys are not functioning normally.

Chronic low exposure can produce irritation of your stomach and intestines, with symptoms such as stomachache, nausea, vomiting and diarrhoea. Other effects associated with swallowing inorganic arsenic include a decreased production of red and white blood cells leading to fatigue, abnormal heart rhythm, blood-vessel damage and impaired nerve function causing a 'pins-and-needles' sensation in the hands and feet.

There is also strong evidence to suggest an association between chronic arsenic exposure and an increased risk of peripheral nervous disorders such as high blood pressure and cardiovascular disease as well as diabetes.

Perhaps the single most characteristic effect of long-term oral exposure to inorganic arsenic (and one widely observed in countries such as Bangladesh, Taiwan and Chile) is a pattern of skin changes. After a few years of continued low-level arsenic exposure, skin disorders such as melanosis (the appearance of white and/or dark patches) and horny growths (papules) on the skin of the hands and feet (known as keratosis) begin to appear. After a latency period of 20–30 years, internal cancers – particularly of the bladder and lung – may also appear.

In fact, arsenic is a recognised carcinogen that is specifically implicated in liver, lung, bladder, kidney and prostate cancers.[68] The risk of lung cancer is particularly high in workers exposed to arsenic at smelters, mines and chemical factories, but also in residents living near such smelters and chemical factories. People who live near waste sites including arsenic may have an increased risk of lung cancer as well.

Similarly, the evidence linking arsenic-based pesticides with skin and lung cancer is both strong and persuasive.[69] This increased cancer risk has not been associated with eating food containing residues, but with inhalation via occupational exposure – for instance, in professional pesticide sprayers and among workers in pesticide-manufacturing plants.

Protect yourself
To avoid arsenic exposure in everyday life, consider the following:

- *Pressure-treated wood* used in playground equipment, decking, picnic tables, park benches and the wooden frames used in garden beds can contain high levels of arsenic, and pose the greatest threat to young children. Avoid these if you can; if you can't, take evasive action. Seal arsenic-treated wood structures every year with polyurethane or some other hard lacquer. Cover picnic tables with a coated tablecloth. Make sure children and adults wash their hands after being in contact with arsenic-treated surfaces, playgrounds or picnic areas, particularly before eating.
- *Workplace exposure* is the most common source of higher-than-average levels of arsenic in adults. Speak to your health and safety officer to make sure that levels in your workplace are monitored and kept at or below permissible levels. In addition, follow guidelines for keeping work clothes separate from other clothes in the home (*see under Lead, page 216*).
- *Check labels* for unexpected arsenic. This includes wood treatment and insecticide/weedkiller products and fireplace logs that produce multicoloured flames. Even if it's not on the label, it may still contain arsenic; this may be the case with wine – older vineyards may

still be contaminated with arsenates – and tobacco products – the plants are sometimes sprayed with arsenic-containing pesticides.

- *Avoid medicines containing arsenic.* Until the 1940s, arsenicals such as Salvarsan and Fowler's solution were widely used in the treatment of various diseases such as syphilis and psoriasis. Arsenic can still be found in some Chinese patented medicines. Arsenic trioxide (Trisenox) is used as a conventional anticancer medicine, and the antiparasitic veterinary drug carbasone also contains arsenic.
- *Measure the arsenic levels* in any groundwater intended for human use. Your local water authority can advise you on how this can be done.

Copper

Copper is naturally present in many foods and is a necessary element in our diet. It is typically found in mineral-rich foods like vegetables (potatoes), legumes (beans and peas), nuts (peanuts and pecans), grains (wheat and rye), fruits (peaches and raisins) and even chocolate.

However, environmental sources are rapidly accumulating and too much copper can be as devastating to health as too little. Natural sources of copper in the environment include windblown dust from native soils, volcanoes, decaying vegetation, forest fires and sea spray. But copper also enters the environment as pollution.

If you work in the copper-mining industry or the processing of copper ore, you are exposed to copper by breathing copper-containing dust or on skin contact. If you grind or weld copper metal, you may breathe in high levels of copper in dust and fumes. Other at-risk occupations include working in industries such as agriculture, water treatment and electroplating, where soluble copper compounds are used. People living near these industries will also be affected.

Some people are exposed to high levels of soluble copper in their drinking water, especially if the water is corrosive, and they have copper plumbing and brass water fixtures. Copper sulphate is often sprayed on crops to kill yeast and fungus, which means higher levels of copper in our foods as well as run-offs that contaminate our water supply. It is also used in the production of phosphate fertilisers.

Copper is often used in intrauterine devices (IUDs) and the women who wear them may experience a steep increase in blood levels of copper. If you swim in pools or use hot tubs, you may be exposed to copper-containing algaecides used to control yeast and bacterial growth. Beer and wine drinkers may also ingest more copper than normal because these drinks are filtered with copper sulphides.

Copper in the body

Minute doses of copper are essential for good health and can even protect against the effects of more toxic metals such as cadmium and lead. Nevertheless, exposure to higher levels can be harmful. If you drink water that contains higher than 30 ppm of copper, you may experience headaches, dizziness, vomiting, diarrhoea, stomach cramps and nausea. Long-term exposure to copper dust in air can irritate the nose, mouth and eyes, and cause headaches, dizziness, nausea and diarrhoea. Excess copper is also associated with brain dysfunction,[70] depression[71] and schizophrenia.[72]

Other, more rare disorders linked to excess copper include gout pain, inflammation of finger and toe joints, restlessness, altered metabolism, oedema, kidney dysfunction, premature birth, hyper- or hypothyroidism, sinusitis, poor hearing, and eye, tongue or limb spasms. Intentionally high intakes of copper can cause liver and kidney damage, and even death.

In younger children, copper toxicity is associated with attention-deficit disorder (ADD), both with and without hyperactivity. Heart-attack patients have been found to have high levels of copper in the blood.[73] It may also have a role to play in the development of Alzheimer's disease.[74]

Although copper has not been classified as a human carcinogen, Japanese studies indicate that high copper levels may create an environment in the body that promotes the growth of some cancers.[75] Research from the US has also implicated excess copper with a twofold increase in liver cancer, possibly due to free-radical damage to the liver.[76]

Protect yourself

Some measures you can take to reduce your exposure to copper include:

- *Run the tap* if you haven't used it for a while. The greatest potential source of copper exposure for most of us is through drinking water, especially in water that is first drawn in the morning after sitting in copper piping and brass faucets overnight. Corrosion can release more copper than is healthy into your home water supply. This is more likely if your house or apartment is less than five years old, the water is soft and it sits in the pipes undisturbed for several hours. To reduce copper in drinking water, run the water for at least 15–30 seconds before using it.
- *How old are your pipes?* Scientific studies show that copper plumbing keeps drinking water clean by keeping down microbial growth, and reduces the need for overly aggressive water treatment to keep the water clean. However, if you are suffering the effects of copper excess, it may be time to replace old copper pipes with plastic ones.
- *Turn down the heat* in the shower or bath. Steam can vaporise copper and other even more dangerous toxins and make them more easily inhaled.
- *Copper pans and kettles* may also be a source of copper. Modern-day copper cookware, which usually has an inner cooking surface of another material like tin or stainless steel, does not release copper and is safe for use in food preparation. However, prolonged contact with older copper pots or cooking utensils, especially if the food is acidic, can dissolve enough copper to cause acute toxicity symptoms such as nausea, vomiting and diarrhoea.
- *Eat organic.* Many insecticides and other sprays that are used in the food industry contain copper, especially those used on fruits and vegetables. Be aware that this is also true of organic foods which can, under certain circumstances, be treated with fungicides such as copper hydroxide, copper oxychloride, copper sulphate and cuprous oxide.

- *Have your copper IUD removed* as it can contribute substantially to higher blood levels of copper. IUDs are also implicated in spreading the bacteria that lead to pelvic inflammatory disease (PID) and other pelvic infections. For these reasons, you may wish to consider another form of contraception.
- *Supplement.* Minerals such as zinc, manganese and iron can prevent copper from being absorbed. Vitamins B6 and folic acid, selenium and cysteine may also be helpful.
- *Copper chelators* are substances that bind to and aid the removal of copper from the body. Useful and relatively non-toxic copper chelators include vitamin C, molybdenum and sulphur-containing amino acids as well as the amino acid glutathione. More powerful chelators may be used, but can have side-effects (*see Chapter 10*).

Manganese

Manganese is another mineral element that is both nutritionally essential and potentially toxic. Like aluminium, it is technically not a 'heavy' metal.

Most reports of manganese toxicity in otherwise healthy people have come from people who inhaled manganese dust at their place of work – for instance, welders, steel workers, railroad workers, miners and those who handle pesticides such as maneb and mancozeb.[77] However, living near a factory, plant or agricultural area that works with manganese can expose average individuals to higher-than-normal levels of manganese.

Other sources of exposure are now recognised. Manganese is found in such everyday items as the common dry-cell battery, fertilisers, welding rods, incandescent light bulbs, magnets and certain bronzes. Manganese ores, and the chemicals made from them, are used as colouring agents for bricks, glass and ceramic products as well as in dyes, paints and varnishes. It is found in fungicides and pharmaceuticals, and many minerals, including carbonates, oxides, silicates and borates, contain manganese. It is added to animal and poultry feeds.

If manganese compounds, either naturally occurring, or from a factory or hazardous waste site, get into the drinking water, you could be exposed to unhealthy levels. You may also be exposed by eating non-organic foods that have been sprayed with manganese-containing pesticides. Patients who are being fed intravenously with total parenteral nutrition (TPN) may receive excessively high levels of manganese[78] as will infants who are bottlefed.

Indeed, studies show that infant formulas, particularly those based on soya, contain substantially (up to 200 times) more manganese than breastmilk. Whether these higher amounts of manganese are unhealthy for the infant is unknown. Some believe that the infant's immature liver simply cannot handle the load, though the long-term effects of this are poorly researched.

The potential role of manganese as an environmental toxin has grown during the last decade since the magnesium-containing additive methylcyclopentadienyl manganese tricarbonyl (MMT) has become an additive in unleaded petrol.[79] You will be exposed to higher levels of MMT if you live in a major urban area where such petrol is used, if you have a job in which you make or have contact with that petrol every day (such as a motor mechanic) or if you are exposed to a high amount of car exhaust on a daily basis (for instance, at bus stops or at petrol stations).

The crucial question is whether manganese exposure from all these sources can lead to toxic effects. Some scientists believe it can.

Manganese in the body

Manganese is present in many foods, including grains and cereals, and is found in high concentrations in tea. Small amounts of manganese each day keep us healthy. However, too much manganese can cause serious illness.

The symptoms of manganese toxicity generally appear slowly over a period of months or years. Exposure to high levels of manganese injures the part of the brain that helps control body movements; miners or steel workers exposed to high levels of manganese dust in air for many years may suffer from a degenerative disease called 'manganism'. This is similar to Parkinson's disease, and includes feelings of weakness and lethargy, and can progress to other symptoms such as speech disturbances, a mask-like face and tremors.[80]

The symptoms of manganism are also similar to those of Creutzfeldt–Jakob disease (CJD), and links have been made between the manganese in animal feeds and the occurrence of what has been dubbed 'mad-cow disease' (*see Chapter 6 for more details*). While some of the symptoms of manganism may improve with treatment, most of the brain injury is permanent.[81] [82]

You don't need to be occupationally exposed to manganese, however, to be harmed by it. Animal evidence suggests that high levels of exposure to environmental manganese (in the soil, water, air or food) may increase the chances of birth defects.[81] Other evidence suggests that children who drink water and eat food with higher-than-usual levels of manganese are less coordinated and do more poorly in school than non-exposed children.[81]

There are also studies showing that people who drink water containing high concentrations of manganese can develop symptoms similar to those seen in manganese miners and steel workers.[83]

Similarly, chronic non-occupational exposure to high levels of manganese by inhalation can also result in nervous system damage.[84] Unlike ingested manganese, inhaled manganese is transported directly to the brain before it can be metabolised in the liver.[85] A recent study showed that older people who inhaled manganese from the air and who had high levels of manganese in their blood showed signs of neurological problems similar to those reported in occupationally exposed individuals.[81]

More distressing is the evidence that this manganese-induced parkinsonism is permanent and progressive; even after the sources of manganese have been withdrawn from the person's environment, the neurological damage continues to increase [86] – a finding that underscores the importance of early avoidance.

Protect yourself

As with all toxic metals, the best protection is to avoid exposure – not easy if you work in an industry that uses or produces this element. To be on the safe side:

- *If you work in an industry that uses manganese,* speak to your health and safety officer to make sure you are being protected.
- *Eat organic* to avoid the pesticides maneb and mancozeb, which are used on a wide variety of produce.
- *Buy a water filter.* This will help filter out a range of heavy metals.
- *Breastfeed your baby.* Paediatricians and other experts agree that human milk is the only milk suitable for human babies. Breastfeeding boosts immunity and helps protect the developing neurological system while protecting against the excessive manganese consumption associated with some formulas.
- *Avoid ceramic dishes* and cookware as these can leach manganese into food.
- *Some commercially available antiseptics* – for instance, potassium permanganate – contain manganese. Use safer alternatives such as natural tea tree, lavender oil or grapefruitseed extract. You can even make a simple, safe and effective saline antiseptic solution by putting two teaspoons of salt into a litre of boiling water, and allowing this to cool before use.

10 A Final Word: Supporting the Process from A to Z

MUCH OF THIS BOOK IS DEVOTED TO EXPOSING THE MAJOR TOXINS that affect health and making recommendations for how best to avoid these. Avoiding toxic exposures is the single most important step to regaining your health. However, if you have been chronically exposed over many years, your body may need additional help to begin functioning optimally again.

Many books have been written on ways to improve your health, including fasting and detox, immune support and diet. Not all the recommendations in these books have been proven to work; indeed, most of them simply reflect the latest fads. Fasting is a good example. While fasting is generally purported to be the best way to energise the body and aid detoxification, this is not necessarily so. Fasting can, under some circumstances, cause harm by releasing large amounts of toxins into the system, where they are free to cause damage to organs such as the kidneys and liver. For most of us, sweaty exercise and saunas are probably better alternatives.

This A to Z looks at the range of therapies and activities you can use to help minimise the effects of toxic exposures. The star ratings (maximum of five) are based on how much evidence there is for their effectiveness as well as how easy they are to incorporate into your life. The more stars the option has, the more likely it will help keep you well and help your body fight off the effects of toxic exposures. Incorporate as many of these activities as you can, as often as you can, into your regular routine to improve your overall health and bolster your body's defences against a toxic world.

Avoidance
★★★★★

The absolute best way to minimise your exposure to environmental toxins is to consciously practice avoidance. This can mean identifying allergies and avoiding those things that trigger them. It can mean not inhaling nicotine or overindulging in caffeine and alcohol. It can include avoiding toxic chemicals like fluoride and the volatile organic compounds found in most cleaning products, toiletries and perfumes. It can mean buying organic, using natural wood in preference to plastic, using natural pest repellents in the home and garden, and seeking out paints and other types of home decoration that are low in toxins. You have more control over this than you probably realise, and doing whatever you can to lower your exposure to toxins will have a greatly beneficial effect on your health in both the short and long term.

Breathe
★★★★☆

Breathing properly can help clear the lungs and bloodstream of toxins. It is also relaxing and so lowers levels of stress hormones, and encourages the immune system to work more efficiently. Getting more oxygen into the lungs is reputed to have the knock-on effect of improving the function of the eliminatory organs such as the liver and kidneys as well as the digestive tract. Oxygen-rich blood also feeds the nervous system, in particular the brain, which requires three times more oxygen to function than other organs in the body.

Unfortunately, most people breathe in a shallow, inefficient way that reduces oxygen consumption and, therefore, the available benefits of breathing.

When the breath is shallow, the lungs are not taking in sufficient oxygen and are not eliminating sufficient carbon dioxide. As a result, the body becomes oxygen-starved, allowing toxins to build up. In addition, shallow breathing does not exercise the lungs enough and so reduces their ability to function optimally, creating a vicious circle of lost vitality.

There are several reasons for the inefficient way most of us breathe. These include:

- *Fast-paced lifestyle.* Where the body goes, the breath will follow. When our bodies and minds are in a rush, our breathing will also be rushed.
- *Stress.* When we are under stress, our fight-or-flight responses cause our breath to become more shallow.
- *Emotions* such as depression, anxiety and fear can affect the rate of breathing, causing it to be fast and shallow.
- *Modern technology* and automation reduces our need for physical activity. Without physical activity, there is little need to breathe deeply.
- *Too much time spent indoors.* We work and spend most of our leisure time indoors and this increases our exposure to pollution. In addition, there is a belief that when the body is in a polluted environment, it instinctively inhales less air – taking in just enough air to tick over – to protect itself from the pollution.

The benefits of breathing correctly are receiving more and more scientific interest. Yogic breathing, or *pranayama*, which is slow, rhythmic and focused on the outbreath, has produced a wide range of benefits in recent studies. Practices that involve breathing through the nostrils have been found to both stimulate and relax the sympathetic nervous system.[1] This type of breathing is also invigorating,[2] and able to increase oxygen consumption and boost metabolism.[3] The practice of yoga can also help with blood-glucose control.[4] Similarly, studies into *qigong* breathing exercises have shown that these promote up to 20 percent better oxygen consumption.[5]

To get the best out of deep breathing, try not to do it somewhere too polluted. Deep breathing on the high street or at the bus stop may not give your lungs the treat they need. Instead, take a walk in the park, get out into the country or go to the seaside. Better yet – and more convenient – make your home a toxin-free zone where you can practice deep-breathing exercises in peace and comfort. With practice, your breathing will become more efficient, naturally, wherever you are.

Chelation

☆☆☆

Chelation (pronounced *key-lay-shun*) therapy uses a variety of substances to remove toxic metals from the body. These substances bind to metals like lead, cadmium and arsenic, as well as other toxic substances, and help remove them from the body. Chelation therapy is extensively documented in the medical literature, and is recognised as a legitimate treatment for lead poisoning. It has also been used to reverse hardening of the arteries.

The body does have its own natural chelation processes – digestion, assimilation, transport of food nutrients, and the formation of enzymes and hormones – as well as its own detoxification channels. However, when the amount of metal in the body becomes too high for the body to deal with by itself, chelation may be necessary.

The most well-known chelator is EDTA (ethylenediaminetetraacetic acid), an amino acid that is generally administered via an intravenous solution. EDTA binds to calcium deposits in the arteries and is used in cases of atherosclerosis, where it has a more than 80 percent success rate. It can also remove lead (but not mercury) from the body. Intravenous EDTA is less expensive and less invasive than surgery, and there is evidence to suggest that EDTA can also be useful for aneurysm, Alzheimer's disease and senile dementia, arthritis, autoimmune disorders, cancer, cataracts, diabetes, emphysema, gallstones, hypertension, kidney stones, Lou Gehrig's disease, osteoporosis, Parkinson's disease, scleroderma, stroke, varicose veins, venomous snake bite, and other conditions involving an interruption in blood flow and diminished oxygen delivery.[6]

Intravenous EDTA is probably best reserved for those whose bodies are very polluted and who need urgent detoxification. Although non-toxic, EDTA can produce side-effects in some people. These include burning, redness and swelling at the injection site, fever, hypotension (low blood pressure), joint pain, skin outbreaks or rashes, upset stomach and, rarely, irritation of the kidneys and liver.[7] People who are debilitated, emaciated, have weak or diseased kidneys, or advanced cardiovascular disease (end stage) are probably not good candidates for intravenous chelation as a sudden, massive infusion of EDTA may put too much stress on the kidneys, liver and detoxification pathways in these individuals. However, there are some therapists that dispute this and say that professionally administered chelation poses little threat.

Stronger metal chelators such as DMPS (2,3-dimercapto-1-propanesulphonic acid) or DMSA should only be used under a doctor's supervision and are even outlawed in some places.

Oral chelation using nutritional food supplements containing chelating agents (such as EDTA, but also numerous natural chelators such as vitamins, minerals, amino acids, antioxidants, phytonutrients and herbs) can also be effective, but will be a slower process. This is because only 4–18 percent of an oral EDTA dose is absorbed (compared with 100 percent of an intravenous dose).[8] Nevertheless, some oral chelation formulas have the ability to chemically bond with and bring about the elimination of mercury and other metals from the body. The addition of vitamins, minerals, enzymes and antioxidants may make oral chelation a less harmful process and more supportive of the body. While taking chelators, you should do all that you can to support the body and avoid unnecessary sources of toxins. (*For more information, see Detox, Exercise, Functional Foods and Juice.*)

Detox and Fasting

☆☆

Detoxification is an ongoing process that removes wastes and toxins from the body whether you are eating or not. In a healthy person, it is the job of the liver and kidneys to detoxify the body. Supported by a healthy lifestyle, these organs are supremely capable of doing their job.

Nevertheless, detox is a major buzzword in the health industry. Go into any healthfood shop and you will find any number of 'detox in a box' products. Most of these are as useless as they are expensive.

If you wish to detox, here are some points to consider that will help you achieve a better result:

- *Why do you want to detox?* Have you been exposed to a specific identifiable toxin, such as dental amalgam? Do you work in a job that regularly exposes you to solvents and other VOCs? If so, over-the-counter products are unlikely to help. You should be detoxing under the supervision of a practitioner who can tailor a regime to suit your individual needs.
- *There's more to detox than loose bowels and an overstimulated bladder.* Most commercial detox mixtures are little more than combinations of laxative and diuretic herbs. While this may aid elimination up to a point, it does little to deal with the deeper problems of accumulated toxins – for instance, those stored in fatty tissues. What's more, long-term use of laxatives and diuretics can substantially skew the normal mineral balance of the body.
- *Think green.* Green foods, rather than fruit-based products, have a better reputation for aiding detox (*see Juice for more information*).
- *Have a regular sauna* – dry or steam saunas heat the body tissues several inches below the skin, enhancing all your metabolic processes. When all of your skin's sweat glands are working well, they can perform as much detoxification as one (or both) kidneys.

Increased sweating increases the elimination of salt and water through the skin as well as of metals (such as nickel, copper, zinc and lead),[9] toxic volatile hydrocarbons (including benzene, styrene, toluene, trichloroethylene and PCBs),[10] pesticides (such as DDT and DDE) and other toxins.[11]

• *Keep it simple.* Vast mixtures of herbs in detox formulas may not be any more effective than a carefully chosen mixture of three or four. If in doubt, always consult a qualified herbalist.

Many people combine fasts with detox regimes. Often, detox in conjunction with fasting is used in clinical practice to treat a range of disorders such as rheumatoid arthritis,[12] high cholesterol[13] and pancreatitis.[14] Detox may also be helpful for some psychiatric disorders such as depression and schizophrenia.[15]

In cases of extreme poisoning such as acute exposure to PCBs, fasting may aid the process of detoxification.[16] However, there is little to suggest that, in a healthy person, fasting is necessary to boost the power of a detox.

Nevertheless, if you choose to fast, it is helpful to know that the success of a fast depends on many factors, including the type and length of fast, and your overall level of health. Contrary to popular belief, fasting is not a good way to lose weight nor a permanent way to detoxify the body. It is a short-term intervention that must be followed-up by good health practices to maintain any benefits.

At best, fasting can provide your body with a physiological break that enables it to divert more energy to the process of removing waste and restoring balance. Under proper supervision, fasting can be constructive and uplifting. Gone into without forethought and for prolonged periods of time, it can weaken and even kill.

Safe fasting

Most people can safely fast for a short period of time without undue harm to the body. If you are considering a short fast of three to five days, there are guidelines that can help it be more beneficial.

- Prepare for your fast the day before by making your last meal one of fruits and vegetables; some authorities recommend that your diet the day before a fast should be vegan.
- Only water should be consumed while fasting, and the quantity of water should be dictated by thirst. You should not consume coffee, tea, juice, soft drinks, cigarettes or anything else by mouth. Herbal teas can be supportive of a fast, but they should not be sweetened.
- Fasting should not be combined with vigorous exercise, though short walks in the fresh air may be beneficial. Conserve your energy to maximise healing. Try to take a nap or two during the day.
- Avoid exposures to chemicals such as those contained in toiletries as these add to your body's toxic burden. Instead, consider washing simply with lukewarm water.
- Try to avoid extremes of temperature. Your body temperature may drop during a fast so make sure that you stay warm.
- If the sun is out, try to get 10–20 minutes a day of exposure.
- When you are ready to break your fast, do so slowly by choosing small quantities of food (fruits and vegetables are ideal) at room temperature. Eat slowly and chew thoroughly.

When not to fast

Most authorities agree that a detox regime with or without fasting is unlikely to harm the body and can even be healthful. However, there are some situations and some people for whom fasting is not recommended. Don't detox or fast when you are stressed or depressed. Similarly, detox of a seriously polluted body can have implications for the health of vital organs such as the kidneys and liver, so find a qualified practitioner before starting.

If you have diabetes, ulcers or liver, kidney, heart or lung disease, advanced cancer or a compromised immune system, you should not fast or take herbal remedies unless advised to do so by a qualified practitioner. Those taking medications should also not fast as this can alter the potency of some drugs.

Detoxification programmes are also not recommended for pregnant or breastfeeding women[17] or for children and infants.[18] The time to detox is before you become pregnant and after your baby has stopped breastfeeding.

Exercise

☆☆☆☆☆

Our bodies are designed to be used. When we don't use them to their optimal extent, muscles deteriorate, metabolism becomes sluggish and breathing becomes shallow. For all these reasons, it is desirable to develop good, sensible habits of exercise – whether they are aerobic routines, an active lifestyle or weight training – that you can easily incorporate into your life for the rest of your life.

Over the years, many studies have documented the positive benefits of regular exercise. For instance, physically active individuals have:

- lower rates of heart disease[19]
- less depression and anxiety[20]
- better blood pressure control[21]
- better glucose control[22]
- reduced joint swelling in those with arthritis[23]
- lower risk of colon cancer[24] and diverticular disease[25] as well as other cancers
- fewer gallstones[26]
- reduced risk of bone fracture[27]
- better sleep quality[28]
- better mental health[29]
- greater enthusiasm for life[30]
- maintenance of ideal weight[31]
- longer life (an average of seven years longer).[32]

Studies also show that regular aerobic exercise can help detoxify the body.[33] For example, in a study of firemen exposed to toxic PCBs, a two- to three-week detox programme which involved diet, daily saunas and 30–60 minutes of exercise twice a week helped remove these highly toxic substances from their bodies more quickly.[34]

Exercise does not have to be onerous. Walking around a shopping mall is just as healthy as walking around the block.[35] Indeed, walking is really an ideal and natural form of exercise that anyone can routinely participate in.[36] Walking also provides direct contact with the elements and nature, which can be calming and refreshing to the senses. Walking is a load-bearing exercise that tones muscles, and improves fitness, circulation, appetite and breathing.

Similarly, gentle regimes such as yoga and *qigong* have shown benefits. In studies, *qigong* practitioners have shown increased immune responses,[37] improved mental concentration and greater calm.

Overdoing It

It is possible to take exercise too seriously. Overtraining can lead to physical injuries, but it can also encourage oxidative stress. The more energetic and long-lasting your exercise, the more oxygen you take into your body. During intense exercise, we can take in up to 20 times the normal volume of oxygen. This is generally considered a good thing, but more oxygen also means increased demands on the body as it struggles to metabolise all this extra oxygen. The result is a well-known, but little publicised, adverse effect of intensive training – oxidative stress and the production of muscle- and organ-damaging free radicals.

Overtraining can also lead to an imbalance in the stress hormone cortisol. Within the normal range, cortisol can be protective. But too much or too little can have important effects on health. When levels are high, strength can start to decrease;[38] when levels are low, there is a marked inability to deal with other stressors.[39] Cortisol metabolism is also a source of free radicals (*see Chapter 3 for more information*).

Functional Foods

☆☆☆

Consider these simple kitchen-cupboard solutions to combat everyday toxins:

- *The pectin found in apple and pear seeds* can protect your body from damage by toxic metals. It works by blocking the absorption of toxins while aiding detoxification. Try making apples or pears stewed with their seeds a regular feature of your diet.

- *Garlic and onions* contain powerful antioxidants that aid the body's natural day-to-day efforts to detox. Use these liberally in cooking. Other sulphur-rich foods like broccoli and bile stimulants such as lemon and bitter greens also assist in detoxification.

- *Peas, beans and lentils* also contain unique antioxidants, and are high in fibre, which can bind to toxins and aid their excretion from the body. Pulses are a good alternative source of protein, so why not substitute a couple of meat meals each week for one based on (organic) pulses.

- *A high-fibre diet* in general is useful for trapping toxins and assisting in the elimination of heavy metals. Fibre helps reduce intestinal permeability, sometimes known as leaky gut – a condition that can lead to allergies and toxic build-up in the bloodstream. It also prevents deactivated oestrogens from being reactivated and reabsorbed. Consider adding water-soluble, mucilaginous fibres such as psyllium seeds and flaxseeds to your diet. These can be ground up, and added to cereals, soups and baked foods.

- *Bananas* have antioxidant qualities.

- *Eggs* protect against lead and mercury contamination.

- *All leafy dark-green vegetables,* especially cruciferous vegetables (belonging to the cabbage family), can inhibit the carcinogenic effects of chemicals. Try to include plenty of kale, spinach, broccoli and brussels sprouts in your diet. Other green foods that contain chlorophyll are also natural chelators that can draw heavy metals out of the system.[6] Herbs like cilantro (coriander) are a good choice. A good way to take your greens is to buy a juicer and use it to make vegetable juices – they are not as sweet as fruit juices, but they pack more punch in the detox stakes.

- *Consider seaweeds.* Seaweeds and alginates can also bind to heavy metals. There is evidence, for instance, that the freshwater green algae *Chlorella* can draw persistent chemicals, such as PCBs, out of the system.[40] Similarly, research stretching back several decades shows that Arctic seaweeds are an aid to detoxification.[41] These

can be taken as supplements or added to your diet.
- *Black tea* is also thought to provide some protection from heavy metal toxicity – but evidence so far is only from animals. Similar results are likely with green tea.

Good Fats

☆☆☆

Forget your fat phobia. Increasing your intake of healthy fats is important to maintaining good health. Good fats can help leach toxins out of your system, prevent inflammation and protect the gut from toxic damage.

While most of us now understand that essential fats are important for health, making sense of them can be difficult. The world of essential fats is like a jumbled alphabet soup of EFAs, ALAs, EPAs and DHAs. Summing it up simply is impossible but, in general, there are two main 'families' of essential fatty acids: omega-6 and omega-3.

In each family of EFAs, there is a particularly important acid: in the omega-6 family, it is linoleic acid, or LA. This is converted in the body to gamma-linolenic acid (GLA) and later into the series 1 and 2 prostaglandins that, in high quantities, can have a deleterious effect on health.

In the omega-3 family, alpha-linolenic acid, or LNA, is the most important. In the body, this is converted to eicosapentaenoic acid (EPA). EPA can also be synthesised in the body from docosahexaenoic acid (DHA). EPA and DHA help keep our arteries clean and our platelets less sticky. EPA is the starting material for making series 3 prostaglandins, which have beneficial effects on blood pressure, cholesterol and blood-fat levels as well as kidney function, the inflammatory response and immune function. Too much or too little of these prostaglandins can leave the body unable to cope with illness.

Generally speaking, we get far too much omega-6s and not nearly enough omega-3s. In a healthy diet, the ratio of omega-6 to omega-3 should be 2:1.

According to fats expert Udo Erasmus,[42] including more of these healthy fats in our diet while avoiding trans fats may encourage the body to lose weight (a good way to also lose stored toxins). In his experience, those who take 45–70 mL of mixed omega-3 and omega-6 fatty acids (the equivalent of 3–5 American-sized tablespoons, 4–7 UK dessertspoons or 2–3 UK tablespoons) will consistently lose weight even if they don't alter their diets. He adds, however, that the results will be better if the EFAs are part of a comprehensive diet regime that includes increasing your intake of greens, cutting down on saturated fats, switching to organic foods wherever possible, and supplementing with digestive enzymes.

Do It Yourself

Humans can manufacture the fatty acids DHA and EPA from red and brown algae in much the same way that fish do. Given that fish oils can spoil quickly and are subject to wide variations in quality, this type of supplementation might be worth considering. Vegetarians, for instance, have been shown to substantially increase their levels of DHA and EPA with algae supplements.[43] But take note that vegetarians – for a variety of reasons not all linked to diet – are generally healthier than the rest of the population. Only optimally nourished people can make their own supplies of DHA and EPA. Likewise, the ability of the body to convert LNA to EPA can be hampered by low levels of vitamins B3, B6 and C, and magnesium and zinc. In addition to nutritional deficiencies, the overconsumption of saturated fat, trans fatty acids and cholesterol all interfere with this conversion.

There is, however, a downside to algae since they are very efficient at absorbing any toxins in their growing environment.[44] If you choose to take algae supplements, make sure that they are manufactured to the highest standards by a reputable company.

To get your daily dose of good fats, British nutritionist Patrick Holford, of the Institute for Optimum Nutrition, suggests:[45]

The best natural sources of omega-3:
LNA: flaxseed, hempseed, canola, soyabean and walnut oils, and dark-green leaves
EPA/DHA: coldwater fish, salmon, mackerel, sardines.

You can get what you need from:
Hempseed oil, 1 tablespoon
Flaxseed oil, 1 tablespoon
Flax seeds, 2 tablespoons
Pumpkin seeds, 4 tablespoons
EPA/DHA supplement, 1000 mg.

The best natural sources of omega-6:
LA: safflower, sunflower, hemp, soybeans, walnut, pumpkin, sesame and flax
GLA: borage seed, blackcurrant seed, evening primrose oil.

You can get what you need from:
Hemp seed, 1 tablespoon
Sunflower seeds, 1 tablespoon
Pumpkin seeds, 2 tablespoons
Sesame seeds, 1.5 tablespoons
Evening primrose oil, 1000 mg
Borage oil, 500 mg.

Choose one source of omega-3 and omega-6 from each list to achieve a good intake of EFAs. Another good source of both types of fatty acids is dried beans such as kidney, haricot and soya. Regularly including these in your diet will ensure your EFA needs are met.

Houseplants

✩✩✩

A two-year study by NASA scientists suggests that the most sophisticated pollution-absorbing device in your home is a potted plant.[46]

Living, green and flowering plants have an amazing ability to remove a number of toxic chemicals from the air, including formaldehyde, benzene and carbon monoxide. You can use plants in your home or office to improve the quality of the air and to make it a more pleasant place to live and work, where people feel better, perform better and enjoy life more. For an area of 1800 square feet, 15–20 plants are required to clean the air.

The top most effective houseplants are:

- English ivy (*Hedera helix*)
- spider plant (*Chlorophytum comosum*)
- golden pothos (*Epipiremnum aureum*)
- peace lily (*Spathiphyllum 'Mauna Loa'*)
- Chinese evergreen (*Aglaonema modestum*)
- bamboo or reed palm (*Chamaedorea sefritzii*)
- snake plant (*Sansevieria trifasciata*)
- heartleaf philodendron (*Philodendron scandens 'oxycardium'*)
- selloum philodendron (*Philodendron selloum*)
- elephant-ear philodendron (*Philodendron domesticum*)
- red-edged dracaena (*Dracaena marginata*)
- cornstalk dracaena (*Dracaena fragrans 'Massangeana'*)
- Janet Craig dracaena (*Dracaena deremensis 'Janet Craig'*)
- Warneck dracaena (*Dracaena deremensis 'Warneckii'*)
- weeping fig (*Ficus benjamina*).

In general, leafy green plants such as philodendron, spider plant and the golden pothos are more effective in removing formaldehyde while flowering plants such as gerbera daisy and chrysanthemum are superior in removing benzene from the atmosphere.

Immune Support

☆☆☆

Many environmental toxins are immune-toxic – in other words, they interfere with the proper function of the immune system. While tip-top immune function is only one aspect of the protection you need in the face of a toxic environment, it is worth cultivating since a healthy immune system will help you fight off diseases that can further run you down, such as colds, flu, fungal infections and parasites.

There's no magic to maintaining a well-functioning immune system; much of the advice in this section can help you achieve it. Specifically, consider *Exercise*, *Nutrition* and *Avoidance* as your best allies in this respect.

Juice

☆☆☆

Fruit juices – even freshly squeezed ones – are tasty, but full of sugar; when it comes to detox, they cannot compare with the powerful effect of vegetable juices. Having said that, you need to be choosey about which vegetables you select. Veggie juices made from carrots and beetroot taste good, but are as full of sugar as most fruit juices.

Mild detox drinks can be made from greens such as celery, fennel (anise) and cucumber. This is a good way to introduce yourself to the taste and effects of veggie juices if you've never had them before.

However, it is the dark-green leafy, though sometimes less palatable, vegetable juices that will benefit you the most. This is partly because of their chlorophyll content and partly because of their high antioxidant content. Once you get used to the milder juices, you can introduce more powerful mixtures made from lettuces such as red leaf, green leaf, romaine and endive as well as other greens like escarole, spinach, cabbage and Chinese cabbage or *bok choy*.

Adding herbs like parsley and cilantro (coriander) to the juices will add flavour as well as further detox benefits. Start with small amounts and monitor your body's responses.

Other types of greens you can use (sparingly because they are very bitter) include kale, collard greens, dandelion greens and mustard greens.

Make sure you wash all your greens thoroughly before juicing and, where possible, buy organic for even more benefit.

Kick the Habit

☆☆☆

Excess use of tobacco products, alcohol and caffeine wreak havoc on your body. They also encourage toxic damage. Cigarette-smoking, for instance, exposes you to cadmium and carcinogenic polycyclic aromatic hydrocarbons (PAHs). Alcohol can alter immune and endocrine functions, and is poisonous to your internal organs, specifically your liver. In this day and age, no one has to justify advice to cut down.

Caffeine, although considered the most benign of the three, can have wide-ranging and debilitating effects on the body, and is just as addictive as nicotine. In excess, it is implicated in as many disorders as alcohol, including hypoglycaemia,[47] heart disease,[48] miscarriage[49] and cancer.[50] Coffee also dehydrates the body[51] and a dehydrated body is less able to function properly, and to fight off infection and the effects of toxic exposures.

Caffeine Kids?

Is giving children a cola drink almost as bad as giving them cigarettes? According to American scientist Dr Roland Griffiths, a psychopharmacologist working at Johns Hopkins University School of Medicine in Baltimore, Maryland, the answer is yes, and the parallels between the marketing of nicotine and caffeine are "pretty stunning". Both, he says, are psychoactive drugs. Until recently, cigarette companies denied nicotine was addictive and claimed it was added merely as a flavour enhancer for cigarettes. Now the same is being said for caffeine.

In 2000, Griffiths published a study accusing the makers of fizzy drinks of pumping extra caffeine into their products to get consumers, especially children, hooked on them. Of course, the soda manufacturers responded as one with a unanimous "hogwash". As anticipated, they claimed that caffeine was only a mild stimulant, added simply to enhance the flavour of their drinks.

The main results of Dr Griffiths' study, however, refute this.[52] Certainly, the majority of adults in the study said they preferred caffeinated colas. This would seem to validate the manufacturers' claim that caffeine enhances a drink's flavour. But when Dr Griffiths' team gave the group of regular cola consumers drinks containing various concentrations of caffeine, few could tell the difference between them. At a caffeine concentration of 0.1 mg/mL, which is the approximate concentration of the majority of soft-drink products, only 8 percent could detect a difference in flavour. The rest could not tell the difference until caffeine levels were raised beyond those legally permitted.

Lose Weight

☆☆☆☆

Keeping your weight down is good for your health in many ways. Excess fat can put a strain on your heart, clog your arteries and encourage a sedentary lifestyle. It also acts as a reservoir for many everyday toxins. Many common toxins are lipophilic – they like to be surrounded by fat.

Some experts even believe that, in some cases, obesity may even be a response to accumulated toxins in the body. As a rule, the body does not like to let the concentration of potentially harmful substances rise too high. However, if the body just can't work quickly enough to do this, its other option is to 'dilute' the toxins. Under these circumstances, some observers believe that fat becomes the body's storage system – a way of controlling and keeping these toxins from circulating to and damaging other parts of the body. The recent discovery that body fat behaves like an organ, storing nutrients, protecting vital organs and helping to regulate immune function, makes this theory all the more probable.[53]

Dr Elson Haas, director of the Preventative Medicine Center of Marin County in San Rafael, California, concurs that obesity is almost always associated with toxicity and that any weight-loss regime should include measures to support the body as toxic chemicals are released.[54] When we lose weight, we reduce our fat and thereby our toxic load. But during weight loss, we also liberate more of these toxins and thus need more protection. While losing weight, greater intakes of water, fibre and antioxidant nutrients such as vitamins C and E, beta-carotene, selenium and zinc, as well as liver-support herbs such as milk thistle may be appropriate means of protection.

Another way in which the body attempts to dilute toxins is through the accumulation of water. Individuals who feel that their extra weight is the result of water retention may also benefit from a sensible detoxification programme.

Monitor

☆☆

Have the levels of electromagnetic fields (EMFs) in your home pro-fessionally tested, particularly if you live in an area near power lines or train tracks. Your local area power company can do this for you. Before buying a home, check that no power lines run directly under the property. If levels are very high, there may be little you can do bar moving. This is not always a viable option, but you can protect chil-dren by making sure that they sleep in the room furthest away from the source of the EMFs.

You could also try measuring levels in and around your home, work and school environments yourself with a portable device such as those available from Powerwatch and Perspective Scientific (in the UK) and Less EMF Inc (in the US) *(see Chapter 11 Useful Contacts for details)*. Remember: EMFs can pass through walls. The EMF level you are detecting on your portable meter could be radiating from the next room, from next door or elsewhere outside of your home. Measure the EMFs from appliances both when they are operating and when they are turned off. Some appliances (like TVs) are still drawing current even when they are turned off. Avoid areas where the field is above 1 mG, and do what you can to reduce levels by getting rid of unnecessary electrical gadgets, and turning off and unplugging appliances when not in use.

If radon is a concern, most countries have radiation protection groups you can turn to if you want advice on measuring levels in your home or elsewhere. In the UK, contact the National Radiological Protection Board; in Ireland, the Radiological Protection Institute of Ireland; in the US, the Environmental Protection Agency's Radiation Protection Division; in Canada, the Canadian Radiation Protection Association; and in Australia, the Australian Radiation Protection Society.

Similarly, if you wish to know what is in your water, the local water board can send someone out to test it for you.

Nutritious Food

☆☆☆

Food is inexorably linked with health. It is the bedrock on which a healthy life is based. It is the body's buffer against the onslaughts of an increasingly toxic environment. Yet today, most of us do not eat food in any reasonable sense of the word.

Instead, we eat an approximation of food. We eat meat byproducts enhanced with meat flavours to make them palatable. We eat processed, quick-cook microwave and oven meals that contain more preservatives and other additives than they do nutrients. Even the healthy cereals we eat for breakfast are so highly processed and nutritionally poor that the manufacturers have to add vitamins to them simply so that they can be classified as foods.

Every day, we put this nutritionally poor, unbalanced stuff into our bodies and then wonder why our bodies don't function properly.

Matters are not helped by the constantly changing advice of dietitians and government bodies. Much of their advice – reduce fat, eat raw foods, follow a 'Mediterranean diet' – has never been researched in detail and some of it is downright damaging. This is not the place for a full discussion of the faddism of nutritionists – however, it would certainly pay any interested individual to do some digging on their own and question whom all this everchanging dietary advice really serves. Chances are, you will find it benefits multinational food-producing companies.

Such companies have massive influence worldwide and have no interests in our eating fresh, unprocessed food. A steak is a steak is a steak. But a prepared meat product, seasoned and formed from "select cuts of beef" is a patented recipe, and patented recipes (which, with a bit of clever marketing, can be sold to the public as healthy, nutritious, quick and easy) are where the profits are. Fresh food is not high on priority lists because there is less profit in it.

What to avoid

Get into the habit of reading food labels in the supermarket. Don't be fooled into thinking that a high pricetag guarantees quality. Some very high-priced name-brand processed foods are full of the worst kinds of additives while some of the more moderately priced non-name brands may be perfectly acceptable. Equally, some organic foods, especially cakes and biscuits, contain more sugar than conventional brands. Generally speaking, you should avoid:

- *Hydrogenated fats*, sometimes known as trans fats, which are harmful to your heart and contribute to obesity.
- *Artificial food colours*, which have been linked to allergies, asthma and hyperactivity in children. Many are made from carcinogenic chemicals.
- *Nitrites and nitrates*, often found in smoked or preserved meats, as these can develop into carcinogenic nitrosamines in the body.
- *Sulphites* such as sulphur dioxide and metabisulphite, which are preservatives implicated in allergic and asthmatic reactions.
- *Sugar*, which tastes nice and may be fine in moderation, but too much can contribute to hypoglycaemia and diabetes, increased blood fats (triglycerides), *Candida* overgrowth, obesity and dental caries.
- *Soya protein isolates*, the type of soya added to your bread and other bakery products, and also used in meat substitutes, dairy products and baby formulas. The only soya that is remotely healthy is fermented soya, which contains the whole plant. Fermenting makes the nutrients in soya products more easily absorbed by the body. Even so, soya can lower the availability of vitamins A, C, B and E and the mineral zinc, and may have an undesirable oestrogenic effect.[55] It can also lower iron levels, which may be why Oriental women balance soya intake with iron-rich seaweed.
- *Artificial sweeteners*, which have been implicated in a range of neurological problems (such as headaches and nervous tics) and

behavioural problems (such as hyperactivity in children). Most artificial sweeteners are potentially carcinogenic, and should especially be avoided by children and pregnant women.

- *MSG*, or monosodium glutamate, a flavour enhancer used in almost all processed foods. It is a relative of the artificial sweetener aspartame (both are known as excitotoxins – chemicals that over-stimulate the nervous system). MSG is a common allergen and can cause neurological symptoms such as headache, dizziness, chest pains, depression and mood swings. It is considered a neurotoxin.
- *Preservatives* such as BHA, BHT and EDTA, which can cause allergic reactions, hyperactivity and cancer. BHT may be toxic to the nervous system and liver.
- *Artificial flavours and aromas*, which are basically perfume ingredients scaled down for oral consumption. These have been linked to allergic, neurological and behavioural problems, and may be associated with asthmatic reactions.
- *Refined flours*, as these are low in nutrients and high in calories. Overconsumption can lead to carbohydrate imbalances, altered insulin production and symptoms such as fatigue and dizziness.
- *Salt*, which, like sugar, has its place in moderation. It is necessary for proper nerve function and maintaining the body's water balance. But too much can lead to fluid retention and increased blood pressure.
- *Olestra*, an artificial fat that can cause diarrhoea and digestive disturbances.

In addition, consider the additives you can't see. Many 'fresh' foods are coated in petroleum-derived waxes to help maintain freshness. The waxes on fruits and vegetables are based on petrochemicals and may trigger allergies. They may also contain a substance called morpholine that, according to World Health Organization reports, turns into the carcinogen *N*-nitrosomorpholine.

Foods that are regularly waxed include thin-skinned produce such as cucumbers, peppers and apples. In addition, all fruits and vegetables are repeatedly sprayed with a multitude of pesticides and fungicides while in storage. Unwanted additives can also seep in from packaging. For example, if the plastic packaging is derived from vinyl chloride – a known carcinogen and endocrine disrupter – this can easily migrate into foods, especially those that are acidic or fatty.

A word about GM foods

Increasingly, news headlines about genetic modification leave many of us anxious and confused about the food we eat. We now have the technology to alter the most basic building blocks of life. Unfortunately, we have not conducted the studies necessary to prove or disprove the safety of GM foods over either the long or short term. We are unaware of whether GM foods can, for instance, cause damage to a vulnerable fetus at certain stages of development.

GM foods don't taste better and are not cheaper to buy; they have, however, been implicated in increased resistance to antibiotics and the growth of 'superbugs'. They have also been linked to an increased incidence of allergies, unpredictable rises of toxins in the body, increased cancer rates and a decline in the nutritional quality of foods. Ironically, studies show that, contrary to most industry reports, US farmers growing GM crops are using just as many toxic pesticides and herbicides as conventional farmers – and in some cases are using more.

Indeed, one of the 'benefits' of these herbicide-resistant crops is that farmers can spray as much of a particular herbicide on their crops as they want, thereby killing the weeds without damaging their crop. Scientists estimate that herbicide-resistant crops planted around the globe will triple the amount of toxic, broad-spectrum herbicides used in agriculture.

Food can either be genetically modified itself or contain genetically modified ingredients. The issues are complex, but if you are concerned, you might consider avoiding or limiting:

- *Tomatoes (and tomato puree)*, the first GM foods to be sold. In the US, you can buy fresh tomatoes which have been genetically modified; in the UK, you can only buy puree made from these tomatoes. Watch out for ready-made foods such as pizza which may use GM tomato puree.

- *Soya*, modified to resist weedkiller. In the US, supplier of most of the world's soya, GM and unmodified soya are not kept separate, and processed foods may contain both. Soya is present in most baked and prepackaged foods in several forms: oil (often just labelled vegetable oil), vegetable fat, flour, lecithin and vegetable protein.
- *Maize*, which has been modified to contain bacteria toxic to a common crop pest. Maize is used as a grain, as corn (or maize) flour, corn meal, corn starch, corn syrup, dextrose, glucose, fructose, xanthan gum, maltodextrin and as corn oil. Be aware of things like chocolate bars and sweet drinks which contain sugars derived from maize.
- *Cheese*, which can be made with a GM enzyme called chymosin instead of traditional rennet. Chymosin is used in many vegetarian cheeses and increasingly in hard cheeses for general consumption.
- *Enzymes*, used in a large number of products including drinks, bakery goods and dairy products. Manufacturers are not obliged to include these on the product information.
- *Canola*, or rapeseed, mainly used as an oil. Some crops now contain human genes.
- *Yeast*, which has been genetically modified and approved for making bread; it is difficult to know the extent to which it is used in bakery products.
- *Vitamin B2,* known as riboflavin, and now widely produced from genetically modified microorganisms. It is generally added to breakfast cereals, soft drinks, baby foods and diet foods.
- *E numbers*, which indicate preservatives, flavourings and colourings. Watch out for E101, E101a, E150, E153, E161c, E322, E471 and E621, all of which may be GM derivatives.

To spot GM foods, you will have to read the labels. But even this will not guarantee that your diet will be GM-free. Labelling laws can be very confusing, and seem to exist mostly to protect the manufacturer rather than the consumer. Certain GM ingredients, such as flavourings and additives, do not need to be listed on the label and very few manufacturers volunteer this information. For the moment, the best way to avoid GM foods is to eat as much organic and freshly prepared (by you in your home) food as possible.

In addition to GM organisms in our food, concerns have recently been expressed that some excipients (inert ingredients) in nutritional supplements may also include genetically modified ingredients. Most health supplements that are not licensed medicines are classed as foods and, as such, are obliged to warn the consumer on the label if they are known to contain GM ingredients. Supplements that are licensed medicines (for instance, some folic acid and cod liver oil supplements) are not required to alert consumers to the presence of GM ingredients or derivatives.

According to Genetic Food Alert (GFA) in the UK, unless expressly denied by the manufacturer, the following excipients may be genetically modified:

- *Derivatives of soya, maize (corn), cotton or rapeseed*, including oils which are used as carriers for vitamins (A, D and E) in supplements; lecithin and vitamin E which are used as antioxidants; and sweeteners such as dextrose, glucose, dextrins, maltodextrins and sorbitol.
- *GM microorganisms or their products*, including some bacteria, brewer's yeast and baker's yeast. Products of GM bacteria can include aspartame and enzymes used as processing aids (which may not be listed on the label) such as alpha-acetolactate decarboxylase, alpha-amylase, catalase, chymosin a, chymosin b, cyclodextrin glucosyltransferase, beta-glucanase, glucose isomerase, glucose oxidase, hemicellulase (xylanase), lipase, triacylglycerol, maltogenic amylase, pectinesterase, protease and pullulanase.
- *Products of GM-fed or -treated animals*, including gelatine, bonemeal and albumen from animals raised on GM ingredients or injected with GM growth hormones such as BST.

The GFA has compiled a list of guaranteed GM-free supplements which can be accessed on their website (*see Chapter 11 Useful Contacts*) along with other information on GM additives in supplements.

Organics

☆☆☆

Pesticides are harmful to people – no one can reasonably dispute that – and eating organic is still the best way to avoid ingesting pesticides.

Unfortunately, organic food can be so expensive that it is beyond some people's reach. This doesn't mean that you need to be resigned to a refrigerator full of toxic food. One way to lower your burden is to prioritise, reserving organic purchases for those foods known to contain high levels of pesticides and other toxins, such as dairy and meat products, and grains.

The level of pesticides in fruits and vegetables can vary enormously, depending on the crop and the season. Research in this area has revealed some startling findings. In 1995, the Environmental Working Group (EWG), a pressure group based in Washington, DC, reviewed studies conducted by the Food and Drug Administration and the Environmental Protection Agency into the pesticide contents of 42 different types of produce in the US.[56] They found that some types of produce had very little pesticide residue. According to their findings, the least to the most polluted were:

- avocados
- corn
- onions
- sweet potatoes
- cauliflower
- brussels sprouts
- grapes (US)
- bananas
- plums
- spring onions

- watermelon
- broccoli.

But, among the most contaminated, there were a few surprises. Strawberries were contaminated with more types of pesticides than any other fruit or vegetable, followed by peppers, spinach, cherries, peaches, celery, cantaloupe, apples, apricots, grapes (non-US), green beans and cucumbers. Pesticide residues cannot easily be washed off and are often absorbed into the flesh of the plant, so even peeling the skin of certain fruits will not reduce your intake by much. Instead, as the chart below shows, the EWG recommended that, if you regularly eat these foods, you might consider substituting other foods of equal or better nutritional value and lower pesticide rating.

Food	Main Nutrients	Alternatives
Strawberries	Vitamin C	Blueberries, raspberries, blackberries, oranges, grapefruit, cantaloupe, kiwis or watermelon
Peppers	Red peppers contain carotenoids (vitamin A), and both green and red peppers are rich in vitamin C	*Alternatives to green peppers:* green peas, broccoli or romaine lettuce; *alternatives to red peppers:* romaine lettuce, carrots, broccoli, brussels sprouts, asparagus or tomatoes
Spinach	Carotenoids (vitamins A), vitamin C and folic acid	Broccoli, brussels sprouts, romaine lettuce or asparagus
Cherries	Vitamin C	Oranges, blueberries, raspberries, blackberries, grapefruit, cantaloupe or kiwis
Peaches	Carotenoids (vitamin A) and vitamin C	Nectarines, cantaloupe, watermelon, tangerines, oranges, or red or pink grapefruit
Cantaloupe	Vitamin A (carotenoids), vitamin C and potassium	Cantaloupe in season (May to December) or watermelon

Food	Main Nutrients	Alternatives
Celery	Some carotenoids, but not a good source of vitamins	Carrots, romaine lettuce, broccoli or radish
Apples	Vitamin C	Pears, oranges, grapefruit, cantaloupe, kiwis, watermelon, nectarines, bananas, tangerines or virtually any fruit not on the most contaminated foods list
Apricots	Carotenoids (vitamin A), vitamin C and potassium	Nectarines, cantaloupe, watermelon, tangerines, oranges, red or pink grapefruit or watermelon
Green beans	Not a particularly rich source of vitamins or carotenoids	Green peas, broccoli, cauliflower, brussels sprouts, potatoes or asparagus
Grapes (Chilean)	Vitamin C	Grapes in season (May to December)
Cucumbers	Not a particularly rich source of vitamins or carotenoids	Carrots, romaine lettuce, broccoli, radish or virtually any vegetable not on the most contaminated foods list

The benefits of eating lots of fruits generally outweighs any potential risks from low-level pesticide residues found in produce. Nevertheless, why voluntarily ingest high levels of pesticides when good alternatives are available either through buying organic or choosing your non-organic produce (and other foodstuffs) carefully?

Pick Your Poison

☆☆☆☆

We are both passive and direct recipients of pollution. Reading through this book, you may find yourself becoming dismayed at the overwhelming number of ways in which the environment can be toxic to the human body. It would be understandable for anyone to feel like giving up before they even began. Many people might reason that as long as they look reasonably healthy, what does it matter if they don't feel so well. The information in this book, however, is geared towards helping you take a longer-term view.

You cannot avoid all poisons in the environment. That is not what this book is about nor is it an idea it cares to promote. It may even be that we have come too far down the road in polluting our planet to ever be able to avoid all environmental toxins. But you do have more power than you think and you can, to a very large and influential extent, pick your poisons.

One way to do this is to be aware of what your particular weak spots are. These may be genetic weak spots, or weak spots developed in your own lifetime. For instance, if you have a family history of cancer, it makes sense to avoid carcinogenic chemicals and metals as far as is possible. If your family has a history of neurological disorders (for instance, multiple sclerosis) or autoimmune diseases (such as arthritis), you should be on the look-out for neurotoxic and immunotoxic chemicals. If you suffer from menstrual problems, chemicals that disrupt your hormonal symptoms may play a part. Get to know what these chemicals are and learn to avoid them.

You can also protect your children – who are the most vulnerable to environmental insults – by keeping your home environment as free from pollutants as possible. You are in control, you have the power and it is your responsibility.

Questions

☆☆

As children, we are brought up to take what we are given and accept it. As adults, we have to break out of this mould and learn to ask more of those around us.

Ask questions of yourself and of the people who supply the goods you buy. Read labels and, if they don't give you the information you need, write to the manufacturer and ask them to supply it. An enquiring mind is one of your best defences against hidden pollutants.

In the same vein, make sure you ask questions of all practitioners and other 'experts' who propose to help you 'detox' or improve your health in other ways. Alternative health is now big business. Many companies have products to sell – and they don't care if they are inferior. Many practitioners have diaries to fill, and the bottom line is often placed before good patient care.

If you don't like the answers you get, buy different products or access your healthcare from a different practitioner.

Relaxation

☆☆☆

Healthy people understand the value of taking a break – not just once a year, but every day and at the weekend. They generally have hobbies and interests that absorb them fully, and schedule time for these in their lives. They also take regular holidays and value – indeed, actively pursue – time with family and friends. These individuals do for themselves what most 'stress management' experts make a lot of money teaching; they learn to spread the load, switch off and recharge their emotional batteries from time to time.

Relaxation lowers levels of stress hormones and boosts immunity. It slows your heart rate and deepens your breathing.[57] Formal types of relaxation, such as Transcendental Meditation, have been shown to reduce hypertension and oxidative stress,[58] raise blood concentrations of the stress-busting hormone dehydroepiandrosterone sulphate (DHEAS)[59] and improve symptoms of chronic pain syndromes.[60]

But you can also relax by simply having a change of scene, by 'vegging out' in front of the TV or going to the movies, or taking a walk in the park. Equally, you can schedule relaxation time, for instance, by having regular massage or sauna sessions. Whichever way you do it, the benefits will be manifold.

Sleep

☆☆☆☆

Sleep is not the same as relaxation. Sleep is an active state that is essential for physical and mental restoration. These days, many of us simply don't get enough of it either because we do not recognise its importance or because we have trouble falling asleep even when we're tired.

Lack of sleep has long been known to impact on heart health,[61] mood and memory.[62] Recently, sleep deprivation has also been shown to adversely affect glucose tolerance[63] as well as glucose and insulin regulation.[64] One US study found that sleep debt, a situation frequently imposed by modern lifestyles, can result in profound metabolic alterations. Researchers found that just one week of sleep deprivation altered subjects' hormone levels (produced lower levels of thyroid hormones and higher levels of stress hormones) as well as their capacity to metabolise carbohydrates.[65]

Under normal circumstances, we spend a third of our lives in bed, so getting the most from your sleep time is possibly the simplest way to improve your health and your resistance to many of the toxic elements you encounter each day. To get a better night's sleep, consider the following:

- *Bedrooms are for sleeping.* Remove all other distractions from your bedroom, including TVs, computers, bills to be paid and any work brought home from the office. In addition, follow the advice in Chapter 7 for making your bedroom an EMF-free zone.
- *Keep your sleep schedule consistent.* Plan regular hours of sleep each day, then stick to the programme.
- *Don't exercise* or involve yourself in difficult mental tasks near bedtime.
- *Don't drink before bedtime.* It is a myth that alcohol helps us sleep. Instead, it temporarily depresses the nervous system and is then rapidly metabolised, causing a rebound stimulation a few hours later. The same goes for caffeine and cigarettes, both of which can keep you awake if you have them too close to bedtime.

- *Keep the bedroom dark* – in fact, the darker the better. Darkness stimulates the nightly production of melatonin, the hormone necessary to regulate our day/night, sleep/wake cycles. Get rid of nightlights, cover lighted clockfaces and make sure your curtains are lined to keep out any light from outside.
- *Open a window* as fresh air can be an aid to refreshing sleep.
- *Is it time to replace the mattress?* Your mattress should provide firm support to your body throughout the night. Soft, sagging mattresses can lead to backache, sleeplessness and stress. Although expensive, the newer varieties of latex rubber mattresses, or those made from space age materials such as Tempur, have many advantages over sprung types including firmness, the ability to mould their shape to the body, lower levels of dust mites and no metal parts to attract EMFs to the bed.
- *Night-waking* can be a sign of nighttime hypoglycaemia. Eat a light snack before bedtime or drink a glass of warm milk, which contains tryptophan, an amino acid known to induce sleep.
- *Snoring* can create poor sleep for both the snorer and his/her partner. If the snorer is overweight, losing weight may help eliminate some of the fat in the throat, thus clearing breathing passages. Allergies can also cause snoring, so you might want to investigate whether the problem is food, dander, chemicals or airborne allergens. Alcohol consumption close to bedtime can also exacerbate snoring.

Tests

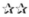

There are a number of tests you can undergo to check levels of metals and other poisons in your body. Hair analysis, which usually involves taking a small sample of recent hair growth from the nape of the neck, is a common way of testing for the presence of heavy metals. A lab analysis can give you fairly accurate information on the presence of calcium, magnesium, sodium, potassium, iron, copper, manganese, zinc, chromium and selenium, but also potentially more damaging metals such as lead, mercury, cadmium and arsenic.

Some practitioners also offer blood and urine testing, though these have been shown to be less effective in the detection of minerals and, especially, toxic-metal exposure. This is because blood shows what is being transported in the body while urine shows what is being eliminated. Stool testing, however, can be useful for diagnosing the presence of parasites in the gut.

To test for allergies, practitioners use either a skin-prick test or blood analysis such as the RAST (radioallergosorbent test) or the ELISA (enzyme-linked immunosorbent assay). These latter two are based on the idea that, when the body registers an allergen in its midst, it produces a variety of immunoglobulin antibodies. Both tests look for the presence of antibodies, although there is continuing debate over how useful either (or, indeed, any) of the current test methods is since different tests performed by different laboratories on the same samples of blood can produce sometimes wildly differ-ent results. Many pharmacies now sell testing over the counter, but this is unlikely to be very accurate. For a better chance of success, you need to visit an allergy specialist who has access to a reliable lab.

Few of these kinds of test are offered on the National Health Service. You will need to seek out a private practitioner to have them performed.

Uncomplicate Your Life

☆☆☆☆

Cultivating simplicity in your life is not just some vague hippie dream.[66] These days, it requires a iron will to resist advertising pres-sure to buy more stuff and consume more than you need. The fact is, the less stuff you have in your life, the less likely you are to come in contact with environmental toxins. If you only use the microwave to heat up coffee or bake potatoes, perhaps the time has come to get rid of this significant source of radiation in your home altogether. If you unclutter your home, chances are you will not need so many plastic boxes to store things – reducing these means less formaldehyde gas in the air. Likewise, if you use fewer cosmetics, toiletries, air fresheners and harsh household cleaners, you will be reducing your exposure to solvents and other VOCs as well as environmental hormone mimics. Many of the toxins we encounter every day are the result of our unbridled consumerism so choose not to buy into this unhealthy addiction.

Vitamins and Minerals

☆☆☆☆

Although they are not panaceas, nutritional supplements can help make up for some of the deficiencies in your diet. Here are some of the best for keeping free radicals under control and maintaining healthy immune function.

Glutathione

Glutathione is a small protein composed of three amino acids: cysteine, glutamic acid and glycine. It is found in high concentrations in liver cells. Studies show that glutathione attaches to toxic compounds in the liver, neutralising them or enabling them to be excreted.[67]

Glutathione is abundant in fresh fruits and vegetables. In this form, it is easily absorbed by the body and may have anticancer effects.[68] While some nutritionists recommend 1–3 g daily, glutathione in the form of supplements is not well absorbed – and studies show that supplementing with glutathione alone is not helpful.[69] If you want to raise levels of glutathione in your body, a more effective way is to increase your intake of nutrients known to help the body manufacture this nutrient. These include nutrients such as vitamin C[70] as well as also alpha-lipoic acid, glutamine, methionine and S-adenosylmethionine (SAMe).

Selenium

Selenium is essential for proper immune function and may have anti-cancer effects.[75] It also helps to make zinc more effective and works closely with vitamin E to maintain not just a healthy liver, but a healthy heart as well. Brazil nuts are the best food source of selenium with yeast, and whole grains and seafood also provide useful amounts. Animal studies have found that selenium from yeast is better absorbed than selenium in the form of selenite.[76] Consider taking 200–300 IU daily to keep healthy.

Vitamin C

Vitamin C, or ascorbic acid, aids the detoxification process in several ways. Adequate vitamin C can strengthen many parts of the body including the blood vessels and muscles. It has a protective effect on the heart[71] and eyes, and can boost immunity and aid wound healing. It may also help protect the body against the accumulation of lead.[72] In the same way that it interacts with glutathione, it also interacts with other antioxidants, including vitamin E, making them more effective. Aim for 1 g daily.

Vitamin E

The major fat-soluble antioxidant in the body, vitamin E is the most-studied free-radical quencher.[73] Vitamin E and water-soluble vitamin C work synergistically in the fight against free radicals. These two vitamins as well as beta-carotene protect the liver from damage and help support detoxification.[74] Vitamin E is believed to be non-toxic even in high doses, but most of us only need to supplement with 400–800 IU every day.

Zinc

This is an important antioxidant and helps to keep the liver functioning well. Adequate zinc can boost immunity, protect against free radical damage, maintain healthy cells and also help guard against copper overload. A great many people do not get enough zinc. A reasonable daily supplement would be 25–50 mg.

Water

☆☆☆

Most of us have grown up with the idea that we should drink eight 8-oz glasses (approximately 1.5 litres) of water a day to stay healthy. Certainly, water is an essential but overlooked nutrient.[77] Yet, outside of the field of sports medicine, it is almost impossible to find good evidence to support the eight-glasses-a-day theory. Few of us are training for the triathlon (endurance sports are probably the only place where overconsumption of water, such as drinking up to a litre of water prior to extreme exertion, may be justified), and information on how much fluid sedentary-to-moderately active individuals need is less clear-cut.[78]

In the same way that adequate nutrition has little to do with how many vitamin pills you take, adequate hydration is not just a matter of drinking lots of water. It is a matter of checks and balances. How much you need depends on various factors such as your level of activity, what kind of foods you regularly consume and even the climate in which you live.

It is estimated that, every day, the body loses approximately 1.5 litres of water through sweating, breathing and urinating. This must be replaced. The good news is that your daily fluid supply doesn't all have to come from a bottle or a glass. Fruits and vegetables supply water in a form that is easily used by the body while providing a high percentage of vitamins and minerals as a bonus.

In addition, we release about one-third of a litre of water into our systems every day when we burn glycogen for energy. When the body digests carbohydrates, they are broken down into glucose – to meet immediate energy needs – and glycogen. Glycogen is stored in the muscles and liver for future use. Each molecule of glycogen holds on to nine molecules of water, which are released during the course of your day and at times when you need it most, like during intense exercise.

Increasing your fluid intake too dramatically can put unnecessary stress on your kidneys and digestive system. So, if you want to increase your daily intake, try adding a half-pint glass of water every other day until you are drinking as much as you need.

You may also wish to consider the following:

- If you find drinking water makes you feel too full, you may be gulping down large quantities of air each time you swallow. To remedy this, try drinking through a straw.
- The idea that you can dilute your digestive juices by drinking water with a meal is a myth. Every day, the body makes about 10 litres of digestive juices. A glass of water with your food won't even make a dent in this.
- Before engaging in vigorous exercise, try drinking at least half a pint of water beforehand. Keep a water bottle with you, and drink 4–8 oz every 15 minutes or so to maintain body temperature and avoid dehydration.
- Lots of people limit the amount of fluids they drink each day because they want to limit the number of times they go to the toilet. But going to the toilet every two to four hours is a sign of good health. After a few weeks, your bladder will adapt, you will go to the toilet less often and, when you do, you will void larger amounts of pale urine.
- While is it sensible to be guided by your appetite where food is concerned, being guided by your thirst is not a good idea. Regardless of your level of activity, by the time you feel thirsty, you are already partially dehydrated. To avoid this, sip water through-out the day and get into the habit of drinking this in preference to potentially drying liquids such as coffee, tea and sodas. This

and increasing you intake of 'watery' foods (*see below*) will ensure that your body is getting what it needs – without having to carry around heavy designer bottles of water.

A single serving of any of the items below can count towards your total daily fluid intake:

Food	Water (%)
Lettuce	95.5
Kale	91.2
Carrots	91.2
Milk	87.5
Porridge	86.5
Apples	84.4
Grapes	81.6
Potatoes baked in their skins	75.1
Brown rice, cooked	70.3
Cooked beans such as kidney or lentils	70.0
Fish or chicken, broiled	64.0

Sports drinks help to replace lost electrolytes and provide useful levels of sodium, potassium and quick energy in the form of glucose. However, unless you are involved in regular and very heavy workouts, you are unlikely to need to replace electrolytes. For moderately active people, sports drinks probably only offer more calories and less benefit. A regular, wholesome diet will provide the average person with all the electrolytes they need as well as essential nutrients.

Those who are taking multivitamin/mineral supplements should make sure they are adequately hydrated as should those who engage in regular sweaty workouts. Do sip water when exercising even if you don't feel thirsty. During a hard workout, by the time you feel thirsty, you may already be dehydrated.

You also need extra water in warmer weather, when you are running a fever and when you have diarrhoea.

What type of water is best?

The quality of water we drink is almost as important as the quantity. As a general recommendation, for the best-quality water, consider installing a reverse-osmosis filter on your own tap (but be careful since some of these use plastic filters, which can leach chemicals into your drinking water). Beyond that, there are benefits and limitations in every type of water you choose to drink. Bottled water contains fluoride. No home-filter process is infallible. Distilled water is pure, but may be lacking in certain minerals. Jug-type water filters have to do what they claim on the label; this means they filter out a substantial amount of contaminants such as chlorine and heavy metals.[79] But with use, they can also become reservoirs for bacteria.[80]

While some local water authorities seem to be able to produce clean drinkable water, others cannot, and contamination with heavy metals, bacteria and parasites such as *Cryptosporidium* are becoming an increasing concern. Nevertheless, if you have confidence in your local water supply, tapwater does have its benefits – the main one being that it is almost always available. In addition, if you get into the habit of drinking only bottled water, you can easily reach a point where you believe that when the bottle is empty, you've run out of water.

Bottled waters can be high in minerals, but chemicals from the plastic container may leach into the water during storage. There is little evidence that bottled waters are substantially healthier to drink than tapwater, though they are (sometimes) more convenient.[81]

Yell

☆☆

Shout, complain, make a fuss, write letters, be a thorn in someone's side. Big businesses, governments, everyone we perceive as being 'in control' can only get away with polluting our environments and our bodies if we let them. Vocal criticism is the only way to let authorities know that the status quo is unacceptable. If you don't like the idea of complaining, then support those environmental organisations that are willing to complain on your behalf. Greenpeace, Friends of the Earth and the Worldwide Fund for Nature are making a difference by keeping the kind of research detailed in this book in front of our politicians and policymakers. Such gargantuan efforts should be supported wherever possible.

Zest for life

☆☆☆

None of the things suggested in this chapter are possible unless you actually enjoy living. Indeed, self-esteem, social ties and life satisfaction are among the things that most influence the way we take care of ourselves over the long haul.[82] Similarly, a sense of productivity and worth, and faith in God have also been shown to be influential.[83]

Curiosity and taking an interest in the world around you may also have an important role to play[84] as does your personality. But contrary to common perceptions, this doesn't necessarily mean that the most cheerful and optimistic personalities survive the longest. In one study, cheerfulness (defined as optimism and a sense of humour) was linked to early death while conscientiousness (attention to details) was related to longevity.[85] Other research along similar lines has shown that stability of personality and a sense of routine may be the most important factors.[86]

These ideas are underscored by the findings of a retrospective study in which the factors influencing 17 long-surviving Civil War nurses, including Louisa Mae Alcott, Dorothea Dix and Clara Barton, were explored. While social and marital status, altruism and religion were all important, more than any other tangible factor, the presence of a pioneering spirit seemed to be at the root of their longevity.[87]

Clearly, when you enjoy life, when you have people around you who you care about and who care about you, when your work is interesting and challenging, and your mind is free to follow its own thoughts, you become interested in living. You will then have a good reason to do all you can to protect yourself and your loved ones from an increasingly toxic environment.

part three

Finding Out More

11 Useful Contacts

THE FOLLOWING INTERNATIONAL CONTACTS MAY PROVIDE USEFUL starting point for consumers who wish to find out more about environmental toxins and how they affect human health.

General Resources

Children's Environmental Health Network
(www.cehn.org)
110 Maryland Avenue NE
Suite 511
Washington, DC 20002
USA
Tel: (202) 543 4033
Fax: (202) 543 8797
E-mail: cehn@cehn.org

A national multidisciplinary organisation with a mission to protect the fetus and the child from environmental health hazards, and promote a healthy environment.

The website provides information on the Network, the issue of children's environmental health, and links to sources of information and resources in the field.

Clinical Toxicology of Commercial Products
(www.cehn.org/cehn/resourceguide/ctcp.html)

A unique Web resource for information on the chemical formulations of commercial products, such as household cleaners and toiletries. There is a trade-name index as well as a lengthy section on general formulations, organised by type of product.

Green Health Watch
(www.greenhealthwatch.com)
Muir of Logie
Forres
Scotland IV36 2QG
UK
Tel: 01309 611 200

A quarterly newsletter with the latest news and research on the impact of environmental pollution, modern technology and lifestyle on health. Published by the Environment-Health Trust.

International Chemical Safety Cards
(www.cdc.gov/niosh/ipcs/ipcs0000.html)

Run by the US Centers for Disease Control (CDC) and the National Institute for Occupational Safety and Health (NIOSH). Click on the links to find safety data on a wide range of everyday chemicals.

National Library of Medicine PubMed
(www.ncbi.nlm.nih.gov/entrez/query.fcgi)

PubMed is an invaluable service of the US National Library of Medicine, providing access to over 12 million medical journal citations dating back to the mid-1960s as well as to additional life-science journals. The site also includes links to many sites providing full-text articles and other related resources.

Rachel's Environmental & Health Weekly
(www.rachel.org)
Environmental Research Foundation
P.O. Box 5036
Annapolis, MD 21403
USA
Tel: (410) 263 1584
Fax: (732) 791 4603

Regular and well-researched e-newsletter with views on environmental issues.

Science and Environmental Health Network (SEHN)
(www.sehn.org)

Network and think tank for the environmental movement, helping environmental organisations use science in their work, guiding scientists to public-interest research and public service, and informing public policy with science grounded in ethics and logic.

Toxicology Sources
(http://scarlett.libs.uga.edu/ref/toxbib.html)

This University of Georgia site provides links to other useful websites with toxicological and chemical information.

Union of Concerned Scientists
(www.ucsusa.org)
2 Brattle Square
Cambridge, MA 02238-9105
USA
Tel: (617) 547 5552
Fax: (617) 864 9405

An independent non-profit alliance of 60,000 concerned citizens and scientists across the USA committed to combining rigorous scientific analysis with innovative thinking and committed citizen advocacy to build a cleaner, healthier environment and a safer world.

World Resources Institute
(www.wri.org)
10 G Street NE
Suite 800
Washington, DC 20002
USA
Tel: (202) 729 7600
Fax: (202) 729 7610

Provides information and resources on environmental issues, biodiversity, climate change, business and industry, governance, sustainable agriculture, forests and health. WRI publications are well researched and often have an international focus.

Electromagnetics

Circuit
P.O. Box 1UZ
Newcastle-on-Tyne NE99 1UZ
UK

UK home-based self-help group for those suffering from electrical sensitivity.

Coghill Research Laboratories Ltd
(www.cogreslab.co.uk)
Lower Race
Pontypool
Gwent
UK
Tel: 01495 752 122

Laboratory that specialises in bioelectromagnetics, the science investigating the interaction of electricity and magnetism with organic life, the effects of which can be both good and bad. Useful website with EMF protection devices for sale.

Electromagnetic and VDU News

P.O. Box 25
Liphook
Hampshire
UK

News and reviews magazine devoted to bioelectromagnetics issues.

Human Radiation Effects Group

(www.electric-fields.bris.ac.uk)
H.H. Wills Physics Laboratory
Tyndall Avenue
Bristol BS8 1TL
UK
Tel: 0117 926 0353
Fax: 0117 925 1723

Professor Denis Henshaw and colleagues provide information on the health effects of exposure to radiation.

Less EMF Inc.

(www.lessemf.com)
141 Soller Heights Road
Ghent, NY 12075
USA
Tel: 1 (888) LESS EMF (USA toll free)
Tel: (518) 672 6668 (outside USA)
E-mail: lessemf@lessemf.com

Everything for electromagnetic safety in the home and office, including meters, shielding devices and low-EMF appliances.

National Radiological Protection Board
(www.nrpb.org)
Chilton
Didcot
Oxon OX11 0RQ
Tel: 01235 831 600

Agency responsible for EMF research and standards of safety in the UK.

Perspective Science
(www.perspective.co.uk)
100 Baker Street
London W1U 6WB
Tel: 020 7486 6837
E-mail: sales@perspective.co.uk

Manufacturer and distributor of hand-held monitors for both ionising/ nuclear and electromagnetic radiation.

Powerwatch
(www.powerwatch.org.uk)
2 Tower Road
Sutton, Ely
Cambridgeshire CB6 2QA

Hires out power-frequency meters and microwave monitors within the UK. Their website is a source of information on EMF issues.

Environmental Groups

Environmental Working Group
(www.ewg.org)
1718 Connecticut Avenue NW
Suite 600
Washington, DC 20009
USA
E-mail: info@ewg.org

News, features and cutting-edge research and publications on health and the environment.

Friends of the Earth
(http://foe.org.uk)
26–28 Underwood Street
London N1 7JQ
UK
Tel: 020 7490 1555
Fax: 020 7490 0881

One of the UK's leading environmental charities that researches, publishes and provides information on a wide range of local, national and international issues.

Greenpeace
(www.greenpeace.org.uk)
Canonbury Villas
London N1 2PN
UK
Tel: 020 7865 8100
Fax: 020 7865 8200

International, independent, environmental pressure group acting against abuse to the natural world. Comprehensive website features its latest campaigns, consumer information and details on how to join.

Women's Environmental Network
(www.wen.org.uk)
P.O. Box 30626
London E1 1TZ
UK
Tel: 020 7481 9004

Innovative campaigning organisation that represents women and issues linking women, environment and health.

Worldwide Fund for Nature UK (WWF)
(www.wwf-ukk.org)
Panda House
Weyside Park
Godalming
Surrey GU7 1XR
UK
Tel: 01483 426444
Fax: 01483 426409

Environmental illness

The Environmental Medicine Foundation
P.O. Box 4523
Bridport
Dorset DT6 6YG
UK
E-mail: info@environmentalmedicinefoundation.co.uk

A charity concerned with the promotion of environmental medicine.

Food

Genetic Food Alert (GFA)
(www.geneticfoodalert.supanet.com)
4 Bertram House
Ticklemore Street
Totnes
Devon TQ9 5EJ
UK
Tel: 01803 868 523

Campaigning UK-based group that provides data on which foods and supplements may contain genetically modified constituents.

Henry Doubleday Research Association (HDRA)
(www.hdra.org.uk)
Ryton Organic Gardens
Coventry CV8 3LG
UK
Tel: 0124 7630 3517
Fax: 0124 7663 9229

Long-established and Europe's largest organic membership organisation campaigning for better organic standards and wider distribution of organic foods.

Organic Update
(www.organic-research.com)
CABI Publishing
Wallingford
Oxfordshire OX10 8DE
UK
Tel: 01491 832 111

News and information related to organic food, farming and legislation. Also publishes Organic Update newsletter – a free monthly e-digest of organic news from around the world.

Soil Association
(www.soilassociation.org)
Bristol House
40–56 Victoria Street
Bristol BS1 6BY
UK
Tel: 0117 929 0661

Site for the UK's leading group working to promote the benefits of organic food, farming and sustainable forestry to human health, animal welfare and the environment.

Weston A. Price Foundation
(http://www.WestonAPrice.org)
PMB 106-380
4200 Wisconsin Avenue NW
Washington, DC 20016
USA

Dedicated to restoring nutrient-dense foods to the human diet through education, research and activism.

Hormones

Environmental Estrogens and Other Hormones
(www.som.tulane.edu/cbr/ecme/eehome/)

Run by the Center for Environmental Research, Tulane and Xavier Universities, New Orleans, Louisiana, this site provides news and information on the whole range of environmental oestrogens, and how they affect human health.

Introduction to Hormone Disrupting Compounds
(http://website.lineone.net/~mwarhurst/index.html)

These pages provide an introduction to the effects of hormone-disrupting chemicals on man and the environment, and the response of governments and industry to the problem. The material in these pages has been written by Dr A. Michael Warhurst, an environmental chemist who works for Friends of the Earth in London, UK.

Our Stolen Future
(www.ourstolenfuture.org)

The official website for the book Our Stolen Future, *which brought world-wide attention to scientific discoveries revealing that common contaminants can interfere with the natural signals controlling the development of the fetus.*

Indoor Air

Aircare
P.O. Box 46
Greenford UB6 7SU
UK
Freephone: 0800 074 5668
E-mail: elanra@aircare.co.uk

Distributors of the Elanra ioniser – the only ioniser in the world currently registered as a therapeutic instrument.

EPA – Indoor Air Quality Information
(www.epa.gov/iaq)

US Environmental Protection Agency site with useful tips and information on improving indoor air quality.

Fragranced Products Information Service
(www.fpinva.org)

In-depth, often startling, information on the risks of fragrance ingredients and perfumed products.

Pesticides

EPA – Pesticides
(http://www.epa.gov/pesticides/)

US Environmental Protection Agency site with useful tips and information on pesticides, including safe use and alternatives.

Pesticide Action Network
(www.pan-uk.org)
Eurolink Centre
49 Effra Road
London SW2 1BZ
UK
Tel: 020 7274 8895

UK arm of a network of over 600 participating non-governmental organisations, institutions and individuals in over 60 countries working to replace the use of hazardous pesticides with ecologically sound alternatives. Its projects and campaigns are coordinated by five autonomous regional centres. The site contains reports, articles and links to other sites, including other PAN sites and resources.

12 References

Introduction – Poisoned and Confused (pages vii–xii)

1 Masters RD. Biology and politics: linking nature and nurture. *Ann Rev Polit Sci*, 2001; 4: 345–69

2 Edelson SB, Cantor DS. Autism: xenobiotics influences. *Toxicol Ind Health*, 1998; 14: 553–63

3 Wakefield AJ, Montgomery S. Measles, mumps, rubella vaccine: through a glass darkly. *Adv Drug React Toxicol Rev*, 2001; 19: 1–19; Hurley DR *et al*. Referee 1, 2, 3 & 4. *Adv Drug React Toxicol Rev*, 2001; 19: 1–2

4 Schettler T *et al*. *Generations at Risk: Reproductive Health and the Environment*. MIT Press, 2000

Chapter 1 – Does This Sound Like You? (pages 3–16)

1 Rea WJ, Mitchell MJ. Chemical sensitivity in the environment. *J Immunol Allergy Pract*, 1982; Sept/Oct: 21–31; Randolph T, Moss RW. *An Alternative Approach to Allergies*. New York: Bantam Books, 1989

2 Melzer D. Genetics and medicalisation. *BMJ*, 2002; 321: 863–4

3 Finch CE, Tanzi RE. Genetics of aging. *Science*, 1997; 278: 407–11

4 Svendsen AJ *et al*. Relative importance of genetic effects in rheumatoid arthritis: historical cohort study of Danish nationwide twin population. *BMJ*, 2002; 324: 264–6

5 Begg CB. On the use of familial aggregation in population-based case probands for calculating penetrance. *J Natl Cancer Inst*, 2002; 94: 1221–6; Haffty BG *et al*. Outcome of conservatively managed early-onset breast cancer by BRCA1/2 status. *Lancet*, 2002; 359: 1471–7

6 Lichtenstein P *et al*. Environmental and heritable factors in the causation of cancer – analyses of cohorts of twins from Sweden, Denmark, and Finland. *N Engl J Med*, 2000; 343: 78–85; Verkasalo PK *et al*. Genetic predisposition,

environment and cancer incidence: a nationwide twin study in Finland, 1976-1995. *Int J Cancer*, 1999; 83: 743–9

7 Rogers SA. Diagnosing the sick building syndrome. *Environ Health Perspect*, 1987; 76: 195–8; Godish T. *Sick Buildings: Definition, Diagnosis and Mitigation*. Boca Raton, FL: Lewis Publications, 1995

8 Cullen MR. Workers with multiple chemical sensitivity. *Occup Med*, 1987; 2: 655–61; Hileman B. Multiple chemical sensitivity. *Chem Eng News*, 1991; 69: 26–42; Rea WJ. *Chemical Sensitivity, Vol 3*. Boca Raton, FL: Lewis Publications, 1996

9 Crinnion WJ. Environmental medicine, Part 1: The human burden of environmental toxins and their common health effects. *Altern Med Rev*, 2000; 5: 52–63

10 Ashford NA, Miller CS. *Chemical Exposures: Low Levels and High Stakes*. New York: Van Nostrand Reinhold, 1991

11 Randolph T. *Human Ecology and Susceptibility to the Chemical Environment*. Springfield, IL: Charles C Thomas, 1962; Randolph T. *Environmental Medicine – Beginnings and Bibliography of Clinical Ecology*. Fort Collins, CO: Clinical Ecology Publications, 1987

12 Schettler T *et al*. *In Harm's Way: Toxic Threats to Child Development*. Greater Boston Physicians for Social Responsibility, June 2000

13 Centers for Disease Control and Prevention. *National Report on Human Exposure to Environmental Chemicals*. Atlanta, GA: CDC, March 2001; www.cdc.gov/nceh/dls/report/

14 Centers for Disease Control and Prevention. *Second National Report on Human Exposure to Environmental Chemicals*. Atlanta, GA, March 2003; www.cdc.gov/exposurereport/

15 Environmental Working Group. *PFCs – A Family of Chemicals That Contaminate the Planet*. EWG, April 2003

16 Thomas P. *Cleaning Yourself to Death*. Dublin: Gill & Macmillan, 2000

Chapter 2 – Who Says Your Environment Makes You Sick? (pages 17–27)

1 Simmons Hotz A. Poison for profit; Chem/pharm has no equal – what a business plan! *Red Flags Weekly*, 15 May 2002; www.redflagsweekly.com/storm_warnings/poison.html

2 National Institutes of Health. *Environmental Diseases from A to Z*. Publication no. 96-4145, US Department of Health and Human Services, 1997

3 Masters RD. Biology and politics: linking nature and nurture. *Ann Rev Polit Sci*, 2001; 4: 345–69

4 Needleman HL *et al*. Bone lead levels and delinquent behavior. *JAMA*, 1996; 275: 363–9; Tong S *et al*. Lifetime exposure to environmental lead and children's intelligence at 11–13 years: the Port Pirie cohort study. *BMJ*, 1996; 312: 1569–75

5 Gottschalk LA *et al.* Abnormalities in hair trace elements as indicators of aberrant behavior. *Compr Psychiatry*, 1991; 32: 229–37

6 Breakey J. The historical development of concepts in the role of diet and hyperactivity from mid 1970s to mid 1980s. *J Paediatr Child Health*, 1997; 33: 190–4

7 Schoenthaler SJ. The Alabama diet–behavior program: an empirical evaluation at the Coosa Valley Detention Center. *Int J Biosoc Res*, 1983; 5: 79–87; Schoenthaler SJ. The Los Angeles probation department diet–behavior program: an empirical analysis of six institutional settings. *Int J Biosoc Res*, 1983; 5: 88–9; Schoenthaler SJ. The northern California diet–behavior program: an empirical evaluation of 3,000 incarcerated juveniles in Stanislaus County juvenile hall. *Int J Biosoc Res*, 1983; 5: 99–106

8 Jacobson JL, Jacobson SW. Intellectual impairment in children exposed to polychlorinated biphenyls in utero. *N Engl J Med*, 1996; 335: 783–9

9 Stallones L, Beseler C. Pesticide poisoning and depressive symptoms among farm residents. *Ann Epidemiol*, 2002; 12: 389–94

10 Mearns J *et al.* Psychological effects of organophosphate pesticides: a review and call for research by psychologists. *J Clin Psychol*, 1994; 50: 286–94

11 Morrow LA *et al.* Psychiatric symptomatology in persons with organic solvent exposure. *J Consult Clin Psychol*, 1993; 61: 171–4

12 Morrow LA *et al.* Neuropsychological assessment, depression, and past exposure to organic solvents. *Appl Neuropsychol*, 2001; 8: 65–73

13 Lindholm P, Kajdacsy-Balla A. *Screening Environmental Chemical Mixtures for Effects on Prostate Cancer Invasion Properties.* EPA grant number: R827152; http://cfpub.epa.gov/ncer_abstracts/index.cfm/fuseaction/display.highlight/abs tract/1040/report/1999/

14 Choffres ER. Neurotoxic effects of pesticides critical to health. *Nation's Health APHA*, April 1987; David ES. The new victims. *Ecological Illness Law Report*, July-October 1985; Saifer P, Saifer M. Clinical detection of sensitivity to preservatives and chemicals. In Brostoff J, Challacombe S (eds). *Food Allergy and Intolerance.* Philadelphia: WB Saunders, 1987: 416–24

15 Greater Boston Physicians for Social Responsibility. *How Chemical Exposures Affect Reproductive Health: Patient Fact Sheet.* GBPSR, 1996

Chapter 3 – Silent Stress (pages 28–42)

1 Brosschot JF *et al.* Influence of life stress on immunological reactivity to mild psychological stress. *Psychosom Med*, 1994; 56: 216–24

2 McEwen BS. Protective and damaging effects of stress mediators. *N Engl J Med*, 1998; 338: 171–9

3 Seeman TE, Robbins RJ. Aging and hypothalamic-pituitary-adrenal response to challenge in humans. *Endocrinol Rev*, 1994; 15: 233–60

4 Betteridge DJ. What is oxidative stress? *Metabolism*, 2000; 49 (2 Suppl 1): 3–8; Halliwell B *et al.* Free radicals, antioxidants, and human disease: where are we now? *J Lab Clin Med*, 1992; 119: 598–620

5 Halliwell B. Free radicals and oxidative damage in biology and medicine. In Reznick L *et al.* (eds). *Oxidative Stress in Skeletal Muscle.* Boston, MA: Birkhäuser Verlag, 1998; Marx JL. Oxygen free radicals linked to many diseases. *Science,* 1985; 235: 529–31

6 Levin B. The oxidative origins of arthritis. *Nutr Sci News,* 1997; 2: 598–600

7 Rajman I *et al.* The oxidative hypothesis of atherosclerosis. *Lancet,* 1994; 334: 1363–4

8 Chan PK *et al.* Brain injury, edema and vascular permeability changes induced by oxygen-derived free radicals. *Neurology,* 1984; 34: 315–20; Beal MF. Aging, energy and oxidative stress in neurodegenerative diseases. *Ann Neurol,* 1995; 38: 356–66

9 Kehrer JP. Free radicals as mediators of tissue injury and disease. *Crit Rev Toxicol,* 1993; 23: 21–48; Klaunig JE *et al.* The role of oxidative stress in chemical carcinogenesis. *Environ Health Perspect,* 1998; 106 (suppl 1): 289–95

10 Harman D. The free-radical theory of aging. In Pryor WA, (ed). *Free Radicals in Biology (Vol 5).* New York: Academic Press, 1982: 255–75; Harman D. Free radical involvement in aging: Pathophysiology and therapeutic implications. *Drugs Aging,* 1993; 3: 0–80; Harman D. Free radicals in aging. *Mol Cell Biochem,* 1988; 84: 155–61; Harman D. The aging process. *Proc Natl Acad Sci USA,* 1981; 78: 7124–8

11 Ames BN *et al.* Oxidants, antioxidants, and the degenerative diseases of aging. *Proc Natl Acad Sci USA,* 1993; 90: 7915–22

12 Pryor WA. Free-radicals in biological systems. In *Readings from Scientific American: Organic Chemistry of Life.* San Francisco: W.H. Freeman, 1973: 429–38

13 Löscher W, Käs G. Conspicuous behavioural abnormalities in a dairy cowherd near a TV and radio transmitting antenna. *Pract Vet Surg,* 1998; 79: 437–44

14 Lee JM *et al.* Studies on melatonin, cortisol, progesterone and interleukin-1 in sheep exposed to EMF from a 500-kv transmission line. In Stevens RG *et al.* (eds). *The Melatonin Hypothesis – Breast Cancer and Use of Electric Power.* Columbus, OH: Battelle Press, 1997

15 Human Society International, Food and Agriculture Organization of the United Nations Regional Office for Asia and the Pacific. *Guidelines for Human Handling and Transport and Slaughter of Livestock.* Publication no. 2001/4, 2001; Apple J *et al.* Influence of repeated restraint and isolation stress and electrolyte administration on pituitary-adrenal secretions,

electrolytes and other blood constituents of sheep. *J Animal Sci*, 1993; 71: 71; Zavy MT *et al*. Effects of initial restraint, weaning, and transport stress on baseline and ACTH-stimulated cortisol responses in beef calves of different genotypes. *Am J Vet Res*, 1992; 53: 551

16 Mack A. Trying to unlock the mysteries of free radicals and antioxidants. *Scientist*, 1996; 10: 13, 16

17 Stampfer MT *et al*. Vitamin E consumption and the risk of coronary heart disease in women. *N Engl J Med*, 1993; 328: 1444–9; Stampfer MT *et al*. Vitamin E consumption and the risk of coronary heart disease in men. *N Engl J Med*, 1993; 328: 1450–6

18 Heinonen OP *et al*. Prostate cancer and supplementation with alpha-tocopherol and beta-carotene: Incidence and mortality. *J Natl Cancer Inst*, 1998; 90: 440–6; Clark LC *et al*. Effects of selenium supplementation for cancer prevention in patients with carcinoma of the skin: A randomized controlled trial. *JAMA*, 1996; 276: 1957–63

19 Masaki KH *et al*. Association of vitamin C and C supplement use with cognitive function and dementia in elderly men. *Neurology*, 2000; 54: 1265–72

20 Losonczy KG *et al*. Vitamin E and vitamin C supplement use and risk of all-cause and coronary heart disease mortality in older persons. *Am J Clin Nutr*, 1996; 64: 190–6

21 Young G *et al*. Recognition of common childhood malignancies. *Am Fam Physician*, 2000; 61: 2144–54

22 *Mortality Statistics – Childhood, Infant and Perinatal*. London: National Statistics, 1999

23 Calle EE *et al*. Cigarette smoking and risk of fatal breast cancer. *Am J Epidemiol*, 1994; 139: 1001–7

24 Miller RW. Special susceptibility of the child to certain radiation-induced cancers. *Environ Health Perspect*, 1995; 103 (Suppl 6): 41–4

25 Roberts RJ. Overview of similarities and differences between children and adults: implications for risk assessment. In Guzelian PS *et al*. (eds). *Similarities and Differences Between Children and Adults*. Washington, DC: ILSI Press, 1992: 1–15

26 Bearer CF. How are children different from adults? *Environ Health Perspect*, 1995; 103 (Suppl 6): 7–12

27 Boyle JP *et al*. Projection of diabetes burden through 2050: impact of changing demography and disease prevalence in the US. *Diabetes Care*, 2001; 24: 1936–40

28 Lawrence RC *et al*. Estimates of the prevalence of arthritis and selected musculoskeletal disorders in the United States. *Arthritis Rheum*, 1998; 41: 778–99

29 Berger GS. Endometriosis: how many women are affected? *Endometriosis Association Newsletter*, 1995; 14: 4–7

30 Henderson BE *et al*. Toward the primary prevention of cancer. *Science*, 1991; 254: 1131–8

31 Rego MA. Non-Hodgkin's lymphoma risk derived from exposure to organic solvents: a review of epidemiologic studies. *Cad Saude Publ*, 1998; 14 (Suppl 3): 41–66

32 Bertazzi A *et al*. Cancer incidence in a population accidentally exposed to 2,3,7,8-tetrachlorodibenzo-para-dioxin. *Epidemiology*, 1993; 4: 398–406

33 Cantor KP *et al*. Pesticides and other agricultural risk factors for non-Hodgkin's lymphoma among men in Iowa and Minnesota. *Cancer Res*, 1992; 52: 2447–55; Blair A *et al*. Non-Hodgkin's lymphoma and agricultural use of the insecticide lindane. *Am J Indust Med*, 1998; 33: 82–7; Hardell L, Eriksson M. A case-control study of non-Hodgkin lymphoma and exposure to pesticides. *Cancer*, 1999; 85: 1353–60

34 Hoar SK *et al*. Agricultural herbicide use and risk of lymphoma and soft-tissue sarcoma. *JAMA*, 1986; 256: 1141–7

35 Woods JS *et al*. Soft tissue sarcoma and non-Hodgkin's lymphoma in relation to phenoxyherbicide and chlorinated phenol exposure in western Washington. *J Natl Cancer Inst*, 1987; 78: 899–910; Rothman N *et al*. A nested case-control study of non-Hodgkin lymphoma and serum organochlorine residues. *Lancet*, 1997; 350: 240–4

36 Hardell L *et al*. Do flame retardants increase the risk of non-Hodgkin lymphoma? The levels of polybrominated diphenyl ethers are increasing in the environment. *Lakartidningen*, 1998; 95: 5890–3

37 Cantor KP *et al*. Hair dye use and risk of leukemia and lymphoma. *Am J Publ Health*, 1988; 78: 570–1

38 Thun MJ *et al*. Hair dye use and risk of fatal cancers in US women. *J Natl Cancer Inst*, 1994; 86: 210–5

39 Holly EA *et al*. Hair-color products and risk for non-Hodgkin's lymphoma: a population-based study in the San Francisco bay area. *Am J Publ Health*, 1998; 88: 1767–73; Grodstein F *et al*. A prospective study of permanent hair dye use and hematopoietic cancer. *J Natl Cancer Inst*, 1994; 86: 1466–70

40 Washburn EP *et al*. Residential proximity to electricity transmission and distribution equipment and risk of childhood leukemia, childhood lymphoma, and childhood nervous system tumors: systematic review, evaluation, and meta-analysis. *Cancer Causes Control*, 1994; 5: 299–309; Floderus B *et al*. Incidence of selected cancers in Swedish railway workers, 1961-79. *Cancer Causes Control*, 1994; 5: 189–94; Meinert R, Michaelis J. Meta-analyses of studies on the association between electromagnetic fields and childhood cancer. *Radiat Environ Biophys*, 1996; 35: 11–8; Savitz DA *et al*. Case-control study of childhood cancer and exposure to 60-Hz magnetic fields. *Am J Epidemiol*, 1988; 128: 21–38

Chapter 4 – Prudence and Precaution (pages 45–50)

1 Starfield B. Is US health really the best in the world? *JAMA*, 2000; 284: 483–5
2 Hubbard B. *The Secrets of the Drug Industry*, London: WDDTY, 2002
3 *IMS World Review 2001, United Nations, World Population Prospects*. Office for National Statistics, APBI
4 Tickner J *et al. The Precautionary Principle in Action - A Handbook*. Science and Environmental Health Network, 1998; Pollan M. Precautionary Principle. *New York Times*, 9 December 2001; Science and Environmental Health Network. *The Precautionary Principle: A Fact Sheet*. March 1998

Chapter 5 – Sick Buildings, Sick People (pages 51–91)

1 Editorial. Climate change the new bioterrorism. *Lancet*, 2001; 358: 1657; Kunzli N. Public-health impact of outdoor and traffic-related air pollution: a European assessment. *Lancet*, 2000; 356: 795–801
2 Wallace LA *et al*. Personal exposure, indoor-outdoor relationships, and breath levels of toxic air pollutants measured for 355 persons in New Jersey. *EPA 0589*; Wallace LA *et al*. Personal exposures, outdoor concentrations, and breath levels of toxic air pollutants measured for 425 persons in urban, suburban and rural areas. *EPA 0589*; presented at the Annual Meeting of Air Pollution Control Association, San Francisco, CA, 25 June 1984; Ott WR, Roberts JW. Everyday exposure to toxic pollutants. *Sci Am*, 1998; Feb: 86–91
3 Aggazzotti G *et al*. Occupational and environmental exposure to perchloroethylene (PCE) in dry cleaners and their family members. *Arch Environ Health*, 1994; 49: 487–93
4 Hill RH Jr *et al*. p-Dichlorobenzene exposure among 1,000 adults in the United States. *Arch Environ Health*, 1995; 50: 277–80
5 IEH. *Indoor Air Quality in the Home: Nitrogen Dioxide, Formaldehyde, Volatile Organic Compounds, House Dust Mites, Fungi and Bacteria (Assessment A2)*. Leicester, UK: Institute for Environment and Health, 1996
6 Brown SK. Exposure to volatile organic compounds in indoor air: a review. In *Proceedings of the International Clean Air Conference of the Clean Air Society of Australia and New Zealand*, 1992; 1: 95–104; Brown SK. Volatile organic pollutants in new and established buildings in Melbourne, Australia. *Indoor Air*, 2002; 12: 55–63
7 Rogers SA. Diagnosing the tight building syndrome. *Environ Health Perspect*, 1987; 76: 195–8; Menzies R *et al*. Impact of exposure to multiple contaminants on symptoms of sick building syndrome. *Proc Indoor Air*, 1993; 1: 363–8
8 Hedge A. Suggestive evidence for a relationship between office design and self-reports of ill-health among office workers in the United Kingdom. *J Architect Plan Res*, 1984; 1: 163–74; Robertson AS *et al*. Comparison of

health problems related to work and environment measurements in two office buildings with different ventilation systems. *BMJ*, 1985; 291: 373–6; Burge PS *et al.* Sick building syndrome: A study of 4373 office workers. *Ann Occup Hygiene*, 1987; 31: 493–504; Hedge A. Environmental conditions and health in offices. *Int Rev Ergonom*, 1989; 3: 87–110; Mendell M, Smith A. Consistent pattern of elevated symptoms in air-conditioned office buildings: A reanalysis of epidemiologic studies. *Am J Publ Health*, 1990; 80: 1193–9; Zweers T *et al.* Health and indoor climate complaints of 7043 office workers in 61 buildings in the Netherlands. *Indoor Air*, 1992; 2: 127–36; Mendell MJ. Non-specific symptoms in office workers: a review and summary of the epidemiologic literature. *Indoor Air*, 1993; 3: 227–36

 9 Middaugh DA *et al.* Sick building syndrome: Medical evaluation of two work forces. *J Occup Med*, 1992; 34: 1197–203

10 World Health Organization. *Indoor Air Pollutants: Exposure and Health Effects*. EURO Reports and Studies 78, WHO, 1983

11 Morris L, Hawkins L. The role of stress in the sick building syndrome. In Siefert B *et al.* (eds). *Indoor Air '87, Proceedings of the 4th International Conference on Indoor Air Quality and Climate*. Berlin (West): Institute for Water, Soil and Air Hygiene, 1987; 2: 566–71

12 Wilson S, Hedge A. *The Office Environment Survey: A Study of Building Sickness*. London: Building Use Studies Ltd, 1987

13 Hedge A *et al.* Effects of personal and occupational factors on sick building syndrome reports in air-conditioned offices. In Quick JC *et al.* (eds). *Work and Well-Being: Assessments and Interventions for Occupational Mental Health*. Washington, DC: American Psychological Association, 1992: 286–98; Hedge A *et al.* Psychosocial correlates of sick building syndrome. *Indoor Air*, 1995; 5: 10–21; Hedge A *et al.* Predicting sick building syndrome at the individual and aggregate levels. *Environ Int*, 1996; 22: 3–19; Ooi PL, Goh KT. Sick building syndrome: an emerging stress-related disorder? *Int J Epidemiol*, 1997; 26: 1243–9

14 Hedge A. Job stress, job satisfaction, and work-related illness in offices. In *Proceedings of the 32nd Annual Meeting of the Human Factors Society*. Santa Monica, CA. Human Factors Society, 1988; 777–9; Hedge A *et al.* Work-related illness in office workers: a proposed model of the sick building syndrome. *Environ Int*, 1989; 15: 143–58; Skov P *et al.* Influence of personal characteristics, job-related factors and psychosocial factors on the sick building syndrome. *Scand J Work Environ Health*, 1989; 15: 286–96; Stenberg B, Wall B. Why do women report "sick building symptoms" more than men? *Soc Sci Med*, 1995; 40: 491–502

15 Dickey JH. *No Room to Breath: Air Pollution and Primary Care Medicine*. Greater Boston Physicians for Social Responsibility; http://www.psr.org/breathe.htm

16 Lundberg P. Proceedings of the International Conference on Organic Solvent Neurotoxicity, Stockholm, 15–17 October 1984. *Scand J Work Environ Health*, 1985; 11: 1–103; Arlien-Sorborg P. *Solvent Neurotoxicity*. Boca Raton, FL: CRC Press; 1992

17 Boekelheide K. 2,5-Hexanedione alters microtubule assembly-II-enhanced polymerization of crosslinked tubulin. *Toxicol Appl Pharmacol*, 1987; 88: 383–96; Morshed KM *et al*. Propylene glycol-mediated cell injury in a primary culture of human proximal tubule cells. *Toxicol Sci*, 1998; 46: 410–7; Verplanke AJ, Herber RF. Effects on the kidney of occupational exposure to styrene. *Int Arch Occup Environ Health*, 1998; 71: 47–52

18 Karakaya A *et al*. Immune function in N-hexane-exposed workers. *Ann NY Acad Sci*, 1997; 837: 122–5

19 Krzyzanowski M *et al*. Chronic respiratory effects of indoor formaldehyde exposure. *Environ Res*, 1990; 52: 117–25

20 International Agency for Research on Cancer. *IARC Monographs on the Evaluation of Carcinogenic Risks to Humans, Vol 62*. IARC, 1995; National Toxicology Program. *Eighth Annual Report on Carcinogens*. US Department of Health and Human Services, 1998

21 Brown SK, Cheng M. Volatile organic compounds (VOCs) in new car interiors. In *Proceedings of the 15th International Clean Air & Environment Conference*. Sydney, Australia, 26–30 November 2000; 1: 464–8

22 EPA Office of Toxic Substances. *Broad Scan Analysis of the FY82 National Human Adipose Tissue Survey Specimens, EPA 560/5-86-035*. Springfield, VA: National Technical Information Service (NTIS) no. PB 87-177218/REB, 1982

23 White RF, Proctor SP. Solvents and neurotoxicity. *Lancet*, 1997; 349: 1239–43

24 Svensson BG *et al*. Neuroendocrine effects in printing workers exposed to toluene. *Br J Ind Med*, 1992; 49: 402–8

25 Sallmen M *et al*. Time to pregnancy among the wives of men exposed to organic solvents. *Occup Environ Med*, 1998; 55: 24–30

26 Kolstad HA *et al*. Change in semen quality and sperm chromatin structure following occupational styrene exposure. *ASCLEPIOS Int Arch Occup Environ Health*, 1999; 72: 135–41

27 Xu X *et al*. Association of petrochemical exposure with spontaneous abortion. *Occup Environ Med*, 1998; 55: 31–6

28 Khattak S *et al*. Pregnancy outcome following gestational exposure to organic solvents: a prospective controlled study. *JAMA*, 1999; 281: 1106–9

29 Kim Y *et al*. Evaluation of exposure to ethylene glycol monoethyl ether acetates and their possible haematological effects on shipyard painters. *Occup Environ Med*, 1999; 56: 378–82

30 Rafnsson V, Gudmundsson G. Long-term follow-up after methyl chloride intoxication. *Arch Environ Health*, 1997; 52: 355–9

31 Luderer U *et al*. Reproductive endocrine effects of acute exposure to toluene in men and women. *Occup Environ Med*, 1999; 56: 657–66; Goh VH *et al*. Effects of chronic exposure to low doses of trichloroethylene on steroid hormone and insulin levels in normal men. *Environ Health Perspect*, 1998; 106: 41–4

32 Bethwaite PB *et al*. Cancer risks in painters: study based on the New Zealand Cancer Registry. *Br J Ind Med*, 1990; 47: 742–6

33 Fisher A *et al*. Allergic contact dermatitis due to ingredients of vehicles. A "vehicle tray" for patch testing. *Arch Dermatol*, 1971; 104: 286–90; Fisher AA. Reactions to popular cosmetic humectants, Part III, Glycerin, propylene glycol, and butylene glycol. *Cutis*, 1980; 26: 243–4, 269; Eun HC, Kim YC. Propylene glycol allergy from ketoconazole cream. *Contact Derm*, 1989; 21: 274–5

34 Wilson KC *et al*. Propylene glycol toxicity in a patient receiving intravenous diazepam. *N Engl J Med*, 2000; 343: 815; Arbour RB. Propylene glycol toxicity related to high-dose lorazepam infusion: case report and discussion. *Am J Crit Care*, 1999; 8: 499–506

35 Wheless JW. Pediatric use of intravenous and intramuscular phenytoin: lessons learned. *J Child Neurol*, 1998; 13 (Suppl 1): S11–4; discussion, S30–2; Yorgin PD *et al*. Propylene glycol-induced proximal renal tubular cell injury. *Am J Kidney Dis*, 1997; 30: 134–9

36 Bedichek E, Kirschbaum B. A case of propylene glycol toxic reaction associated with etomidate infusion. *Arch Intern Med*, 1991; 151: 2297–8; Kelner MJ, Bailey DN. Propylene glycol as a cause of lactic acidosis. *J Anal Toxicol*, 1985; 9: 40–2; Demey H *et al*. Propylene glycol intoxication due to intravenous nitroglycerin. *Lancet*, 1984; i: 1360

37 Anttila A *et al*. Cancer incidence among Finnish workers exposed to halogenated hydrocarbons. *J Occup Environ Med*, 1995; 37: 797–806

38 Spirtas R *et al*. Retrospective cohort mortality study of workers at an aircraft maintenance facility. *Br J Ind Med*, 1991; 48: 515–30

39 Ashford N, Miller C. *Chemical Exposures: Low Levels and High Stakes*. New York: Wiley & Sons, 1998; Wallace LA *et al*. *Identification of Polar Organic Compounds in Consumer Products and Common Microenvironment*. EPA, 1991

40 Report by the Committee on Science and Technology. *Neurotoxins: At Home and the Workplace*. US House of Representatives, Report no. 99-827, 16 September 1986

41 Anderson RC, Anderson JH. Acute toxic effects of fragrance products. *Arch Environ Health*, 1998; 53: 138–46; Millqvist E, Lowhagen O. Placebo-controlled challenges with perfume in patients with asthma-like symptoms.

Allergy, 1996; 51: 434–9; Anderson RC, Anderson JH. Toxic effects of air freshener emissions. *Arch Environ Health*, 1997; 52: 433–41; Hastings L *et al.* Olfactory primary neurons as a route of entry for toxic agents into the CNS. *Neurotoxicology*, 1991; 12: 707–14; Kumar P *et al.* Inhalation challenge effects of perfume scent strips in patients with asthma. *Ann Allergy Asthma Immunol*, 1995; 75: 429–33; Daughton CG, Ternes TA. Pharmaceuticals and personal care products in the environment: agents of subtle change? *Environ Health Perspect*, 1999; 107 (Suppl 6): 907–38; Buchbauer G *et al.* Fragrance compounds and essential oils with sedative effects upon inhalation. *J Pharm Sci*, 1993; 82: 660–4; Spencer PS *et al.* Neurotoxic properties of musk ambrette. *Toxicol Appl Pharmacol*, 1984; 75: 571–5; Spencer PS *et al.* Neurotoxic fragrance produces ceroid and myelin disease. *Science*, 1979; 204: 633–5

42 Candida Research and Information Foundation. *Perfume Survey.* Winter 1989–1990

43 Wainman T *et al.* Ozone and limonene in indoor air: A source of submicron particle exposure. *Environ Health Perspect*, 2000; 108: 1139

44 Fisher BE. Scent and sensitivity. *Environ Health Perspect*, 1998; 106: 109–11

45 Lin TC *et al.* Environmental exposure to polycyclic aromatic hydrocarbons and total suspended particulates in a Taiwanese temple. *Bull Environ Contam Toxicol*, 2001; 67: 332–8

46 National Research Council. *Environmental Tobacco Smoke: Measuring Exposures and Assessing Health Effects.* Washington, DC: National Academy Press, 1986

47 US Department of Health and Human Services. *The Health Consequences of Involuntary Smoking – A Report of the Surgeon General.* Washington, DC: DHHS, Publication no. PHS 87-8398, 1986

48 UK Department of Health and Social Security. *Fourth Report of the Independent Scientific Committee on Smoking and Health.* London: HMSO, 1988

49 Australian National Health and Medical Research Council. *Effects of Passive Smoking on Health – Report of the NHMRC Working Party on the Effects of Passive Smoking on Health.* Canberra: Australia Government Publishing Service, 1987

50 Hackshaw AK *et al.* The accumulated evidence on lung cancer and environmental tobacco smoke. *BMJ*, 1997; 315: 980–8

51 Repace J. *A Killer on the Loose.* Action on Smoking and Health, April 2003

52 Law MR *et al.* Environmental tobacco smoke exposure and ischaemic heart disease: an evaluation of the evidence. *BMJ*, 1997; 315: 973–80

53 Lewis RG *et al.* Distribution of pesticides and polycyclic aromatic hydrocarbons in house dust as a function of particle size. *Environ Health Perspect*, 1999; 107: 721–6

54 Schneider A, Smith C. Major brands of kids' crayons contain asbestos, tests show. *Seattle Post-Intelligencer*, 23 May 2000; http://seattlepi.nwsource.com/national/cray23.shtml

55 Won D *et al*. Indoor carpet as an adsorptive reservoir for volatile organic compounds. In *Proceedings of the 92nd Annual Meeting of the Air & Waste Management Association*. St Louis, MO, June 1999

56 Duehring C. Carpet – EPA stalls and industry hedges while consumers remain at risk. *Informed Consent*, 1993; 1: 6–32

57 Whitemore RW *et al*. Non-occupational exposures to pesticides for residents of two U.S. cities. *Arch Environ Contam Toxicol*, 1994; 26: 47–59

58 Allsopp M *et al*. *Hazardous Chemical in Carpets*. Greenpeace Research Laboratories/University of Exeter, January 2001

59 Marin V *et al*. Effects of ionization of the air on some bacterial strains. *Ann Ig*, 1989; 1: 1491–500

60 Gabbay J *et al*. Effect of ionization on microbial air pollution in the dental clinic. *Environ Res*, 1990; 52: 99–106

61 Hawkins LH. The possible benefits of negative-ion generators. In Pearse BG (ed). *Health Hazards of VDTs?* Chichester: John Wiley & Sons, 1984

62 Terman M, Terman JS. Treatment of seasonal affective disorder with a high-output negative ionizer. *J Alt Complement Med*, 1995; 1: 87–92; Terman M *et al*. A controlled trial of timed bright light and negative air ionisation for treatment of winter depression. *Arch Gen Psychiatry*, 1988; 55: 875–82

63 Brown GC, Kirk RE. Geophysical variables and behavior: XXXVIII. Effects of ionized air on the performance of a vigilance task. *Percept Motor Skills*, 1987; 64: 951–62; Nakane H *et al*. Effect of negative air ions on computer operation, anxiety and salivary chromogranin A-like immunoreactivity. *Int J Psychophysiol*, 2002; 46: 85

64 Daniell W *et al*. Trial of a negative ion generator device in remediating problems related to indoor air quality. *J Occup Med*, 1991; 33: 681–7

65 Kellogg E *et al*. Long-term biological effects of air ions and DC electric fields on NAMRU mice: first year report. *Int J Biometeorol*, 1985; 29: 253–68; Krueger AP, Reed EJ. Biological impact of small air ions. *Science*, 1976; 24: 1209–13; Krueger AP *et al*. Further observations on the effect of air ions on influenza in the mouse. *Int J Biometeorol*, 1974; 18: 46–56

66 Sulman FG. The impact of weather on human health. *Rev Environ Health*, 1984; 4: 83–119; Sulman FG. Migraine and headache due to weather and allied causes and its specific treatment. *Ups J Med Sci*, 1980; 31 (Suppl): 41–4; Sulman FG *et al*. New methods in the treatment of weather sensitivity. *Fortschr Med*, 1977; 95: 746–52

67 Wolverton BC *et al*. *Interior Landscape Plants for Indoor Air Pollution Abatement*. National Aeronautics and Space Administration, 1989

68 Thomas P. *Cleaning Yourself to Death*. Dublin: Newleaf, 2001

Chapter 6 – The Bug Stops Here (pages 92–129)

1 Carson R. *Silent Spring* (reprint edition), Mariner Books, 1994
2 Grossman J. Dangers of household pesticides. *Environ Health Perspect*, 1995; 103: 550–4
3 PAN UK. Survey of home and garden pesticide use. *News Release: 20 August 2001*
4 Winegar K. Pesticides on domestic flights may be a health hazard. *Conscious Choice: The Journal of Ecology & Natural Living*, 1998; 11: 33
5 McCance RA, Widdowson EM. *The Chemical Composition of Foods, 1st edn.* Special Report Series no: 235, UK: Royal Society of Chemistry/MAFF, 1940
6 McCance RA, Widdowson EM. *The Composition of Foods, 5th edn.* UK: Royal Society of Chemistry/MAFF, 1991
7 Thomas D. Mineral depletion in foods over the period 1940 to 1991. *Nutr Pract*, 2001; 2: 27–9
8 Mayer AM. Historical changes in the mineral content of fruits and vegetables; A cause for concern? *Br Food J*, 1997; 99: 207–11
9 No author listed. Vegetables without vitamins. *Life Extension*, March 2001; www.lef.org/magazine/mag2001/mar2001_report_vegetables.html
10 Fedtke C. Plant physiological adaptations induced by low rates of photosynthesis. *Z Naturforsch*, 1979; 34c: 932–5
11 Sandmann G *et al*. Phytoene desaturase, the essential target for bleaching herbicides. *Weed Sci*, 1991; 39: 474–9
12 Stidham MA. Herbicides that inhibit acetohydroxyacid synthase. *Weed Sci*, 1991; 39: 428–34
13 Kevan PG, Phillips TP. The economic impacts of pollinator declines: an approach to assessing the consequences. *Conserv Ecol*, 2001; 5(1): 8; http://www.consecol.org/vol5/iss1/art8; Cane JH, Tepedino VJ. Causes and extent of declines among native North American invertebrate pollinators: detection, evidence, and consequences. *Conserv Ecol*, 2001; 5(1): 1; http://www.consecol.org/vol5/iss1/art1
14 Gunderson EL. *FDA Total Diet Study*, April 1982–April 1984; Dietary intakes of pesticides, selected elements, and other chemicals. *J Assoc Off Anal Chem*, 1988; 71: 1200–9
15 Food and Drug Administration. *Total Diet Study, Summary of Residues Found Ordered by Food, Market Baskets*. 91-3-99-1, FDA, September 2000
16 *Working Party on Pesticide Residues – 1999 Report*. London: MAFF Publications, 1999
17 Australia New Zealand Food Authority. *The 19th Australian Total Diet Survey*. ANZFA, April 2001

18 Cressey P *et al. 1997/98 New Zealand Total Diet Survey, Part 1: Pesticide Residues.*
    Ministry of Health, 2000; White A. *Pesticides in Food: Why Go Organic?* Pesticide
    Action Network NZ/Safe Food Campaign NZ PAN, New Zealand, 1999

19 Kilthau GF. Cancer risk in relation to radioactivity in tobacco. *Radiol Technol*,
    1996; 67: 217–22

20 Watter RL, Hansen WR. The hazards and implications of the transfer of un-
    supported 210 Po from alkaline soil to plants. *Health Phys J*, 1970; 18: 409–13

21 Office of Environment Health and Safety, Utah State University. Cigarettes
    are a major source of radiation exposure. *SafetyLine*, 1996; Issue 33

22 Marmorstein J. Lung cancer: is the increasing incidence due to radioactive
    polonium in cigarettes? *South Med J*, 1986; 79: 145–50; Winters TH, Franza
    JR. Radioactivity in cigarette smoke. *N Engl J Med*, 1982; 306: 364–5

23 Ames BN *et al.* Ranking possible carcinogenic hazards. *Science*, 1987; 236:
    271–80

24 Wiles R, Campbell C. *Pesticides in Children's Food*. Washington, DC:
    Environmental Working Group, 1993; Wiles R *et al. Tap Water Blues*.
    Washington, DC: Environmental Working Group, 1994

25 Cohen B *et al. Weed Killers by the Glass: A Citizens' Tap Water Monitoring
    Project in 29 Cities*. Washington, DC: Environmental Working Group, 1995

26 US Department of Agriculture. *USDA Pesticide Data Program: Annual
    Summary Calendar Year 1993*. Washington, DC: USDA Agricultural
    Marketing Service, 1995

27 Arnold SF *et al.* Synergistic activation of estrogen receptor with combinations
    of environmental chemicals. *Science*, 1996; 272: 1489–92

28 Gray L *et al.* Chronic nitrosamine ingestion in 1040 rodents: the effect of the
    choice of nitrosamine, the species studies, and the age of starting exposure.
    Cancer Res, 1991; 51: 6470–90; McConnell EE. Comparative responses in
    carcinogenesis bioassays as a function of age at first exposure. In Guzelian PS
    et al. (eds). *Similarities and Differences Between Children and Adults:
    Implications for Risk Assessment*. Washington, DC: International Life Sciences
    Institute, 1992: 66–78

29 Whitemore RW *et al.* Non-occupational exposures to pesticides for residents
    of two U.S. cities. *Arch Environ Contam Toxicol*, 1994; 26: 47–59

30 Environmental Protection Agency. *List of Pesticide Product Inert Ingredients*.
    Washington, DC: Office of Prevention, Pesticides and Toxic Substances, 6
    October 1993

31 US EPA Office of the Inspector General. *Inert Ingredients of Pesticides (Audit
    Report no. E1EPF1-05-0117-1100378*. Washington, DC: Environmental
    Protection Agency, 27 September 1991

32 Briggs SA, The Rachel Carson Council Inc. *Basic Guide To Pesticides*.
    Hemisphere Publishing, 1992

33 Zwick D. *Water Wasteland: Ralph Nader's Study Group Report on Water Pollution.* New York: Bvikin Press, 1971

34 Barbash JE, Resek EA. *Pesticides in Ground Water.* Chelsea, Michigan: Ann Arbor Press, 1996; Wiles R *et al. Tap Water Blues.* Washington, DC: Environmental Working Group 1994; Cohen BA, Wiles R. *Tough to Swallow.* Washington, DC: Environmental Working Group, 1997; Environmental Working Group. *Pouring it On; Nitrate Contamination of Drinking Water.* Washington, DC: Environmental Working Group, 1996; Solomon GM, Mott L. *Trouble on the Farm; Growing Up With Pesticides in Agricultural Communities.* New York: Natural Resources Defense Council, October, 1998

35 *What are the Heath Effects of Contaminants in Drinking Water?* EPA Office of Water; http://www.epa.gov/safewater/dwh/health.html

36 Hignite C, Azarnoff DL. Drugs and drug metabolites as environmental contaminants: chlorophenoxyisobutyrate and salicyclic acid in sewage water effluent. *Life Sci,* 1977; 20: 337–41

37 Daughton CG, Ternes TA. Pharmaceuticals and personal care products in the environment: agents of subtle change. *Environ Health Perspect,* 1999; 107 (Suppl 6): 907–38; Raloff J. Drugged waters. *Sci News,* 1998; 153: 187–9

38 Buser HR, Muller MD. Occurrence of the pharmaceutical drug clofibric acid and the herbicide mecoprop in various Swiss lakes and in the North Sea. *Environ Sci Technol,* 1998; 32: 188–92

39 Andelman JB. Human exposures to volatile halogenated organic chemicals in indoor and outdoor air. *Environ Health Perspect,* 1985; 62: 313–8

40 Brown HS *et al.* The role of skin absorption as a route of exposure for volatile organic compounds (VOCs) in drinking water. *Am J Publ Health,* 1984; 74: 479–84; Maxwell NI *et al.* Trihalomethanes and maximum contaminant levels: the significance of inhalation and dermal exposures to chloroform in household water. *Regul Toxicol Pharmacol,* 1991; 14: 297–312; Jo WK *et al.* Routes of chloroform exposure and body burden from showering with chlorinated tap water. *Risk Anal,* 1990; 10: 575–80

41 Fayer R. Effect of sodium hypochlorite on infectivity of *Cryptosporidium parvum* for neonatal BALB/c mice. *Appl Environ Microbiol,* 1995; 61: 844–6

42 Le Chevallier MW *et al. Giardia* and *Cryptosporidium* spp. in filtered drinking water supplies. *Appl Environ Microbiol,* 1991; 57: 2617–21

43 Crane RI, Wilkinson MJ. *Review of Human Exposure to Water Contaminants.* Foundation for Water Research Report no. FR0290, March 1992

44 Morris RD. Drinking water and cancer. *Environ Health Perspect,* 1995; 103: 225–31; Dunnick JK, Melnick RI. Assessment of the carcinogenic potential of chlorinated water: experimental studies of chlorine, chloramine, and trihalomethanes. *J Natl Cancer Inst,* 1993; 85: 817–22

45 EWG/USPIRG. *Consider the Source – Farm Runoff, Chlorination By-products,*

and Human Health. Washington, DC: Environmental Working Group/US Public Interest Research Group, January 2002

46 Swan SH *et al.* A prospective study of spontaneous abortion: relation to amount and source of drinking water consumed in early pregnancy. *Epidemiology,* 1998; 9: 126–33

47 Waller K *et al.* Trihalomethanes in drinking water and spontaneous abortion. *Epidemiology,* 1998; 9: 134–40

48 Bove FJ *et al.* Public drinking water contamination and birth outcomes. *Am J Epidemiol,* 1995; 141: 850–62

49 Cantor KP *et al.* Drinking water source and chlorination by-products, I – Risk of bladder cancer. *Epidemiology,* 1998; 9: 21–8; Morris RD. Drinking water and cancer. *Environ Health Perspect,* 1995; 103: 225–31

50 McGeehin MA *et al.* Case-control study of bladder cancer and water disinfection methods in Colorado. *Am J Epidemiol,* 1993; 138: 492–501

51 Cantor KP *et al.* Bladder cancer, drinking water source, and tap water consumption: a case-control study. *J Natl Cancer Inst,* 1987; 79: 1269–79

52 Brunelle JA, Carlos J. Recent trends in dental caries in U.S. children and the effect of water fluoridation. *J Dent Res,* 1990; 69: 723–7

53 Burt BA *et al.* The effects of a break in water fluoridation on the development of dental caries and fluorosis. *J Dent Res,* 2000; 79: 761–9; Kunzel W *et al.* Decline in caries prevalence after the cessation of water fluoridation in former East Germany. *Commun Dent Oral Epidemiol,* 2000; 28: 382–9; Maupome G *et al.* Patterns of dental caries following the cessation of water fluoridation. *Commun Dent Oral Epidemiol,* 2001; 29: 37–47; Seppa L *et al.* Caries trends 1992–98 in two low-fluoride Finnish towns formerly with and without fluoride. *Caries Res,* 2000; 34: 462–8

54 Griffin SO *et al.* Esthetically objectionable fluorosis attributable to water fluoridation. *Commun Dent Oral Epidemiol,* 2002; 30: 199–209

55 Beltran-Aguilar ED *et al.* Prevalence and trends in enamel fluorosis in the United States from the 1930s to the 1980s. *J Am Dent Assoc,* 2002; 133: 157

56 Foulkes RG. Case report: mass fluoride poisoning, Hooper Bay, Alaska, a review of the final report of the Alaska Department of Health and Human Services, April 12, 1993. *Fluoride,* 1994; 27: 1, 32–6

57 Danielson C *et al.* Hip fractures and fluoridation in Utah's elderly population. *JAMA,* 1992; 268: 746–8; Jacobsen SJ *et al.* Regional variation in the incidence of hip fracture. US white women aged 65 years and older. *JAMA,* 1990; 264: 500–2; Cooper C *et al.* Water fluoridation and hip fracture. *JAMA,* 1991; 266: 513–4

58 Whitford GM. Fluoride in dental products: safety considerations. *J Dent Res,* 1987; 66: 1056–60; Hodge HC. *The Safety of Fluoride Tablets or Drops in Continuing Evaluation of the Use of Fluorides.* Boulder, CO: Westview Press, 1979

59 Shulman JD, Wells LM. Acute fluoride toxicity from ingesting home-use dental products in children, birth to 6 years of age. *J Publ Health Dent*, 1997; 57: 150–8

60 World Resources Institute. *World Resources 1998-1999*. Oxford: Oxford University Press, 1998

61 Moses M. Pesticide-related health problems and farmworkers. *AAOHN J*, 1989; 37: 115–30

62 National Research Council. *Carcinogens and Anticarcinogens in the Human Diet – a comparison of naturally occurring and synthetic substances*. Washington, DC: National Academy Press, 1996

63 Ritter L. Report of a panel on the relationship between public exposure to pesticides and cancer. Ad Hoc Panel on Pesticides and Cancer, National Cancer Institute of Canada. *Cancer*, 1997; 80: 2019–33

64 World Wildlife Fund. *Chemical Trespass – A Toxic Legacy*. WWF-UK, 1999

65 Natural Resources Defences Council. *Intolerance Risk: Pesticides in our Children's Food*. Washington, DC: NRDC, 1989

66 Daniels JL *et al*. Pesticides and childhood cancers. *Environ Health Perspect*, 1997; 105: 1068–77; Meinert R *et al*. Leukemia and non-Hodgkin's lymphoma in childhood and exposure to pesticides: results of a register-based case-control study in Germany. *Am J Epidemiol*, 2000; 151: 639–46; 647–50 (discussion); Buckley JD *et al*. Pesticide exposures in children with non-Hodgkin lymphoma. *Cancer*, 2000; 89: 2315–21; Meinert R *et al*. Childhood leukaemia and exposure to pesticides: results of a case-control study in northern Germany. *Eur J Cancer*, 1996; 32A: 1943–8; Unger M, Olsen J. Organochlorine compounds in the adipose tissue of deceased people with and without cancer. *Environ Res*, 1980; 23: 257–63

67 Davis JR *et al*. Family pesticide use and childhood brain cancer. *Arch Environ Contam Toxicol*, 1993; 24: 87–92

68 Zahm SH, Ward MH. Pesticides and childhood cancer. *Environ Health Perspect*, 1998; 106 (Suppl 3): 893–908

69 Lowengart RA *et al*. Childhood leukemia and parents' occupational and home exposures. *J Natl Cancer Inst*, 1987; 79: 39–46

70 Leiss J, Savitz D. Home pesticide use and childhood cancer: A case control study. *Am J Publ Health*, 1995; 85: 249–52

71 Buckley JD *et al*. Pesticide exposures in children with non-Hodgkin lymphoma. *Cancer*, 2000; 89: 2315–21

72 National Research Council. *Environmental Neurotoxicology*. Washington, DC: National Academy Press, 1992; National Research Council. *Pesticides in the Diets of Infants and Children*. Washington, DC: National Academy Press, 1993

73 Walkowiak J *et al*. Environmental exposure to polychlorinated biphenyls and quality of the home environment: effects on psychodevelopment in early childhood. *Lancet*, 2001; 358: 1602–7

74 Guillette EA *et al.* An anthropological approach to the evaluation of pre-school children exposed to pesticides in Mexico. *Environ Health Perspect*, 1998; 106: 347–53

75 Jacobson JL, Jacobson SW. Intellectual impairment in children exposed to polychlorinated biphenyls in utero. *N Engl J Med*, 1996; 335: 783–9

76 Purdey M. BSE – Dying to know the truth. *Ecologist*, November: 2002; Bounias M, Purdey M. Transmissible spongiform encephalopathies: a family of etiologically complex diseases – a review. *Sci Total Environ*, 2002; 297: 1–19

77 Purdey M. Ecosystems supporting clusters of sporadic TSEs demonstrate excesses of the radical-generating divalent cation manganese and deficiencies of antioxidant cofactors Cu, Se, Fe, Zn. *Med Hypoth*, 2000; 54: 278–306; Brown DR *et al.* Consequences of manganese replacement of copper for prion protein function and proteinase resistance. *EMBO J*, 2000; 19: 1180–6

78 Kogevinas M *et al.* Soft tissue sarcoma and non-Hodgkin's lymphoma in workers exposed to phenoxy herbicides, chlorophenols, and dioxins: two nested case-control studies. *Epidemiology*, 1995; 6: 396–402; Morrison HI *et al.* Herbicides and cancer. *J Natl Cancer Inst*, 1992; 84: 1866–74; Smith JG, Christophers AJ. Phenoxy herbicides and chlorophenols: a case control study on soft tissue sarcoma and malignant lymphoma. *Br J Cancer*, 1992; 65: 442–8; Hoar Zahm S *et al.* A case-referent study of soft-tissue sarcoma and Hodgkin's disease. Farming and insecticide use. *Scand J Work Environ Health*, 1988; 14: 224–30

79 Hoar SK *et al.* Agricultural herbicide use and risk of lymphoma and soft-tissue sarcoma. *JAMA*, 1986; 256: 1141–7

80 Eriksson M, Karlsson M. Occupational and other environmental factors and multiple myeloma: a population based case-control study. *Br J Ind Med*, 1992; 49: 95–103

81 Fleming L *et al.* Aplastic anemia and pesticides, an etiologic association? *J Occup Med*, 1993; 35: 1106–15

82 Bosma H *et al.* Pesticide exposure and risk of mild cognitive dysfunction. *Lancet*, 2000; 356: 912–3

83 Compaton JE *et al.* Reduced bone formation after exposure to organophosphates. *Lancet*, 1999; 354: 1791–2

84 No authors listed. Disease associated with exposure to certain herbicide agents: type 2 diabetes. Final rule. *Fed Regist*, 2001; 66: 23166–9

85 Longnecker MP *et al.* Polychlorinated biphenyl serum levels in pregnant subjects with diabetes. *Diabetes Care*, 2001; 24: 1099–101

86 Longnecker MP, Michalek JE. Serum dioxin levels in relation to diabetes mellitus among Air Force veterans with background levels of exposure. *Epidemiology*, 2000; 11: 44–8

87 Barsano CP, Thomas JA. Endocrine disorders of occupational and environmental origin. *Occup Med*, 1992; 7: 479–502

88 Repetto R, Baliga S. *Pesticides and the Immune System: the Public Health Risks.* Washington, DC: World Resources Institute, 1996

89 Steenland K *et al.* Thyroid hormones and cytogenetic outcomes in backpack sprayers using ethylene-bis (dithiocarbamate) (EBDC) fungicides in Mexico. *Environ Health Perspect*, 1997; 105: 1126–30

90 Rae WJ. *Chemical Sensitivity vols 1-4.* Boca Raton: Lewis Publishers, 1992

91 Dunstan RH *et al.* A preliminary investigation of chlorinated hydrocarbons and chronic fatigue syndrome. *Med J Aust*, 1995; 163: 294–7

92 Behan PO. Chronic fatigue syndrome as a delayed reaction to chronic low-dose organophosphate exposure. *J Nutr Environ Med*, 1996; 6: 341–50

93 Hornick SB. Factors affecting the nutritional quality of crops. *Am J Alt Agric*, 1992; 7: 63–8

94 Worthington V. Effects of agricultural methods on nutritional quality: a comparison of organic with conventional crops. *Alt Ther Health Med*, 1998; 4: 58–69

95 Knorr D *et al.* Quantity and quality determination of ecologically grown foods. In *Sustainable Food Systems.* Westport, CN: AVI Publishing, 1983: 352–81

96 Bentley EM *et al.* Fluoride ingestion from toothpaste by young children. *Br Dent J*, 1999; 186: 460–2

Chapter 7 – Turn on, Plug in, Get Sick (pages 130–162)

1 Brodeur P. *Currents of Death: Powerlines, Computer Terminals, and the Attempt to Cover Up Their Threat to Your Health.* New York: Simon & Schuster, 1989; Becker R. *Cross Currents: The Promise of Electromedicine, the Perils of Electropollution.* Los Angeles: Jeremy P Tarcher, 1990; Coghill R. *Something in the Air.* Gwent: Coghill Research Laboratories, 1997

2 Miller AB *et al.* Leukaemia following occupational exposure to 60 Hz electric and magnetic fields among Ontario electric utility workers. *Am J Epidemiol*, 1996; 144: 150–60

3 Reiser H-P *et al.* The influence of electromagnetic fields on human brain activity. *Eur J Med Res*, 1995; 1: 27–32; Borbely AA *et al.* Pulsed high-frequency electromagnetic field effects on human sleep and sleep electro-encephalogram. *Neurosci Lett*, 1999; 275: 207–10

4 Freuda G *et al.* Effects of microwaves emitted by cellular phones on human slow brain potentials. *Bioelectromagnetics*, 1998; 19: 384–7; Krause CM *et al.* Effects of electromagnetic fields emitted by cellular telephones on t EEG during a memory task. *Neuro Rep*, 2000; 11: 761–4

5 Braune S *et al.* Resting blood pressure increase during exposure to radio-frequency electromagnetic field. *Lancet*, 1998; 351: 1857–8

6 Lai H *et al.* Effects of low-level microwave irradiation on amphetamine hyperthermia are blockable by naloxone and classically conditionable. *Psychopharmacology,* 1986: 88: 354–61; Lai H *et al.* A review of microwave irradiation and actions of psychoactive drugs. *IEEE Engineer Med Biol,* 1987; March: 31–6; Lai H. Research on the neurological effects of nonionizing radiation at the University of Washington. *Bioelectromagnetics,* 1992; 13: 513–26; Lai H. Neurological effects of radiofrequency electromagnetic radiation. In Lin JC (ed). *Advances in Electromagnetic Fields in Living Systems.* New York: Plenum Press, 1994

7 Cutz A. Effects of microwave radiation on the eye: the occupational health perspective. *Lens Eye Toxic Res,* 1989; 6: 379–86

8 Stang A *et al.* The possible role of radiofrequency radiation in the development of uveal melanoma. *Epidemiology,* 2001; 12: 7–12; Inskip PD. Frequent radiation exposures and frequency-dependent effects: the eyes have it. *Epidemiology,* 2001; 12: 1–4; Johansen C *et al.* Mobile phones and malignant melanoma of the eye. *Br J Cancer,* 2002; 86: 348–9

9 Hall SC *et al.* Effects of microwaves on isolated eyes. *Proceedings of the Bioelectromagnetics Conference,* Bologna, Italy, 1997; Silk AC. Mobile phones and human exposure. *Optometry Today,* 1999; 23 April: 24–31

10 WHO. *Environmental Health Criteria 137: Electromagnetic Fields (300 Hz to 300 GHz).* Geneva, Switzerland: WHO, 1993

11 Chen G *et al.* Effect of electromagnetic field exposure on chemically induced differentiation of friend erythroleukemia cells. *Environ Health Perspect,* 2000; 108: 967–72

12 Fröhlich H. The biological effects of microwaves and related questions. *Adv Electronics Electron Phys,* 1980; 53: 85–152; Grundler W, Kaiser F. Experimental evidence for coherent excitations correlated with cell growth. *Nanobiology,* 1992; 1: 163–76; Hyland GJ. Non-thermal bioeffects induced by low-intensity microwave irradiation of living systems. *Engineer Sci Edu J,* 1998; 7: 261–9; Fröhlich H (ed). *Biological Coherence and Response to External Stimuli.* Berlin: Springer-Verlag, 1988

13 Frey AH (ed). *On the Nature of Electromagnetic Field Interactions with Biological Systems* Austin, TX: RG Landes, 1994

14 Persson BRR *et al.* Blood-brain barrier permeability in rats exposed to electromagnetic fields used in wireless communication. *Wireless Networks,* 1997; 3: 455–61

15 Winkler T *et al.* Impairment of blood-brain barrier function by serotonin-induced desynchronization of spontaneous cerebral cortical activity: experimental observations in the anaesthetized rat. *Neuroscience,* 1995; 68: 1097–104; Barbanti P *et al.* Increased density of dopamine D5 receptor in peripheral blood lymphocytes of migraineurs: a marker of migraine? *Neurosci Lett,* 1996; 207: 73–6

16 Youbicier-Simo BJ, Bastide M. Pathological effects induced by embryonic and postnatal exposure to EMF radiation by cellular mobile phones (written evidence to IEGMP). *Radiat Protect*, 1999; 1: 218–23

17 Mann K, Roschke J. Effects of pulsed high-frequency electromagnetic fields on human sleep. *Neuropsychobiology*, 1996; 33: 41–7; Akerstedt T *et al*. A 50-Hz electromagnetic field impairs sleep. *J Sleep Res*, 1999; 8: 77–81

18 No author. Defining the EMF–melatonin relationship: real-world and lab findings diverge. *Microwave News*, 1997; Mar/Apr: 3–4

19 Liburdy RP *et al*. ELF magnetic fields, breast cancer, and melatonin: 60 Hz fields block melatonin's oncostatic action on ER+ breast cancer cell proliferation. *J Pineal Res*, 1993; 14: 89–97

20 Fews AP *et al*. Increased exposure to pollutant aerosols under high-voltage power lines. *Int J Radiat Biol*, 1999; 75: 1505–21; Fews AP *et al*. Corona ions from powerlines and increased exposure to pollutant aerosols. *Int J Radiat Biol*, 1999; 75: 1523–31

21 Henshaw DL *et al*. Enhanced deposition of radon daughter nuclei in the vicinity of power frequency electromagnetic fields. *Int J Radiat Biol*, 1996; 69: 25–38; Henshaw DL *et al*. Radon: A causative factor in the induction of myeloid leukaemia and other cancers in adults and children? *Lancet*, 1990; 335: 1008–12

22 University of Bergen. *Meteorological Report Series*. Report no. 101994, ISBN 82-90569-61-0

23 Preece AW *et al*. *Radon, Skin Cancer and Interaction With Power Lines*. US Department of Energy Contractors Review Meeting, San Antonio, Texas, November 17–21, 1996

24 Kallen B *et al*. Delivery outcome among physiotherapists in Sweden: is non-ionizing radiation a fetal hazard? *Arch Environ Health*, 1982; 37: 815; Nordstrom S *et al*. Reproductive hazards among workers at high-voltage substations. *Bioelectromagnetics*, 1983; 4: 91–101

25 Kieler H *et al*. Routine ultrasound screening in pregnancy and the children's subsequent handedness. *Early Hum Dev*, 1998; 50: 233–45; Paneth N. Prenatal sonography – safe or sinister? *Lancet*, 1998; 352: 5–6; Visser GH *et al*. Effects of frequent ultrasound during pregnancy. *Lancet*, 1993; 342: 1359–60

26 Hande MP, Devi PU. Teratogenic effects of repeated exposures to x-rays and/or ultrasound in mice. *Neurotox Teratol*, 1995; 17: 179–88

27 Campbell JD *et al*. Case-control study of prenatal ultrasonography exposure in children with delayed speech. *Can Med Assoc J*, 1993; 149: 1435–40

28 Stark CR. Short- and long-term risks after exposure to diagnostic ultrasound in utero. *Obstet Gynecol*, 1984; 63: 194–200

29 Tarantal AF, Hendricks AG. Evaluation of the bioeffects of prenatal ultrasound exposure in the cynomolgus macaque (*Macaca fascicularis*): II. Growth and behaviour during the first year. *Teratology*, 1989; 39: 149–62

30 Tarantal AF *et al.* Evaluation of the bioeffects of prenatal ultrasound exposure in the cynomolgus macaque (*Macaca fascicularis*): III. Developmental and hematologic studies. *Teratology*, 1993; 47: 159–70

31 Mole R. Possible hazards of imaging and Doppler ultrasound in obstetrics. *Birth*, 1986; 13: 29–37; Boswar KL *et al.* Heating of guinea-pig fetal brain during exposure to pulsed ultrasound. *Ultrasound Med Biol*, 1993; 19: 415–24; Edwards R. Shadow of a doubt. *New Sci*, 1999; 12 June: 23

32 Reif JS *et al.* Residential exposure to magnetic fields and risk of canine lymphoma. *Am J Epidemiol*, 1995; 14: 352–9

33 Lee JM *et al.* Studies on melatonin, cortisol, progesterone and interleukin-1 in sheep exposed to EMF from a 500-kV transmission line. In Stevens RG *et al.* (eds). *The Melatonin Hypothesis – Breast Cancer and Use of Electric Power.* Columbus, OH: Battelle Press, 1997

34 Löscher W, Käs G. Conspicuous behavioural abnormalities in a dairy cowherd near a TV and radio transmitting antenna. *Pract Vet Surg*, 1998; 79: 437–44

35 Wiltscho W *et al.* A magnetic pulse leads to a temporary deflection in the magnetic orientation of migratory birds. *Experimentia*, 1994; 50: 97–700

36 Hitchock R *et al. Radio Frequency and ELF Electromagnetic Energies: A Handbook for Health Professionals.* New York: Van Nostrand Reinhold, 1995

37 Rea WJ. Electromagnetic field sensitivity. *J Bioelectr*, 1991; 10: 241–56

38 National Research Council. *Multiple Chemical Sensitivities: Addendum to Biological Markers in Immunotoxicology.* Washington, DC: National Academy Press, 1992

39 Smith CW. Electrical sensitivities in allergy patients. *Clin Ecol*, 1986; 4: 93–102

40 Persinger M *et al.* Psychophysiological effects of extremely low-frequency electromagnetic fields: a review. *Percept Motor Skills*, 1973; 36: 1131–59

41 Petrucci N. Exposure of the critically ill patient to extremely low-frequency electromagnetic fields in the intensive care environment. *Intensive Care Med*, 1999; 25: 847–51

42 Valerio BC *et al.* Exposure of nursing personnel to electromagnetic fields in neonatal intensive care. *Assist Inferm Ric*, 2002; 21; 28–31

43 McGowan P. Masts hidden in petrol station signs. *London Evening Standard*, 2002; 8 October

44 Dendy PP. Mobile phones and the illusory pursuit of safety. *Lancet*, 2000; 356: 1782

45 Rothman KJ. Epidemiological evidence on the health risks of cellular telephones. *Lancet*, 2000; 356: 1837–40

46 Hyland GJ. Physics and biology of mobile telephony. *Lancet*, 2000; 356: 1833–6

47 Eulitz C *et al.* Mobile phones modulate response patterns of human brain activity. *Neuroreport*, 1998; 9: 3229–32

48 Braune S *et al.* Resting blood pressure increase during exposure to a radio-frequency electromagnetic field. *Lancet*, 1998; 351: 1857–8

49 Frey AH. Headaches from cellular telephones: are they real and what are the implications? *Environ Health Perspect*, 1998; 106: 101–3

50 Senior K. Mobile phones: are they safe? *Lancet*, 2000; 355: 1793

51 von Klitzing L. *Clinically Relevant Events of Bioeffects by Pulsed EM-Fields According to GSM- and DECT-Technique at Extremely Low Energy Levels.* Presented at Mobile Phones and Health Symposium, October 25–28, 1998, University of Vienna, Austria; Best S. Mobile phone protection devices. *PROOF!*, 2000; 5(1): 10–3

52 Gandhi OP *et al.* Electromagnetic absorption in the human head and neck for mobile telephones at 835 and 1900 MHz. *IEEE Trans MTT*, 1996; 44: 1884–97

53 Feychting M *et al.* Magnetic fields and childhood cancer – a pooled analysis of two Scandinavian studies. *Eur J Cancer*, 1995; 31A: 2035–9; Ahlbom A *et al.* Electromagnetic fields and childhood cancer. *Lancet*, 1993; 342: 1295–6; London SJ *et al.* Exposure to residential electric and magnetic fields and risk of childhood leukaemia. *Am J Epidemiol*, 1991; 134: 923–37; Savitz DA *et al.* Case-control study of childhood cancer and exposure to 60-Hz magnetic fields. *Am J Epidemiol*, 1988; 128: 21–38

54 National Radiation Protection Board. *ELF Electromagnetic Fields and the Risk of Cancer: Report of an Advisory Group on Non-Ionizing Radiation.* Chilton, Didcot: Documents of the NRPB 12, 2001

55 Linet ME *et al.* Residential exposure to magnetic fields and acute lymphoblastic leukemia in children. *N Engl J Med*, 1997; 337: 1–7; McBride ML *et al.* Power-frequency electric and magnetic fields and risk of childhood leukemia in Canada. *Am J Epidemiol*, 1999; 149: 831–42; Ahlbom A *et al.* A pooled analysis of magnetic fields and childhood leukaemia. *Br J Cancer*, 2000; 83: 692–8; Greenland S *et al.* A pooled analysis of magnetic fields, wire codes, and childhood leukaemia. *Epidemiology*, 2000; 11: 624–34

56 Wertheimer N, Leeper E. Electrical wiring configurations and childhood cancer. *Am J Epidemiol*, 1979; 109: 273–84

57 Feychting M, Ahlbom A. Magnetic fields and cancer in children residing near Swedish high-voltage powerlines. *Am J Epidemiol*, 1993; 138: 467–81

58 UK Childhood Cancer Study Investigators. Exposure to power frequency magnetic fields and the risk of childhood cancer: a case-control study. *Lancet*, 1999; 354: 1925–31

59 Dockerty JD *et al.* Electromagnetic field exposures and childhood leukaemia in New Zealand. *Lancet*, 1999; 354: 1967–8

60 Eckert EE. Magnetic influences on fetus and infant as reason for sudden infant death syndrome: a new testable hypothesis. *Med Hypoth*, 1992; 38: 66–9

61 Coghill RW. The electric railway children: an electromagnetic aetiology for cot death? *Hosp Equip Suppl*, 1989; June: 9

62 Coghill RW *et al*. ELF electric and magnetic fields in the bedplace of children diagnosed with leukaemia: a case-control study. *Eur J Cancer Prev*, 1996; 5: 153–8

63 Hardell L *et al*. Ionizing radiation, cellular telephones and the risk of brain tumours. *Eur J Cancer Prev*, 2001; 10: 523–9

64 Hardell L *et al*. Cellular and cordless telephones and the risk for brain tumours. *Eur J Cancer Prev*, 2002; 11: 377–86; Hardell L *et al*. Case-control study on the use of cellular and cordless phones and the risk for malignant brain tumours. *Int J Radiat Biol*, 2002; 78: 931–6

65 Hardell L *et al*. Case-control study on radiology work, medical x-ray investigations, and use of cellular telephones as risk factors for brain tumors. *Medscape Gen Med*, 2000; 4 May; http://www.medscape.com/viewarticle/408055

66 Demers PA *et al*. Occupational exposure to electromagnetic fields and breast cancer in men. *Am J Epidemiol*, 1991; 134: 340–7; Matanoski GM *et al*. Electromagnetic field exposure and male breast cancer. *Lancet*, 1991; 337: 737; Tynes T, Anderson A. Electromagnetic fields and male breast cancer. *Lancet*, 1990; 336: 1596

67 Wertheimer N, Leeper E. Magnetic field exposure related to cancer subtypes. *Ann NY Acad Sci*, 1987; 502: 43–53; Loomis DP *et al*. Breast cancer mortality among female electrical workers in the United States. *J Natl Cancer Inst*, 1994; 86: 921–5; Coogan P *et al*. Occupational exposure to 60Hz magnetic fields and risk of breast cancer in women. *Epidemiology*, 1996; 7: 459–64

68 Stevens RG. Electric power use and breast cancer: a hypothesis. *Am J Epidemiol*, 1987; 125: 556–61; Stevens RG *et al*. Electric power pineal function, and the risk of breast cancer. *Fed Am Soc Exp Bio J*, 1992; 6: 853–60

69 Selmaoui B *et al*. Magnetic fields and pineal function in humans: evaluation of nocturnal exposure to extremely low frequency magnetic fields on serum melatonin and urinary 6-sulfatoxymelatonin circadian rhythms. *Life Sci*, 1996; 58: 1539–49

70 Reiter RJ. Static and extremely low frequency electromagnetic field exposure: reported effects on the circadian production of melatonin. *J Cell Biochem*, 1993; 51: 394–403; Hill SM, Blask DE. Effects of the pineal hormone melatonin on the proliferation and morphological characteristics of human breast cancer cells (MCF-7) in culture. *Cancer Res*, 1988; 48: 6121–6

71 Guenel P *et al*. Incidence of cancer in persons with occupational exposure to electromagnetic fields in Denmark. *Br J Ind Med*, 1993; 50: 758–64; Loomis

D. Cancer of breast among men in electrical occupations. *Lancet*, 1991; 339: 1482–3; Rosenbaum PF *et al*. Occupational exposures associated with male breast cancer. *Am J Epidemiol*, 1994; 139: 30–6; Theriault G *et al*. Cancer risks associated with occupational exposure to magnetic fields among electric utility workers in Ontario and Quebec, Canada, and France: 1970-1989. *Am J Epidemiol*, 1994; 139: 550–72; MacDowall ME. Mortality of persons resident in the vicinity of electricity transmission facilities. *Br J Cancer*, 1986; 53: 271–9; Schreiber GH *et al*. Cancer mortality and residence near electricity transmission equipment: a retrospective cohort study. *Int J Epidemiol*, 1993; 22: 9–15; Cantor KP *et al*. Re: Breast cancer mortality among female electrical workers in the United States. *J Natl Cancer Inst*, 1995; 87: 227–8

72 Savitz DA *et al*. Update on methodological issues in the epidemiology of electromagnetic fields and cancer. *Epidemiol Rev*, 1994; 15: 558–66

73 Etherington DJ *et al*. An ecological study of cancer incidence and radon levels in South West England. *Eur J Cancer*, 1996; 32A: 1189–97

74 Preece AW *et al*. *Radon, Skin Cancer and Interaction With Power Lines*. US Department of Energy Contractors Review Meeting, San Antonio, Texas, November 17–21, 1996

75 Armstrong B *et al*. Association between exposure to pulsed electromagnetic fields and cancer in electric utility workers in Quebec, Canada and France. *Am J Epidemiol*, 1994; 140: 805–20; Vagero D, Olin R. Incidence of cancer in the electronics industry: using the new Swedish Cancer Environment Registry as a screening instrument. *Br J Ind Med*, 1983; 40: 188–92; Wertheimer N, Leeper E. Magnetic field exposure related to cancer subtypes. *Ann NY Acad Sci*, 1987; 502: 43–54

76 Erren T. Re: Association between exposure to pulsed electromagnetic fields and cancer in electrical utility workers in Quebec, Canada and France. *Am J Epidemiol*, 1996; 143: 841

77 McDowall ME. Mortality of persons resident in the vicinity of electricity transmission facilities. *Br J Cancer*, 1986; 53: 271–9

78 Washburn EP *et al*. Residential proximity to electricity transmission and distribution equipment and risk of childhood leukemia, childhood lymphoma, and childhood nervous system tumors: systematic review, evaluation, and meta-analysis. *Cancer Causes Control*, 1994; 5: 299–309; Floderus B *et al*. Incidence of selected cancers in Swedish railway workers, 1961-79. *Cancer Causes Control*, 1994; 5: 189–94; Meinert R, Michaelis J. Meta-analyses of studies on the association between electromagnetic fields and childhood cancer. *Radiat Environ Biophys*, 1996; 35: 11–8; Savitz DA *et al*. Case-control study of childhood cancer and exposure to 60-Hz magnetic fields. *Am J Epidemiol*, 1988; 128: 21–38

79 Verkasalo PK *et al*. Magnetic fields of transmission lines and depression. *Am J Epidemiol*, 1997; 146: 1037–45

80 van Wijngaarden E *et al.* Exposure to electromagnetic fields and suicide among electric utility workers: a nested case-control study. *Occup Environ Med*, 2000; 57: 258–63

81 Lyle B *et al.* Suppression of T-lymphocyte cytotoxicity following exposure to sinusoidally amplitude-modified fields. *Bioelectromagnetics*, 1983; 4: 281–92

82 Beale IL *et al. Chronic Health Problems in Adults Living Near High-Voltage Transmission Lines: Evidence for a Dose-Response Relation With Magnetic Field Exposure.* Presented at the 2nd World Conference on Electricity and Magnetism in Biology & Medicine, Bologna, Italy, June 1997; Beale I *et al.* Psychological effects of chronic exposure to 50 Hz magnetic fields in humans living near extra-high-voltage transmission lines. *Bioelectromagnetics*, 1997; 18: 584–94

83 Bonhomme-Faivre L *et al.* Study of human neurovegetative and hematologic effects of environmental low-frequency (50-Hz) electromagnetic fields produced by transformers. *Arch Environ Health*, 1998; 53: 87–92

84 Wertheimer N, Leeper E. Possible effects of electric blankets and heated waterbeds on fetal development. *Bioelectromagnetics*, 1986; 7: 13–22; Belanger K *et al.* Spontaneous abortion and exposure to electric blankets and heated water beds. *Epidemiology*, 1998; 9: 36–42

85 Li DK *et al.* A population-based prospective cohort study of personal exposure to magnetic fields during pregnancy and the risk of miscarriage. *Epidemiology*, 2002; 13: 9–20; Lee GM *et al.* A nested case-control study of residential and personal magnetic fields measures and miscarriages. *Epidemiology*, 2002; 13: 21–31

86 Becker R. *Cross Currents: The Promise of Electromedicine, the Perils of Electropollution.* Los Angeles: Jeremy P Tarcher, 1990

87 Hondou T. Rising level of public exposure to mobile phones: accumulation through additivity and reflectivity. *J Phys Soc Jpn*, 2002; 71: 432–7

88 Charlton A, Bates C. Decline in teenage smoking with rise in mobile phone ownership: hypothesis. *BMJ*, 2000; 321: 1155

89 Harris C *et al.* Survey of physical ergonomics issues with school children's use of laptop computers. *Int J Indust Ergonom,* 2000; 26: 337–46

Chapter 8 – Fooling the Body (pages 163–203)

1 Committee on Hormonally Active Agents in the Environment, National Research Council. *Hormonally Active Agents in the Environment.* National Academy of Sciences, 2000; European Workshop on the Impact of Endocrine Disrupters on Human Health and Wildlife, 2–4 December 1996, Weybridge, UK. *Proceedings, Report No. EUR 17549.* Copenhagen, Denmark: European Commission DG XII, April 1997

2 Harrison PTC. Endocrine disrupters and human health. *BMJ*, 2001; 323: 1317–8; Harrison PTC *et al.* Reproductive health in humans and wildlife: are

adverse trends associated with environmental chemical exposure? *Sci Total Environ*, 1997; 205: 97–106

3 Biles JE *et al*. Determination of bisphenol A in re-usable polycarbonate food contact plastics and migration to food-simulating liquids. *J Agric Food Chem*, 1997; 45: 3541–4; Lambert C, Larroque M. Chromatographic analysis of water and wine samples for phenolic compounds released from food contact expoxy resins. *J Chromatogr Sci*, 1997; 35: 57–62

4 Brotons JA *et al*. Xenoestrogens released from lacquer coatings in food cans. *Environ Health Perspect*, 1995; 103: 608–12

5 Yoshida T *et al*. Determination of bisphenol A in canned vegetables and fruit by high performance liquid chromatography. *Food Addit Contam*, 2001; 18: 69–75

6 Barrett JR. Soy and children's health: a formula for trouble. *Environ Health Perspect*, 2002; 110: A294–6

7 Strom BL. Exposure to soy-based formula in infancy and endocrinological and reproductive outcomes in young adulthood. *JAMA*, 2001; 286: 807–14

8 Eklund G, Oskarsson A. Exposure of cadmium from infant formulas and weaning foods. *Food Addit Contam*, 1999; 16: 509–19

9 Worldwide Fund for Nature. *Bisphenol A – A Known Endocrine Disruptor. A WWF European Toxics Programme Report*, April 2000

10 Santodonato J. Review of the estrogenic and antiestrogenic activity of poly-cyclic aromatic hydrocarbons: Relationship to carcinogenicity. *Chemosphere*, 1997; 34: 835–48; Arcaro KF *et al*. Antiestrogenicity of environmental poly-cyclic aromatic hydrocarbons in human breast cancer cells. *Toxicology*, 1999; 133: 115–27

11 Routledge EJ *et al*. Some alkyl hydroxy benzoate preservatives (parabens) are estrogenic. *Toxicol Appl Pharmacol*, 1998; 153: 12–9

12 Schlumpf M *et al*. In vitro and in vivo estrogenicity of UV screens. *Environ Health Perspect*, 2001; 109: 239–44; Nakagawa Y *et al*. Metabolism and toxic-ity of benzophenone in isolated rat hepatocytes and estrogenic activity of its metabolites in MCF-7 cells. *Toxicology*, 2000; 156: 27–36

13 Ford RA *et al*. 90-day dermal toxicity study and neurotoxicity evaluation of nitromusks in the albino rat. *Food Chem Toxicol*, 1990; 28: 55–6

14 Geldof AA *et al*. Estrogenic action of commonly used fragrant agent citral induces prostatic hyperplasia. *Urol Res*, 1992; 20: 139–44

15 Sharma-Wagner S *et al*. Occupation and prostate cancer risk in Sweden. *J Occup Environ Med*, 2000; 42: 517–25

16 Seinen W *et al*. AHTN and HHCB show weak estrogenic – but no uterotrophic activity. *Toxicol Lett*, 1999; 111: 161–8

17 Blount BC *et al*. Levels of seven urinary phthalate metabolites in a human reference population. *Environ Health Perspect*, 2000; 108: 979–82

18 Environmental Health Network of California. *FDA Petition no. 99P-1340.* Filed May 1999

19 Ilonka A *et al.* Potent competitive interactions of some brominated flame retardants and related compounds with human transthyretin in vitro. *Toxicol Sci,* 2000; 56: 95–104

20 Barsano CP, Thomas J. Endocrine disorders of occupational and environmental origin. *Occup Med,* 1992; 7: 479–502; Birnbaum LS. Developmental effects of dioxins and related endocrine disrupting chemicals. *Toxicol Lett,* 1995; 82/83: 743–50; Chemically-induced alterations in sexual and functional development: The wildlife/human connection. In Colborn T, Clement C (eds). *Advances in Modern Environmental Toxicology, vol 21.* Princeton, NJ: Princeton Scientific Publishing, 1992; US Environmental Protection Agency Risk Assessment Forum. *Special Report on Environmental Endocrine Disruption: An Effects Assessment and Analysis.* 1997; http://www.epa.gov/ORD/WebPubs/endocrine/; McLachlan JA, Arnold SF. Environmental estrogens. *Sci Am,* 1996; September-October; http://www.americanscientist.org/articles/96articles/McLachla.html

21 Davis DL *et al.* Medical hypothesis: bifunctional genetic-hormonal pathways to breast cancer. *Environ Health Perspect,* 1997; 105 (Suppl 3): 571–6

22 Peat R. Estriol, DES, DDT, etc. *Townsend Lett Docs,* 1997; 162: 53–7

23 Epstein S. *The Breast Cancer Prevention Program.* London: John Wiley & Sons, 1998

24 Hirose T *et al.* Estrogenic/antiestrogenic activities of benzo[a]pyrene monohydroxy derivatives. *J Health Sci,* 2001; 47: 552–8; Fertuck KC *et al.* Interaction of polyaromatic hydrocarbon (PAH)-related compounds with the alpha and beta isoforms of the estrogen receptor. *Toxicol Lett,* 2001; 121: 167–77

25 MAFF. *Food Surveillance Information Sheet, Number 82: Phthalates in Food.* London: Ministry of Agriculture, Fisheries and Food, 1996

26 Geldof AA *et al.* Estrogenic action of commonly used fragrant agent citral induces prostatic hyperplasia. *Urol Res,* 1992; 20: 139–44

27 Gray LE Jr. Xenoendocrine disrupters: laboratory studies on male reproductive effects. *Toxicol Lett,* 1998; 102–3: 331–5

28 Schlumpf M *et al.* In vitro and in vivo estrogenicity of UV screens. *Environ Health Perspect,* 2001; 109: 239–44

29 Nakagawa Y *et al.* Metabolism and toxicity of benzophenone in isolated rat hepatocytes and estrogenic activity of its metabolites in MCF-7 cells. *Toxicology,* 2000; 156: 27–36

30 Toppari J *et al.* Trends in the incidence of cryptorchidism and hypospadias, and methodological limitations of registry-based data. *Hum Reprod Update,* 2001; 7: 282–6; Pierik FH *et al.* A high hypospadias rate in The Netherlands. *Hum Reprod,* 2002; 17: 1112–5

31 Klip H *et al.* Hypospadias in sons of women exposed to diethylstilbestrol in utero: a cohort study. *Lancet,* 2002; 359: 1102–7

32 Mocarelli P *et al.* Paternal concentrations of dioxin and sex ratio of offspring. *Lancet,* 2000; 355: 1858–63

33 Moshammer H, Neuberger M. Sex ratio in the children of the Austrian chloracne cohort. *Lancet,* 2000; 356: 1271–2

34 Den Hond E *et al.* Sexual maturation in relation to polychlorinated aromatic hydrocarbons: Sharpe and Skakkebaek's hypothesis revisited. *Environ Health Perspect,* 2002; 110: 771–6

35 Herman-Giddens ME *et al.* Secondary sexual characteristics and menses in young girls seen in office practice: a study from the Pediatric Research in Office Settings network. *Pediatrics,* 1997; 99: 505–12; Partsch CJ, Sippell WG. Pathogenesis and epidemiology of precocious puberty – effects of exogenous oestrogens. *Hum Reprod Update,* 2001; 7: 292–302

36 Blanck HM *et al.* Age at menarche and tanner stage in girls exposed in utero and postnatally to polybrominated biphenyl. *Epidemiology,* 2000; 11: 641–7

37 Saenz de Rodriguez CA *et al.* An epidemic of precocious development in Puerto Rican children. *J Pediatr,* 1985; 107: 393–6

38 Colon I *et al.* Identification of phthalate esters in the serum of young Puerto Rican girls with premature breast development. *Environ Health Perspect,* 2000; 108: 895–900

39 Eskenazi B *et al.* Serum dioxin concentrations and endometriosis: a cohort study in Seveso, Italy. *Environ Health Perspect,* 2002; 110: 629–34

40 Eskenazi B *et al.* Serum dioxin concentrations and menstrual cycle characteristics. *Am J Epidemiol,* 2002; 156: 383–92

41 Yu ML *et al.* Menstruation and reproduction in women with polychlorinated biphenyl (PCB) poisoning: long-term follow-up interviews of the women from the Taiwan Yucheng cohort. *Int J Epidemiol,* 2000; 29: 672–7

42 Cooper GS *et al.* Organochlorine exposure and age at natural menopause. *Epidemiology,* 2002; 13: 729–33

43 Wolff MS, Weston MA. Breast cancer risk and environmental exposures. *Environ Health Perspect,* 1997; 105 (Suppl 4): 891–6

44 Wasserman M *et al.* Organochlorine compounds in neoplastic and adjacent apparently normal breast tissue. *Bull Environ Contam Toxicol,* 1976; 15: 478–84

45 Warner M *et al.* Serum dioxin concentrations and breast cancer risk in the Seveso Women's Health Study. *Environ Health Perspect,* 2002; 110: 625–8

46 Hoyer AP *et al.* Organochlorine exposure and risk of breast cancer. *Lancet,* 1998; 352: 1816–20

47 Wolff MS *et al.* Blood levels of organochlorine residues and risk of breast cancer. *J Natl Cancer Inst,* 1993; 85: 648–52

48 Mussalo-Rauhamaa H. Occurrence of beta-hexachlorocyclohexane in breast cancer patients. *Cancer*, 1990; 66: 2124–8; Falck F. Pesticides and polychlorinated biphenyl residues in human breast lipids and their relation to breast cancer. *Arch Environ Health*, 1992; 47: 143–6

49 Romieu I *et al*. Breast cancer, lactation history, and serum organochlorines. *Am J Epidemiol*, 2000; 152: 363–70

50 Gladen BC, Rogan WJ. DDE and shortened duration of lactation in a northern Mexican town. *Am J Publ Health*, 1995; 85: 504–8

51 Bell EM *et al*. A case-control study of pesticides and fetal death due to congenital anomalies. *Epidemiology*, 2001; 12: 148–56

52 Pastore LM *et al*. Risk of stillbirth from occupational and residential exposures. *Occup Environ Med*, 1997; 54: 511–8

53 Raloff J. Macho waters. *Sci News*, 2001; 159: 8

54 Watanabe N, Kurita M. The masculinization of the fetus during pregnancy due to inhalation of diesel exhaust. *Environ Health Perspect*, 2001; 109: 111–9

55 Editorial. Male reproductive health and environmental oestrogens. *Lancet*, 1995; 345: 933–5; Toppari J *et al*. *Male Reproductive Health and Environmental Chemicals with Estrogenic Effects*. Copenhagen, Denmark: Danish Environmental Protection Agency, April 1995; Toppari J *et al*. Changes in male reproductive health and effects of endocrine disruptors in Scandinavian countries. *Cad Saude Publ*, 2002; 18: 413–20

56 Sultan C *et al*. Environmental xenoestrogens, antiandrogens and disorders of male sexual differentiation. *Mol Cell Endocrinol*, 2001; 178: 99–105

57 Carlsen L *et al*. Evidence for decreasing quality of semen during last 50 years. *BMJ*, 1992; 305: 609–13

58 Swan SH *et al*. Have sperm densities declined? A reanalysis of global trend data. *Environ Health Perspect*, 1997; 105: 1228–32

59 Swan SH *et al*. The question of declining sperm density revisited: an analysis of 101 studies published 1934–1996. *Environ Health Perspect*, 2000; 108: 961–6

60 Jensen TK *et al*. Do environmental estrogens contribute to the decline in male reproductive health? *Clin Chem*, 1995; 41: 1896–901

61 Oliva A *et al*. Contribution of environmental factors to the risk of male infertility. *Hum Reprod*, 2001; 16: 1768–76

62 Tielemans E *et al*. Pesticide exposure and decreased fertilisation rates in vitro. *Lancet*, 1999; 354: 484–5

63 Guo YL *et al*. Semen quality after prenatal exposure to polychlorinated biphenyls and dibenzofuran. *Lancet*, 2000; 356: 1240–1

64 Skakkebaek NE. Endocrine disrupters and testicular dysgenesis syndrome. *Horm Res*, 2002; 57 (Suppl 2): 43; Norgil Damgaard I *et al*. Impact of expo-

sure to endocrine disrupters in utero and in childhood on adult reproduction. *Best Pract Res Clin Endocrinol Metab*, 2002; 16: 289–309

65 Skakkebaek NE *et al.* Germ cell cancer and disorders of spermatogenesis: an environmental connection? *APMIS*, 1998; 106: 3–11, 12

66 Toppari J *et al.* Male reproductive health and environmental xenoestrogens. *Environ Health Perspect*, 1996; 104 (Suppl 4): 741–803

67 Hardell L *et al.* Increased concentrations of polychlorinated biphenyls, hexa-chlorobenzene and chlordanes in mothers to men with testicular cancer. *Environ Health Perspect*, 2003; 111: 930–4
http://ehpnet1.niehs.nih.gov/docs/2003/5816/abstract.html

68 Ekbom A, Akre O. Increasing incidence of testicular cancer – birth cohort effects. *APMIS*, 1998; 106: 225–9, 229–31 (discussion)

69 Ohlson CG, Hardell L. Testicular cancer and occupational exposures with a focus on xenoestrogens in polyvinyl chloride plastics. *Chemosphere*, 2000; 40: 1277–82

70 Griffiths K *et al.* Phytoestrogens and diseases of the prostate gland. *Baillière's Clin Endocrinol Metab*, 1998; 12: 625–47; Mitchell JH *et al.* Effects of phy-toestrogens on growth and DNA integrity in human prostate tumor cell lines: PC-3 and LNCaP. *Nutr Cancer*, 2000; 38: 223–8

71 Bosland MC. The role of steroid hormones in prostate carcinogenesis. *J Natl Cancer Inst Monogr*, 2000; 27: 39–66

72 Wetherill Y *et al.* The xenoestrogen bisphenol A induces inappropriate andro-gen receptor activation and mitogenesis in prostatic adenocarcinoma cells. *Mol Cancer Ther*, 2002; 1: 515–24

73 Golden RJ *et al.* Environmental endocrine modulators and human health: an assessment of the biological evidence. *Crit Rev Toxicol*, 1998; 28: 109–227

74 Santti R *et al.* Phytoestrogens: potential endocrine disruptors in males. *Toxicol Ind Health*, 1998; 14: 223–37

75 Warhurst M. *Introduction to Hormone Disrupting Compounds*;
http://website.lineone.net/~mwarhurst/

76 Colbin T *et al.* *Our Stolen Future.* http://www.ourstolenfuture.org

77 Boyd CA *et al.* Behavioral and neurochemical changes associated with chronic exposure to low-level concentration of pesticide mixtures. *J Toxicol Environ Health*, 1990; 30: 209–21

78 Porter WP *et al.* Groundwater pesticides: interactive effects of low concentra-tions of carbamates aldicarb and methamyl and the triazine metribuzin on thyroxine and somatotropin levels in white rats. *J Toxicol Environ Health*, 1993; 40: 15–34; Porter WP *et al.* Toxicant-disease-environment interactions associated with suppression of immune system, growth, and reproduction. *Science*, 1984; 224: 1014–7

79 Porter WP *et al.* Endocrine, immune and behavioral effects of aldicarb (carbamate), atrazine (triazine) and nitrate (fertilizer) mixtures at groundwater

concentrations. *Toxicol Ind Health*, 1999; 15: 133–50

80 Laisi A *et al.* The effect of maneb, zineb, and ethylenethiourea on the humoral activity of the pituitary-thyroid axis in rat. *Arch Toxicol Suppl*, 1985; 8: 253–8

81 Brechner RJ *et al.* Ammonium perchlorate contamination of Colorado River drinking water is associated with abnormal thyroid function in newborns in Arizona. *J Occup Environ Med*, 2000; 42: 777–82

82 Thayer KA *et al.* Altered prostate growth and daily sperm production in male mice exposed prenatally to subclinical doses of 17-alpha-ethinyl oestradiol. *Hum Reprod*, 2001; 16: 988–96

83 Water supplier owes no duty towards ultra-sensitive plants. *Times Law Reports*, 2 March 2002

84 Ouellet M *et al.* Hindlimb deformities (ectromelia, ectrodactyly) in free-living anurans from agricultural habitats. *J Wildlife Dis*, 1997; 33: 95–104; Chow G. Pesticides and the mystery of deformed frogs. *J Pesticide Reform*, 1997; 17: 14; Doyle R. Amphibians at risk. *Sci Am*, 1998; August: 27

85 La Clair JJ *et al.* Photoproducts and metabolites of a common insect growth regulator produce developmental deformities in *Xenopus*. *Environ Sci Technol*, 1998; 32: 1453–61

86 Kaltreider RC *et al.* Arsenic alters the function of the glucocorticoid receptor as a transcription factor. *Environ Health Perspect*, 2001; 109: 245

87 Strauss L *et al.* Dietary phytoestrogens and their role in hormonally dependent cancers. *Toxicol Lett*, 1998; 102–103: 349–54

88 Boulet MJ *et al.* Climacteric and menopause in seven Southeast Asian countries. *Maturitas*, 1994; 19: 157–76; Tang GW. Menopausal symptoms. *J Hong Kong Med Assoc*, 1993; 45: 249–54

89 Albertazzi P *et al.* Dietary soy supplementation and phytoestrogen levels. *Obstet Gynecol*, 1999; 94: 229–31

90 Washburn S *et al.* Effect of soy protein supplementation on serum lipoproteins, blood pressure, and menopausal symptoms in perimenopausal women. *Menopause*, 1999; 6: 7–13; Albertazzi P *et al.* The effect of dietary soy supplementation on hot flushes. *Obstet Gynecol*, 1998; 91: 6–11

91 Albertazzi P *et al.* Dietary soy supplementation and phytoestrogen levels. *Obstet Gynecol*, 1999; 94: 229–31; Knight DC *et al.* The effect of Promensil, an isoflavone extract, on menopausal symptoms. *Climacteric*, 1999; 2: 79–84; Baber RJ *et al.* Randomized placebo-controlled trial of an isoflavone supplement and menopausal symptoms in women. *Climacteric*, 1999; 2: 85–92

92 Knight DC *et al.* 1999, op cit; Baber RJ *et al.* 1999, op cit; Quella SK *et al.* Evaluation of soy phytoestrogens for the treatment of hot flashes in breast cancer survivors: A North Central Cancer Treatment Group Trial. *J Clin Oncol*, 2000; 18: 1068–74

93 Crouse JR III *et al*. A randomized trial comparing the effect of casein with that of soy protein containing varying amounts of isoflavones on plasma concentrations of lipids and lipoproteins. *Arch Intern Med*, 1999; 159: 2070–6; Anderson JW *et al*. Meta-analysis of the effects of soy protein intake on serum lipids. *N Engl J Med*, 1995; 333: 276–82; Arora A *et al*. Antioxidant activities of isoflavones and their biological metabolites in aliposomal system. *Arch Biochem Biophys*, 1998; 356: 133–41; Kapiotis S *et al*. Genistein, the dietary-derived angiogenesis inhibitor, prevents LDL oxidation and protects endothelial cells from damage by atherogenic LDL. *Arterioscler Thromb Vasc Biol*, 1997; 17: 2868–74; Raines EW, Ross R. Biology of atherosclerotic plaque formation: possible role of growth factors in lesion development and the potential impact of soy. *J Nutr*, 1995; 125 (3 Suppl): 624S–30S

94 Anderson JW *et al*. Meta-analysis of the effects of soy protein intake on serum lipids. *N Engl J Med*, 1995; 333: 276–82

95 Wilcox JN, Blumenthal BF. Thrombotic mechanisms in atherosclerosis: potential impact of soy proteins. *J Nutr*, 1995; 125 (3 Suppl): 631S–8S; Anthony MS *et al*. Soybean isoflavones improve cardiovascular risk factors without affecting the reproductive system of peripubertal rhesus monkeys. *J Nutr*, 1996; 126: 43–50

96 Jenkins DJ *et al*. Effect of soy protein foods on low-density lipoprotein oxidation and ex viva sex hormone receptor activity – a controlled crossover trial. *Metabolism*, 2000; 49: 537–43

97 Hodgson JM *et al*. Supplementation with isoflavonoid phytoestrogens does not alter serum lipid concentrations: a randomized controlled trial in humans. *J Nutr*, 1998; 128: 728–32

98 Anderson JJ, Garner SC. Phytoestrogens and bone. *Baillière's Clin Endocrinol Metab*, 1998; 12: 543–57; Potter SM *et al*. Soy protein and isoflavones: their effects on blood lipids and bone density in postmenopausal women. *Am J Clin Nutr*, 1998; 68 (6 Suppl): 1375S–9S

99 Scheiber MD, Rebar RW. Isoflavones and postmenopausal bone health: a viable alternative to estrogen therapy? *Menopause*, 1999; 6: 233–41; Barnes S. Evolution of the health benefits of soy isoflavones. *Proc Soc Exp Biol Med*, 1998; 217: 386–92

100 Arjmandi BH *et al*. Dietary soybean protein prevents bone loss in an ovariectomized rat model of osteoporosis. *J Nutr*, 1996; 126: 161–7

101 Adlercreutz CH *et al*. Soybean phytoestrogen intake and cancer risk. *J Nutr*, 1995; 125 (3 Suppl): 757S–70S

102 Messina MJ *et al*. Soy intake and cancer risk: a review of the in vitro and in vivo data. *Nutr Cancer*, 1994; 21: 113–31

103 Zava DT *et al*. Estrogen and progestin bioactivity of foods, herbs and spices. *Proc Soc Exp Biol Med*, 1998; 217: 369–78

104 McMichael-Phillips DF *et al.* Effects of soy-protein supplementation on epithelial proliferation in the histologically normal human breast. *Am J Clin Nutr*, 1998; 68 (6 Suppl): 1431S–5S

105 Ingram D *et al.* Case-control study of phyto-oestrogens and breast cancer. *Lancet*, 1997; 350: 990–4; Wu AH *et al.* Tofu and risk of breast cancer in Asian-Americans. *Cancer Epidemiol Biomarkers Prev*, 1996; 5: 901–6; Peterson G, Barnes S. Genistein inhibition of the growth of human breast cancer cells: independence from estrogen receptors and the multi-drug resistance gene. *Biochem Biophys Res Commun*, 1991; 179: 661–7; Fotsis T *et al.* Genistein, a dietary-derived inhibitor of in vitro angiogenesis. *Proc Natl Acad Sci USA*, 1993; 90: 2690–4

106 Deutch B *et al.* Menstrual discomfort in Danish women reduced by dietary supplements of omega-3 PUFA and B_{12} (fish oil or seal oil capsules). *Nutr Res,* 2000; 20: 621–31

107 Canaris GJ *et al.* The Colorado thyroid disease prevalence study. *Arch Intern Med*, 2000; 160: 526–34

108 McCallum KA, Reading C. Hot flushes are induced by thermogenic stimuli. *Br J Urol*, 1989; 64: 507–10

109 Winterich JA, Umberson D. How women experience menopause: the importance of social context. *J Women Aging*, 1999; 11: 57–73

110 Adler ST. Conceptualizing menopause and midlife Chinese American and Chinese women in the US. *Maturitas*, 2000; 35: 11–23

111 Neilsen FH *et al.* Effect of dietary boron on mineral, estrogen, and testosterone metabolism in postmenopausal women. *FASEB J*, 1987; 1: 394–7

112 Neilsen FH. Studies on the relationship between boron and magnesium which possibly affects the formation and maintenance of bones. *Magnes Trace Elem*, 1990; 9: 61–9

113 Miksicek RJ. Commonly occurring plant flavonoids have estrogenic effect. *Mol Pharmacol*, 1993; 44: 37–43

114 Kuiper GG *et al.* Interaction of estrogenic chemicals and phytoestrogens with estrogen receptor. *Endocrinology*, 1998; 139: 4252–63

115 National Institutes of Health. *International Position Paper on Women's Health and Menopause.* NIH Publication no. 02-3284; Rossouw JE *et al.* Risks and benefits of estrogen plus progestin in healthy postmenopausal women: principal results from the Women's Health Initiative randomized controlled trial. *JAMA*, 2002; 288: 321–33; Fletcher SW, Colditz GA. Failure of estrogen plus progestin therapy for prevention. *JAMA*, 2002; 288: 366–8

116 Hilakivi-Clarke L *et al.* Maternal exposure to genistein during pregnancy increases carcinogen-induced mammary tumorigenesis in female rat offspring. *Oncol Rep*, 1999; 6: 1089–95

117 Schiff I *et al.* Effect of estriol administration on the hypogonadal woman.

Fertil Steril, 1978; 30: 278–82

118 Lippman M *et al*. Effects of estrone, estradiol, and estriol on hormone-responsive human breast cancer in long-term tissue culture. *Cancer Res*, 1977; 37: 1901–7

119 Nwannenna AI *et al*. Clinical changes in ovariectomized ewes exposed to phytoestrogens and 17-beta-estradiol implants. *Proc Soc Exp Biol Med*, 1995; 208: 92–7

120 Miksicek RJ. Estrogenic flavonoids: structural requirements for biological activity. *Proc Soc Exp Biol Med*, 1995; 208: 44–50

121 Bennetts H *et al*. A breeding problem of sheep in the southwest division of Western Australia. *J Dept Agric West Aust*, 1946; 23: 1–12

122 Adams N. A changed responsiveness to oestrogen in ewes with Dover disease. *J Reprod Fertil*, 1981; Suppl 30: 223–30

123 Vining RF, McGinley RA. The measurement of hormones in saliva: possibilities and pitfalls. *J Steroid Biochem*, 1987; 27: 81–94; Stevenson JC, Purdie DW. Use of Pro-Gest cream in postmenopausal women. *Lancet*, 1998; 352: 905–6; Grimes DA. Progestins, breast cancer, and the limitations of epidemiology. *Fertil Steril*, 1992; 57: 492–4; Keshgegian AA, Cnaan A. Estrogen receptor-negative, progesterone receptor-positive breast carcinoma: poor clinical outcome. *Arch Pathol Lab Med*, 1996; 120: 970–3; Cooper A *et al*. Systemic absorption of progesterone from Progest cream in postmenopausal women. *Lancet*, 1998; 351: 1255–6; Cundy T *et al*. Bone density in women receiving depot medroxyprogesterone acetate for contraception. *BMJ*, 1991; 303: 13–6

124 National Toxicology Program. *10th Report on Carcinogens*. US Department of Health and Human Services, December 2002

125 Rockhill B *et al*. A prospective study of recreational physical activity and breast cancer risk. *Arch Intern Med*, 1999; 159: 2290–6

Chapter 9 – Metallica (pages 204–243)

1 Harte J *et al*. *Toxics A to Z: A Guide to Everyday Pollution Hazards*. Berkeley, CA: University of California Press, 1991

2 Kellas B, Dworkin A. *Surviving the Toxic Crisis*. Olivenhain, CA: Professional Preference Publishing, 1996

3 Casdorph H, Walker M. *Toxic Metal Syndrome*. Garden City Park, NY: Avery Publishing, 1995

4 National Institute of Environmental Health Sciences. Toxic and essential metal interactions. *Ann Rev Nutr*, 1997; 17: 37–50; Goyer RA. Nutrition and metal toxicity. *Am J Clin Nutr*, 1995; 61 (Suppl 3): 646S–50S; Spivey-Fox MR. Nutritional influences on metal toxicity. *Environ Health Perspect*, 1979; 29: 95–104

5 David OJ *et al*. Lead and hyperactivity. Behavioral response to chelation: a pilot study. *Am J Psychiatry*, 1976; 133: 1155; Leviton A *et al*. Pre- and post-natal low-level lead exposure and children's dysfunction in school. *Environ Res*, 1993; 60: 30–43; Eppright TD *et al*. ADHD, infantile autism, and elevated blood level: a possible relationship. *Mol Med*, 1996; 93: 136–8; Brockel BJ, Cory-Slechta DA. Lead, attention, and impulsive behavior. *Pharmacol Biochem Behav*, 1998; 60: 545–52; Wecker L *et al*. Trace element concentrations in hair from autistic children. *Defic Res*, 1985; 29: 15–22; Capel ID *et al*. Comparison of concentrations of some trace, bulk, and toxic metals in the hair of normal and dyslexic children. *Clin Chem*, 1981; 27: 879–81

6 Gottschalk LA *et al*. Abnormalities in hair trace elements as indicators of aberrant behavior. *Compr Psychiatry*, 1991; 32: 229–37; Schauss AG. Comparative hair mineral analysis in a randomly selected "normal" population and violent criminal offenders. *Int J Biosoc Res*, 1981; 1: 21–41

7 Bowdler NC, Beasley DS. Behavioral effects of aluminum ingestion. *Pharmacol Biochem Behav*, 1979; 10: 505–12; Trapp GA, Miner GD. Aluminum levels in brain in Alzheimer's disease. *Biol Psychiatry*, 1978; 13: 709–18

8 Casdorph HR. *Toxic Metal Syndrome*. Avery Publishing Group, 1995; Levick SE. Dementia from aluminum pots? *N Engl J Med*, 1980; 303: 164; Rodier PM. Developing brain as a target of toxicity. *Environ Health Perspect*, 1995; 103 (Suppl 6): 73–6; Rice DC. Issues in developmental neurotoxicology: interpretation and implications of the data. *Can J Publ Health*, 1998; 89 (Supp1): S31–40

9 Weiss B. The scope and promise of behavioral toxicology. In Russell R *et al*. (eds). *Behavioral Measures of Neurotoxicity: Report of a Symposium*. National Research Council, National Academy Press, 1990: 395–413

10 Klinghardt D. Metal toxicity. *Explore*, 2000; 10 (1); www.explorepub.com/articles/klinghardt.html

11 Kaplan GA *et al*. Social connections and mortality from all causes and from cardiovascular disease: prospective evidence from eastern Finland. *Am J Epidemiol*, 1988; 128: 370–80; Berkman LF, Syme SL. Social networks, host resistance, and mortality: a nine-year follow-up study of Alameda County residents. *Am J Epidemiol*, 1979; 109: 186–204

12 Bahnson C. Stress and cancer: The state of the art. *Psychosomatics*, 1980; 21: 975–80; Temoshok L. Personality, coping style, emotions and cancer: towards an integrative model. *Cancer Surv*, 1987; 6: 545–67

13 Lane JD *et al*. Personality correlates of glycemic control in type 2 diabetes. *Diabetes Care*, 2000; 23: 1321–5

14 Clark HR. *The Cure for All Diseases*. New Century, 1996

15 Barry PSI. A comparison of concentrations of lead in human tissue. *Br J Ind*

Med, 1975; 32: 119–39

16 Rosen JF *et al.* Reduction in 1,25-dihydroxy vitamin D in children with increased lead absorption. *N Engl J Med*, 1980; 302: 1128–31; Mahaffey KR *et al.* Association between age, blood lead concentrations and serum 1,25-dihydroxycholecalciferol levels in children. *Am J Clin Nutr*, 1982; 35: 1327–31

17 Ruff HA *et al.* Declining blood lead levels and cognitive changes in moderately lead-poisoned children. *JAMA*, 1993; 269: 1641–6

18 Bellinger D *et al.* Longitudinal analysis of prenatal and postnatal lead exposure and early cognitive development. *N Engl J Med*, 1987; 316: 1037–43

19 Lewendon G *et al.* Should children with developmental and behavioural problems be routinely screened for lead? *Arch Dis Child*, 2001; 85: 286–8

20 Tong S *et al.* Lifetime exposure to environmental lead and children's intelligence at 11-13 years: the Port Pirie cohort study. *BMJ*, 1996; 312: 1569–75

21 Needleman HL *et al.* Deficits in psychologic and classroom performance in children with elevated dentine lead levels. *N Engl J Med*, 1979; 300: 584–695

22 Needleman HL *et al.* Bone lead levels and delinquent behavior. *JAMA*, 1996; 275: 363–9

23 Needleman HL *et al.* Long-term effects of childhood exposure to lead at low doses: an eleven-year follow-up report. *N Engl J Med*, 1990; 322: 83–8

24 Mahaffey KR. Environmental lead toxicity: nutrition as a component of intervention. *Environ Health Perspect*, 1990; 89: 75–8; Agency for Toxic Substances and Disease Registry (ATSDR). *Case Studies in Environmental Medicine: Lead Toxicity*. US Department of Health and Human Services, 1992

25 Wasson SJ *et al.* Lead in candle emissions. *Sci Total Environ*, 2002; 296: 159–74; Nriagu JO, Kim MJ. Emissions of lead and zinc from candles with metal-core wicks. *Sci Total Environ*, 2000; 250: 37–41; van Alphen M. Emission testing and inhalational exposure-based risk assessment for candles having Pb metal wick cores. *Sci Total Environ*, 1999; 243–244: 53–65

26 Sobel HL *et al.* Lead exposure from candles. *JAMA*, 2000; 284: 180

27 *National Report on Human Exposure to Environmental Chemicals*. Atlanta, GA: Centers for Disease Control and Prevention, March 2001; www.cdc.gov/nceh/dls/report/

28 Huggins HA. *It's All in Your Head: Diseases Caused by Silver-Mercury Fillings, 4th edn*. Life Sciences Press, 1990

29 Richardson GM. *Assessment of Mercury Exposure and Risks from Dental Amalgam*. Ottawa, Ontario: Medical Devices Bureau, Environmental Health Directorate, Health Canada, 18 August 1995

30 Goering PL *et al.* Symposium overview: Toxicity assessment of mercury vapor from dental amalgams. *Fund Appl Toxicol*, 1992; 19: 319–29

31 Svare CW *et al.* The effect of dental amalgams on mercury levels in expired air. *J Dent Res*, 1981; 60: 1668–71; Vimy MJ, Lorscheider FL. Serial measurements of intra-oral air mercury: estimation of daily dose from dental amalgam. *J Dent Res*, 1985; 64: 1072–5

32 Levenson J. *Menace in the Mouth*. London: WDDTY, 2000

33 Ehmann WD *et al.* Brain trace elements in Alzheimer's disease. *Neurotoxicology*, 1986; 7: 197–206; Thompson CM *et al.* Regional brain trace-element studies in Alzheimer's disease. *Neurotoxicology*, 1988; 9: 1–8; Wenstrup D *et al.* Trace element imbalances in isolated subcellular reactions of Alzheimer's disease brains. *Brain Res*, 1990; 533: 125–31

34 Schettler T. Toxic threats to neurologic development of children. *Environ Health Perspect*, 2001; 109 (Suppl 6): 813–6; Grandjean P *et al.* Cognitive deficit in 7-year-old children with prenatal exposure to methylmercury. *Neurotoxicol Teratol*, 1997; 19: 417–28

35 Drasch G *et al.* Mercury burden of human fetus and infant tissues. *Eur J Pediatr*, 1994; 153: 607–10

36 *The Merck Index, 12th edn.* 1996; 9451: 1590

37 Sainio EL *et al.* Metals and arsenic in eye shadows. *Contact Derm*, 2000; 42: 5–10

38 Friberg L *et al. Environmental Health Criteria 134: Cadmium.* Geneva: World Health Organization, 1992

39 Agency for Toxic Substances and Disease Registry. *Public Health Statement: Cadmium.* ATSDR, March 1989; http://atsdr1.atsdr.cdc.gov:8080/ToxProfiles/phs8808.html

40 Kabelitz L. Heavy metals in herbal drugs. *Eur J Herbal Med*, 1998; 4: 25–33

41 Kaneta M *et al.* Chemical form of cadmium (and other heavy metals) in rice and wheat plants. *Environ Health Perspect*, 1986; 65: 33–7

42 Friberg L *et al.* (eds). *Handbook of the Toxicology of Metals, Vols I, II, Second Edition.* Amsterdam: Elsevier Science Publishers BV, 1986

43 Bar-Sela S *et al.* Medical findings in nickel-cadmium battery workers. *Isr J Med Sci*, 1992; 28: 578–83

44 Carroll RE. The relationship of cadmium in the air to cardiovascular disease death rates. *JAMA*, 1966; 198: 267–9

45 Webber MM. Selenium prevents the growth stimulatory effects of cadmium on human prostatic epithelium. *Biochem Biophys Res Commun*, 1985; 127: 871–7

46 Salonen JT *et al.* Intake of mercury from fish, lipid peroxidation, and the risk of myocardial infarction and coronary, cardiovascular and any death in Eastern Finnish men. *Circulation*, 1995; 91: 645–55; Foulke JE. Mercury in fish: Cause for concern? *FDA Consumer*, September, 1994

47 Egeland GM, Middaugh JP. Balancing fish consumption benefits with mercury exposure. *Science*, 1997; 278: 1904–5

48 No author listed. Aluminium in the brain: new data. *Chem Ind*, 8 June 1988: 346

49 Flaten TP, Odegard M. Tea, aluminium and Alzheimer's disease. *Food Chem Toxicol*, 1988; 26: 959–60

50 French P *et al*. Dietary aluminium and Alzheimer's disease. *Food Chem Toxicol*, 1989; 27: 495–8

51 Coriat AM, Gillard RD. Beware the cups that cheer. *Nature*, 1986; 321: 570

52 Slanina P *et al*. Dietary citric acid enhances absorption of aluminum in antacids. *Clin Chem*, 1986; 32: 539–41

53 Tamari GM. Aluminum: Toxicity and Prevention. *Townsend Lett Docs*, 1999; 187/188: 98–100

54 Scheibner V. Adverse effects of adjuvants in vaccines. *Nexus*, 2000; 8 (1, 2, 3); www.whale.to/vaccine/adjuvants.html

55 Polizzi S *et al*. Neurotoxic effects of aluminium among foundry workers and Alzheimer's disease. *Neurotoxicology*, 2002; 23: 761–74

56 Zapatero MD *et al*. Serum aluminum levels in Alzheimer's disease and other senile dementias. *Biol Trace Elem Res*, 1995; 47: 235–40; Martyn CN *et al*. Geographical relation between Alzheimer's disease and aluminum in drinking water. *Lancet*, 1989; *i*: 59–62

57 Crapper DR *et al*. Brain aluminum distribution in Alzheimer's disease and experimental neurofibrillary degeneration. *Science*, 1973; 180: 511–3

58 Neri LC, Hewitt D. Aluminium, Alzheimer's disease, and drinking water. *Lancet*, 1991; 338: 390

59 Graves AB *et al*. The association between aluminium-containing products and Alzheimer's disease. *J Clin Epidemiol*, 1990; 43: 35–44

60 Spencer H, Kramer I. Osteoporosis: calcium, fluoride, and aluminum interactions. *J Am Coll Nutr*, 1985; 4: 121–8

61 Wills MR, Savory J. Water content of aluminum, dialysis dementia, and osteomalacia. *Environ Health Perspect*, 1985; 63: 141–7

62 Jacqmin-Gadda H *et al*. Silica and aluminum in drinking water and cognitive impairment in the elderly. *Epidemiology*, 1996; 7: 281–5; Bellia JP *et al*. The role of silicic acid in the renal excretion of aluminium. *Ann Clin Lab Sci*, 1996; 26: 227–33

63 Foster HD. *Health, Disease and the Environment*. Boca Raton, FL: CRC Press, 1992: 311–6; Durlach J. Magnesium depletion and pathogenesis of Alzheimer's disease. *Magnes Res*, 1990; 3: 217–8; Wenk GL, Stemmer KL. Suboptimal dietary zinc intake increases aluminum accumulation into the rat brain. *Brain Res*, 1983; 288: 393–5

64 Werbach MR. *Foundations of Nutritional Medicine: Common Nutritional Deficiencies*. Tarzana, CA: Third Line Press, 1997

65 Prasad AS. Clinical, biochemical and pharmacological role of zinc. *Ann Rev Pharmacol Toxicol*, 1979; 19: 393–426; Sanstead HH *et al*. Zinc nutriture in

the elderly in relation to taste acuity, immune response and wound healing. *Am J Clin Nutr*, 1982; 36: 1046–59

66 Xu J, Thornton I. Arsenic in garden soils and vegetable crops in Cornwall, England: implications for human health. *Environ Geochem Health*, 1985; 7: 131–3; Kavanagh P *et al.* Urinary arsenic concentrations in a high arsenic area of southwest England. *Occup Environ Med*, 1997; 54: 840

67 Peryea FJ. Historical use of lead arsenate insecticides, resulting soil contamination and implications for soil remediation. *Proceedings of the 16th World Congress of Soil Science*. Montpellier, France, 20–26 August 1998: 1–4

68 Guo HR *et al.* Arsenic in drinking water and incidence of urinary cancers. *Epidemiology*, 1997; 8: 545–50; Chen CJ *et al.* Cancer potential in liver, lung, bladder and kidney due to ingested inorganic arsenic in drinking water. *Br J Cancer*, 1992; 66: 888–92; Bates MN *et al.* Arsenic ingestion and internal cancers: a review. *Am J Epidemiol*, 1992; 135: 462–76

69 Pershagen G. The carcinogenicity of arsenic. *Environ Health Perspect*, 1981; 40: 93–100; Mabuchi K *et al.* Lung cancer among pesticide workers exposed to inorganic arsenicals. *Arch Environ Health*, 1979; 34: 312–20; Spiewak R. Pesticides as a cause of occupational skin diseases in farmers. *Ann Agric Environ Med*, 2001; 8: 1–5; Jackson R, Grainge JW. Arsenic and cancer. *Can Med Assoc J*, 1975; 113: 396–401

70 Nolan KR. Copper toxicity syndrome. *J Orthomolec Psychiatr*, 1983; 12: 270–82

71 Narang RL *et al.* Levels of copper and zinc in depression. *Ind J Physiol Pharmacol*, 1991; 35: 272–4

72 Bowman MB, Lewis MS. The copper hypothesis of schizophrenia: a review. *Neurosci Biobehav Rev*, 1982; 6: 321–8

73 Salonen JT *et al.* Serum copper and the risk of acute myocardial infarction: a prospective population study in men in eastern Finland. *Am J Epidemiol*, 1991; 134: 268–76

74 Multhaup G. Amyloid precursor protein, copper and Alzheimer's disease. *Biomed Pharmacother*, 1997; 51: 105–11

75 Sawaki M *et al.* Role of copper accumulation and metallothionein induction in spontaneous liver cancer development in LEC rats. *Carcinogenesis*, 1994; 15: 1833–7

76 Eagon PK *et al.* Hepatic hyperplasia and cancer in rats: alterations in copper metabolism. *Carcinogenesis*, 1999; 20: 1091–6

77 Ferraz HB *et al.* Chronic exposure to the fungicide maneb may produce symptoms and signs of CNS manganese intoxication. *Neurology*, 1988; 38: 550–3

78 Nagatomo S *et al.* Manganese intoxication during total parenteral nutrition: report of two cases and review of the literature. *J Neurol Sci*, 1999; 162: 102–54. Ejima A *et al.* Manganese intoxication during total parenteral nutrition. *Lancet*, 1992; 339: 426; Fell JM *et al.* Manganese toxicity in children

receiving long-term parenteral nutrition. *Lancet,* 1996; 347: 1218–21

79 Normandin L *et al.* Manganese neurotoxicity: behavioral, pathological, and biochemical effects following various routes of exposure. *Rev Environ Health,* 2002; 17: 189–217

80 Chia SE *et al.* Neurobehavioral functions among workers exposed to manganese ore. *Scand J Work Environ Health,* 1993; 19: 264–70

81 Agency for Toxic Substances and Disease Registry (ATSDR). *Toxicological Profile for Manganese.* Atlanta, GA: US Department of Health and Human Services, Public Health Service, 2000

82 Wennberg A *et al.* Manganese exposure in steel smelters a health hazard to the nervous system. *Scand J Work Environ Health,* 1991; 17: 255–62

83 Kawamura R *et al.* Intoxication by manganese in well water. *Kisasato Arch Exp Med,* 1941; 18: 145–69; Kondakis XG *et al.* Possible health effects of high manganese concentrations in drinking water. *Arch Environ Health,* 1989; 44: 175–8; Pal PK. *et al.* Manganese neurotoxicity: a review of clinical features, imaging and pathology. *Neurotoxicology,* 1999; 20: 227–38

84 Keen CL *et al.* Nutritional aspects of manganese from experimental studies. *Neurotoxicology,* 1999; 20: 213–24

85 Davis JM. Methylcyclopentadienyl manganese tricarbonyl: health risk uncertainties and research directions. *Environ Health Perspect,* 1998; 106 (Suppl 1): 191–201

86 Huang CC *et al.* Progression after chronic manganese exposure. *Neurology,* 1993; 43: 1479–83

Chapter 10 – A Final Word: Supporting the Process from A to Z (pages 244–283)

1 Telles S *et al.* Physiological measures of right nostril breathing. *J Alt Complement Med,* 1996; 2: 479–84; Telles S *et al.* Breathing through a particular nostril can alter metabolism and autonomic activities. *Ind J Physiol Pharmacol,* 1994; 38: 133–7

2 Wood C. Mood change and perceptions of vitality: a comparison of the effects of relaxation, visualization and yoga. *J Roy Soc Med,* 1993; 86: 254–8

3 Telles S. Oxygen consumption during pranayamic type of very slow-rate breathing. *Ind J Med Res,* 1991; 94: 357–63

4 Bhatnagar SO, Jain SC. A study of response pattern on non-insulin-dependent diabetics to yoga therapy. *Diabetes Res Clin Pract,* 1993; 19: 69–74

5 Boone T, Flarity JR. Effects of *qigong* on cardiorespiratory changes: a preliminary study. *Am J Chin Med,* 1993; 21: 1–6

6 Pouls M. Oral chelation and nutritional replacement therapy for chemical and heavy metal toxicity and cardiovascular disease. *Townsend Lett Docs,* 1999; 192: 82–91

7 Foreman H. Toxic side effects of EDTA. *J Chron Dis*, 1963; 16: 319–23

8 Halstead B. The scientific basis of EDTA chelation therapy. *Life Enhancement*, 1998; February: 8

9 Hohnadel DC *et al.* Atomic absorption spectrometry of nickel, copper, zinc, and lead in sweat collected from healthy subjects during sauna bathing. *Clin Chem*, 1973; 19: 1288–92

10 Rea WJ *et al.* Clearing of toxic volatile hydrocarbons from humans. *Bol Asoc Med PR*, 1991; 83: 321–4; Kilburn KH *et al.* Neurobehavioral dysfunction in firemen exposed to polychlorinated biphenyls (PCBs): possible improvement after detoxification. *Arch Environ Health*, 1989; 44: 345–50; Tretjak Z *et al.* PCB reduction and clinical improvement by detoxification: an unexploited approach? *Hum Exp Toxicol*, 1990; 9: 235–44

11 Czarnowski D, Gorski J. Excretion of nitrogen compounds in sweat during a sauna. *Pol Tyg Lek*, 1991; 46: 186–7

12 Kroker GA *et al.* Fasting and rheumatoid arthritis: a multicenter study. *Clin Ecol*, 1984; 3: 137–44; Kjeldsen-Kragh J *et al.* Controlled trial of fasting and one-year vegetarian diet in rheumatoid arthritis. *Lancet*, 1991; 338: 899–902; Skoldstam L *et al.* Effects of fasting and lactovegetarian diet on rheumatoid arthritis. *Scand J Rheumatol*, 1979; 8: 249–55; Lithell H *et al.* A fasting and vegetarian diet treatment trial on chronic inflammatory disorders. *Acta Derm Venereol*, 1983; 63: 397–403

13 Duncan TG *et al.* Contraindications and therapeutic results of fasting in obese patients. *Ann NY Acad Sci*, 1965; 131: 632–6; Gresham GA. Is atheroma a reversible lesion? *Atherosclerosis*, 1976; 23: 379–91; Maislos M *et al.* Gorging and plasma HDL-cholesterol – the Ramadan model. *Eur J Clin Nutr*, 1998; 52: 127–30

14 Navarro S *et al.* Comparison of fasting, nasogastric suction and cimetidine in treatment of acute pancreatitis. *Digestion*, 1984; 30: 224–30

15 Boheme DL. Preplanned fasting in the treatment of mental disease: survey of the current Soviet literature. *Schizophren Bull*, 1977; 3: 288–96

16 Imamura M, Tung T. A trial of fasting cure for PCB poisoned patients in Taiwan. *Am J Ind Med*, 1984; 5: 147–53

17 Haas E. *The Detox Diet*. Berkeley, CA: Celestial Arts, 1996: 115

18 Perical M, Percival S. *Infant Nutrition*. New Hamburg, Ontario: Health Coach Systems International, 1995

19 Blair SN *et al.* Changes in physical fitness and all-cause mortality. A prospective study of healthy and unhealthy men. *JAMA*, 1995; 273: 1093–8; Manson JE *et al.* A prospective study of walking as compared with vigorous exercise in the prevention of coronary heart disease in women. *N Engl J Med*, 1999; 341: 650–8

20 Steptoe A *et al.* The effects of exercise training on mood and perceived coping ability in anxious adults from the general population. *J Psychosom Res*, 1989;

33: 537–47; Blumenthal JA *et al.* Effects of exercise training on older patients with major depression. *Arch Intern Med*, 1999; 159: 2349–56; Young RJ. The effect of regular exercise on cognitive functioning and personality. *Br J Sports Med*, 1979; 13: 110–7

21 Arroll B, Beaglehole R. Does physical activity lower blood pressure: a critical review of the clinical trials. *J Clin Epidemiol*, 1992; 45: 439–47

22 Hu FB *et al.* Walking compared with vigorous physical activity and risk of type 2 diabetes in women: a prospective study. *JAMA*, 1999; 282: 1433–9

23 Ettinger WH Jr *et al.* A randomized trial comparing aerobic exercise and resistance exercise with a health education program in older adults with knee osteoarthritis. The Fitness Arthritis and Seniors Trial (FAST). *JAMA*, 1997; 277: 25–31

24 Martinez ME *et al.* Leisure-time physical activity, body size, and colon cancer in women. Nurses' Health Study Research Group. *J Natl Cancer Inst*, 1997; 89: 948–55; Giovannucci E *et al.* Physical activity, obesity, and risk for colon cancer and adenoma in men. *Ann Intern Med*, 1995; 122: 327–34

25 Aldoori WH *et al.* Prospective study of physical activity and the risk of symptomatic diverticular disease in men. *Gut*, 1995; 36: 276–82

26 Leitzmann LF *et al.* Recreational physical activity and the risk of cholecystectomy in women. *N Engl J Med*, 1999; 341: 777–84

27 Campbell AJ *et al.* Randomised controlled trial of a general practice programme of home-based exercise to prevent falls in elderly women. *BMJ*, 1997; 315: 1065–9

28 King AC *et al.* Moderate-intensity exercise and self-rated quality of sleep in older adults. A randomized controlled trial. *JAMA*, 1997; 277: 32–7; Montgomery P, Dennis J. Physical exercise for sleep problems in adults aged 60+ (Cochrane Review). *Cochrane Database Syst Rev*, 2002; (4): CD003404

29 Biddle S. Exercise and psychosocial health. *Res Q Exerc Sport*, 1995; 66: 292–7; Glenister D. Exercise and mental health: a review. *J Roy Soc Health*, 1996; 116: 7–13

30 Collingwood TR, Willett L. The effects of physical training upon self-concept and body attitude. *J Clin Psychol*, 1971; 27: 411–2

31 Skender ML *et al.* Comparison of 2-year weight loss trends in behavioral treatments of obesity: diet, exercise, and combination interventions. *J Am Diet Assoc*, 1996; 96: 342–6; Phinney SD. Exercise during and after very-low-calorie dieting. *Am J Clin Nutr*, 1992; 56 (1 Suppl): 190S–4S; Safer DJ. Diet, behavior modification, and exercise: a review of obesity treatments from a long-term perspective. *South Med J*, 1991; 84: 1470–4

32 Pentimone F, Del Corso L. Why regular physical activity favors longevity. *Minerva Med*, 1998; 89: 197–201

33 Vistisen K *et al.* Cytochrome-P450 IA2 activity in man measured by caffeine

metabolism: effect of smoking, broccoli and exercise. *Adv Exp Med Biol*, 1991; 283: 407–11; Moochhala SM *et al*. Effects of acute physical exercise on aryl hydrocarbon hydroxylase activity in human peripheral lymphocytes. *Life Sci*, 1990; 47: 427–32

34 Kilburn KH *et al*. Neurobehavioral dysfunction in firemen exposed to polychlorinated biphenyls (PCBs): possible improvement after detoxification. *Arch Environ Health*, 1989; 44: 345–50

35 Dunn AL *et al*. Comparison of lifestyle and structured interventions to increase physical activity and cardiorespiratory fitness: a randomized trial. *JAMA*, 1999; 281: 327–34

36 Spelman CC *et al*. Self-selected exercise intensity of habitual walkers. *Med Sci Sports Exerc*, 1993; 25: 1174–9

37 Choi BM, Chung HT. Effect of *qigong* training on proportions of T lymphocyte subsets in human peripheral blood. *Am J Chin Med*, 1995; 23: 27–36; Choi BM, Chung HT. Delayed cutaneous hypersensitivity reactions in *qigong* trainees by multi-test, cell-mediated immunity. *Am J Chin Med*, 1995; 23: 139–44

38 MacIntosh A. Exercise therapeutics update & commentary: exercise and cortisol. *Townsend Lett Docs*, 1998; 184: 38–40

39 Urhausen A *et al*. Impaired pituitary hormonal response to exhaustive exercise in overtrained endurance athletes. *Med Sci Sports Exerc*, 1998; 30: 407–14

40 Morita K *et al*. *Chlorella* accelerates dioxin excretion in rats. *J Nutr*, 1999; 129: 1731–6

41 Tanaka Y *et al*. Studies on the inhibition of intestinal absorption of radioactive strontium, VI: Alginate degradation products as potent in vivo sequestering agents of radioactive strontium. *Can Med Assoc J*, 1968; 98: 1179–82

42 Erasmus U. *Fats that Heal, Fats that Kill*. Burnaby, BC, Canada: Alive Books, 1994

43 Conquer JA, Holub BJ. Supplementation with an algae source of docosahexaenoic acid increases (omega-3) fatty acid status and alters selected risk factors for heart disease in vegetarian subjects. *J Nutr*, 1996; 126: 3032–9

44 McPartland J. Why blue-green algae makes me tired. *Townsend Lett Docs*, 1997; 167: 94–6

45 Holford P. *The Optimum Nutrition Bible*. London: Piatkus, 1998

46 Wolverton BC *et al*. A study of interior landscape plants for indoor air pollution abatement. *NASA*, July 1989; Wolverton BC. *How to Grow Fresh Air: 50 Houseplants to Purify Your Home or Office*. New York: Penguin Books, 1997

47 Kerr D *et al*. Effect of caffeine on the recognition of and responses to hypoglycemia in humans. *Ann Intern Med*, 1993; 119: 799–804

48 Tverdal A *et al*. Coffee consumption and death from coronary heart disease in middle aged Norwegian men and women. *BMJ*, 1990; 300: 566–9; Klatsky AL *et al*. Coffee, tea, and mortality. *Ann Epidemiol*, 1993; 3: 375–81

49 Klebanoff MA *et al.* Maternal serum paraxanthine, a caffeine metabolite, and the risk of spontaneous abortion. *N Engl J Med*, 1999; 341: 1639–44

50 Slattery ML *et al.* Intake of fluids and methylxanthine-containing beverages: association with colon cancer. *Int J Cancer*, 1999; 81: 199–204

51 Neuhauser-Bethold BS. Coffee consumption and total body water homeostasis as measured by fluid balance and bioelectrical impedance analysis. *Ann Nutr Metab*, 1997; 41: 29–36

52 Griffiths RR, Vernotica EM. Is caffeine a flavoring agent in cola soft drinks? *Arch Fam Med*, 2000; 9: 727–34

53 Vines G. Adipose is OK. *New Sci*, 1995; 146: 34–6; Pond CM. *The Fats of Life*. Cambridge University Press, 1998

54 Haas E. *Staying Healthy With Nutrition*. Celestial Arts, 1992

55 Fallon S, Enig M. Not so healthy eating: the trouble with soy. *PROOF!*, 2000; 4(4): 2–6

56 Environmental Working Group. *A Shopper's Guide to Pesticides in Produce*. Washington, DC: EWG, 1995

57 Morse DR *et al.* A physiological and subjective evaluation of meditation, hypnosis, and relaxation. *Psychosom Med*, 1977; 39: 304–24; Morse DR *et al.* Physiological responses during meditation and rest. *Biofeedback Self Reg*, 1984; 9: 181–200

58 Schneider RH *et al.* A randomised controlled trial of stress reduction for hypertension in older African Americans. *Hypertension*, 1995; 26: 820–7; Schneider RH *et al.* Lower lipid peroxide levels in practitioners of the Transcendental Meditation program. *Psychosom Med*, 1998; 60: 38–41; Ornish D *et al.* Can lifestyle changes reverse atherosclerosis? *Lancet*, 1990; 336; 129–33; Gould KL *et al.* Changes in myocardial perfusion abnormalities by positron emission tomography after long-term, intense risk factor modification. *JAMA*, 1995; 27: 894–901; Gould KL *et al.* Improved stenosis geometry by quantitative coronary arteriography after vigorous risk factor modification. *Am J Cardiol*, 1992; 69: 845–53

59 Glaser JL *et al.* Elevated serum dehydroepiandrosterone sulfate levels in practitioners of the Transcendental Meditation (TM) and TM-Sidhi programs. *J Behav Med*, 1992; 15: 327–41

60 Kaplan KH *et al.* The impact of a meditation-based stress reduction program on fibromyalgia. *Gen Hosp Psychiatry*, 1993; 15: 284–9; Taylor DN. Effects of a behavioral stress-management program on anxiety, mood, self-esteem and T-cell count in HIV positive men. *Psychol Rep*, 1995; 76: 451–7

61 Ayas NT *et al.* A prospective study of sleep duration and coronary heart disease in women. *Arch Intern Med*, 2003; 163: 205–9

62 Boethel CD. Sleep and the endocrine system: new associations to old diseases. *Curr Opin Pulm Med*, 2002; 8: 502–5

63 Sheen AJ *et al.* Relationships between sleep quality and glucose regulation in normal humans. *Am J Physiol*, 1996; 271 (2 Pt 1): E261–70

64 Van Cauter E *et al.* Modulation of glucose regulation and insulin secretion by circadian rhythmicity and sleep. *J Clin Invest*, 1991; 88: 934–42

65 Spiegel K *et al.* Impact of sleep debt on metabolic and endocrine function. *Lancet*, 1999; 354: 1435–9

66 Elgin D. *Voluntary Simplicity*. William Morrow, 1993

67 Odelye O *et al.* Alcohol ingestion and lipoperoxidation: role of glutathione in antioxidant defense and detoxification. *J Optim Nutr*, 1993; 2: 173–89

68 Sen CK. Nutritional biochemistry of cellular glutathione. *Nutr Biochem*, 1997; 8: 660–72; Flagg EW *et al.* Dietary glutathione intake and the risk of oral and pharyngeal cancer. *Am J Epidemiol*, 1994; 139: 453–65

69 Jones DP. Glutathione distribution in natural products: absorption and tissue distribution. In Packer L (ed). *Biothiols Methods in Enzymology, Vol. 252*. San Diego, CA: Academic Press, 1995

70 Johnston CJ *et al.* Vitamin C elevates red blood cell glutathione in healthy adults. *Am J Clin Nutr*, 1993; 58: 103–5

71 Wilkinson IB *et al.* Oral vitamin C reduces arterial stiffness and platelet aggregation in humans. *J Cardiovasc Pharmacol*, 1999; 34: 690–3; Valkonen MM, Kuusi T. Vitamin C prevents the acute atherogenic effects of passive smoking. *Free Radic Biol Med*, 2000; 28: 428–36

72 Simon JA, Hudes ES. Relationship of ascorbic acid to blood lead levels. *JAMA*, 1999; 281: 2289–93

73 Meydani M *et al.* Protective effect of vitamin E on exercise-induced oxidative damage in young and older adults. *Am J Physiol*, 1993; 264: R992–8

74 Shakman RA. Nutritional influences on the toxicity of environmental pollutants: a review. *Arch Environ Health*, 1974; 28: 105–33

75 Clark LC *et al.* Effects of selenium supplementation for cancer prevention in patients with carcinoma of the skin. *JAMA*, 1996; 276: 1957–63; Yoshizawa K *et al.* Study of prediagnostic selenium levels in toenails and the risk of advanced prostate cancer. *J Natl Cancer Inst*, 1998; 90: 1219–24

76 Yoshida M *et al.* An evaluation of the bioavailability of selenium in high-selenium yeast. *J Nutr Sci Vitaminol*, 1999; 45: 119–28

77 Kleiner SM. Water: an essential but overlooked nutrient. *J Am Diet Assoc*, 1999; 99: 200–6

78 Valtin H. Drink at least eight glasses of water a day. Really? Is there scientific evidence for "8 x 8"? *Am J Physiol Reg Integr Comp Physiol*, 2002; 283: R993–1004

79 Tobin RS *et al.* Effects of activated carbon and bacteriostatic filters on microbiological quality of drinking water. *Appl Environ Microbiol*, 1981; 41: 646–51

80 Daschner FD *et al.* Microbiological contamination of drinking water in a commercial household water filter system. *Eur J Clin Microbial Infect Dis*, 1996; 15: 233–7

81 No author listed. Bottling out. *Ecologist*, 2003; February: 46

82 Hurst DF *et al.* The relationship of self-esteem to the health-related behaviors of the patients of a primary care clinic. *Arch Fam Med*, 1997; 6: 67–70

83 Pascucci MA, Loving GL. Ingredients of an old and healthy life. A centenarian perspective. *J Holist Nurs*, 1997; 15: 199–213

84 Swan GE, Carmelli D. Curiosity and mortality in aging adults: a 5-year follow-up of the Western Collaborative Group Study. *Psychol Aging*, 1996; 11: 449–53

85 Friedman HS *et al.* Does childhood personality predict longevity? *J Pers Soc Psychol*, 1993; 65: 176–85

86 Lawton MP *et al.* A two-factor model of caregiving appraisal and psychological well-being. *J Gerontol*, 1991; 46: 181–9

87 Woodward W. New surprises in very old places: Civil War nurse leaders and longevity. *Nurs Forum*, 1991; 26: 9–16

Index